PROZAC

PANACEA OR PANDORA?

"THE REST OF THE STORY"

ON THE NEW SSRI ANTIDEPRESSANTS

(PROZAC, ZOLOFT, PAXIL, LOVAN,
LUVOX, ETC.)

by

ANN BLAKE TRACY

AUTHOR'S NOTE: My hope is that what I have been able to discover from this in depth investigation will be of great assistance to both victims and their physicians in recognizing and understanding these adverse drug reactions. I have attempted to present this material in such a way that patients as well as their physicians will be able to glean much critical information. It has been my attempt to write on a layman's level in plainness and simplicity and yet include critical medical documentation for professionals as well. Although I feel it is essential to include documentation by leading experts in many fields of study, I hope that it will not detract from the readability of the book.

PROZAC: PANACEA OR PANDORA? is not intended as medical advice. Its intent is solely informational and educational in nature. Consult a health professional should the need be indicated.

Cover Art by Chase Shephard

Layout, Design & Typesetting by George Wm. Phillips

Published in Salt Lake City, Utah by Cassia Publications

For additional copies

CASSIA PUBLICATIONS
P.O. Box 1044
West Jordan, Utah 84088
1-800-280-0730

WARNING:

It is not advisable to abruptly stop using psychiatric drugs. If you are considering discontinuing the use of Prozac or any of the other SSRIs, it is advisable to do so under the supervision of a physician. Patients are reporting that abrupt discontinuation, rather than tapering off these drugs, can have very serious physical and psychological repercussions. For some individuals this "cold turkey" approach is proving to be extremely dangerous, including seizures, "crashing" into severe rebound depression, mania, and suicidal or violent behavior. (Refer to the section in this text which discusses the serious and often delayed withdrawal involving severe rebound depression - depression which is often more intense than the original depression and which many experience even though they were not originally prescribed these drugs for symptoms of depression.) There are doctors who will assist you in withdrawing from these drugs. If yours is not willing to do so, find one who will. Tapering onto the SSRIs and tapering off the drugs are proving to be among the most critical safety measures.

DEDICATION

...George, for his persistent requests that I investigate Prozac...without his questioning this book would never have been written and many more lives would have been lost or shattered...He has amazed me with the unbelievable strength and courage he has demonstrated in overcoming his five year Prozac induced pandora...and to all those who mean so much to me who have suffered this chemically-induced nightmare...their intensely painful experiences have given me the motivation to search out this information and alert others so that they might avoid this ordeal in their own lives...and to those who have often stood by my side encouraging me to continue - those who have given their lives that we might learn through their tragic experiences.

...My great-great grandfather Charles A. Thomas, for passing on to me the kind of courage it took for him to serve as the mayor of one of the wildest western towns, Tombstone, Arizona, during the era of Johnny Ringo, Wyatt Earp, Doc Holliday, the O.K. Corral, the Bird Cage, etc.

...My children, Jesse and Adrianne, for patiently listening to months and years of Prozac, Prozac, Prozac, and for providing the childlike wisdom that the best remedy for depression is not Prozac, but a puppy. (Whether the problem be physical, mental, emotional or spiritual, *love is the most powerful healing force there is.*)

ACKNOWLEDGEMENTS

Dr. Peter R. Breggin: Psychiatrist, psycho-therapist, for his input and assistance in being gracious enough to agree to be a part of this work by writing a foreword for this second edition, and above and beyond that, for his sacrifice of over twenty years of battling the injustices inflicted upon psychiatric patients and for the great love he possesses for his fellow human beings. **Dr. Michael Decaria:** Psychopharmacologist, for his continued praise of my insight into this issue and for his encouragement and support in my research on Prozac. **Dr. Bruce Wooley:** Neuropsychopharmacologist, for his advice and contributions in the area of psychopharmacology, drawing upon years of experience with PCP and Darvon addiction and teaching and lecturing psychiatrists on the use of psychoactive drugs. **Dr. Ray Smith:** Physiological psychologist, Life Balance International, Inc., for his contribution in the area of addictions, brain wave patterns and CES (cranial electrical stimulation) research and treatment. **Hugh Nibley:** One of the greatest minds in our time and one of my greatest inspirations throughout my life. **The Media:** Those who have demonstrated courage and integrity by alerting an unsuspecting public to the problems arising from the use of Prozac and various other mind-altering drugs. **Others: Guy McConnell,** the national director of the Prozac Survivor's Support Group, **Bonnie Leitsch,** past president of the Prozac Survivor's Support Group, **Coralie Reid, Larry Verbeck, Dwight Harlor,** and **J.C. Gardner** for their assistance in gathering medical information. All those authors whose works have contributed so much to assist me in gathering such an incredible amount of information from so many different areas of study. Your work has given me a joy of learning and understanding as pieces of this puzzle have come together to form this text. I hope that those who read this will be encouraged to immerse themselves in your writings as I have and learn to the extent you have taught me. Also to all those from around the world, from all walks of life who have contributed in so many ways to make this publication possible. I wish there was room to name all of you individually. You know who you are, many of you have had your lives changed forever through your own private experience with one of the new Serotonin Reuptake Inhibitors. I thank you all from the bottom of my heart.

FOREWORD

DR. PETER R. BREGGIN

Why is this such an important book? Why is it imperative for psychiatric survivors and their supporters to begin reporting the damaging effects of psychiatric drugs based on their own experience and perspective?

First of all, the data produced by consumers and victims of psychiatric drugs are an invaluable source of information. But secondly, survivor-generated reports become all the more important because information on the negative effects of psychiatric drugs is not reliably available through drug company and psychiatric channels. It is well known, for example, that it took twenty years before the drug companies and the psychiatric profession began to officially recognize tardive dyskinesia, even though it is an obvious neurological disorder that afflicts up to 50% or more of long-term patients who receive neuroleptic drugs like Haldol and Thorazine. Even today, there is far too much professional resistance to appreciating the size and severity of the tardive dyskinesia epidemic. As I document in *TOXIC PSYCHIATRY* (St. Martin's Press, 1991), the dangerous effects of most psychiatric drugs continue to receive too little attention within the profession.

Only a few days before writing this foreword, I participated in the annual meeting of the American Psychiatric Association in Washington, D.C. Within the Washington Convention Center, a giant hall was devoted to the promotion of books, texts and other products related to psychiatry. By far the overwhelming amount of space was taken over by companies pushing their drugs. It was a virtual Disneyland of Drugs, with towering displays, multi-media demonstrations, and the obligatory attractive salespersons. The free gifts were legion: books, coffee mugs, laminated ID tags - all emblazoned with drug company logos and names.

Among these various pharmaceutical displays, the largest and most outrageous was Eli Lilly's huge pavilion, really a shrine, devoted exclusively to Prozac. It was as spacious as a modern hotel lobby and better appointed. I paced it off and it measured approximately 18 by 36 yards. To enter or exit, you passed beneath great arches and in front of TV screens touting Prozac. In the center, high in the air, a giant moon-like logo turned slowly around. There were many couches, tables and chairs for your convenience. It was as if you had stepped inside a living multi-color 3-dimensional advertisement for Prozac, right out of the pages of the *AMERICAN JOURNAL OF PSYCHIATRY*.

Nowhere within the Prozac pavilion did I find any reference to the controversy

controversy surrounding Prozac. It was as if it did not exist. Glancing around, one would never know the drug had anything but the most miraculous effects.

The American Psychiatric Association showed no shame about promoting the drug companies. The Eli Lilly logo actually appeared on the zippered carrying case given to each psychiatrist attending the convention! It held the various registration and convention materials and nearly every participant carried one about each day.

Some of the most important data in Ann Tracy's book are based on anecdotes and personal experiences rather than controlled, scientific studies. This has some built-in limitations. But what about the data collected by the Food and Drug Administration (FDA), the federal organization that is supposed to be monitoring the dangerous effects of drugs like Prozac? The initial controlled trials for FDA approval last only a few weeks - usually less than two months - and from then on the FDA relies largely on anecdotal reports sent to it by drug companies and individual doctors. Are these more reliable than the reports generated by survivors? I think not. I myself have learned more about the dangerous effects of Prozac from Prozac survivors than from the drug company promotional materials.

Publications by psychiatric survivors offer a healthy balance to the often biased reports that are now available from the drug companies and the psychiatric profession. Ann Tracy's book is a valuable contribution to consumers and professionals alike.

PETER R. BREGGIN, M.D., Director
Center for the Study of Psychiatry
Bethesda, Maryland

CONTENTS

CONTENTS CONT.

PROLOGUE

THE PANDORA'S BOX

"All at once, every evil and spiteful thing flew out, like a swarm of insects infesting the earth with pain and sorrow...thanks to Pandora, life on earth was never quite so joyful ever again." From the story of Pandora's Box

On September 14, 1989, Joseph Wesbecker literally blew the lid off the Pandora's box unveiling one of the most terrible of the paradoxical reactions to Prozac when he walked into his former place of employment, Louisville, Kentucky's Standard Gravure Corp., took the elevator to the third floor and as the elevator doors opened, started firing with an AK-47 semiautomatic assault rifle. In what authorities called a "blood bath you don't get over" Wesbecker took eight lives and wounded twelve others before taking his own life.

Unfortunately, the first medical letter to be published on the relation of Prozac to suicidal ideation and violence came too late for Joseph Wesbecker and twenty of his former co-workers. Although he had been placed on permanent medical disability the previous year after being diagnosed as "manic depressive," he was described as never having had a history of violence. He had never struck his wife or children and in thirty-two years had never had an argument on the job. He had never tried to hurt anyone else and everyone who worked with him described him as your average "nice Joe." Yet one of his victims described the same man, as he turned a gun on her, as "totally devoid of any human element, and human soul...He was just 'gone.' There wasn't anything there." (Friends, family and acquaintances describing the individual who is in trouble on Prozac often refer to them as "gone". There seems to be no other way to describe the complete change in personality that takes place.)

What was the catalyst that turned this gentle man into a savage bloodthirsty murderer almost overnight? His psychiatrist was shocked by his patient's obvious deterioration. Two days before the shooting spree the doctor took Wesbecker off Prozac after a five week period of usage and wrote these notes:

"Patient seems to have deteriorated. Tangential thought.

"Weeping in session. Increased agitation and anger.

11

"Question (?) from Prozac.

"Because of deterioration I encouraged patient to go into the hospital for stabilization but he refused.

"Plan - Discontinue Prozac which may be cause. Return to clinic in two weeks."

He didn't return in two weeks. He walked into the annals of history two days later as one of the most notorious mass murderers ever.

Wesbecker had for many years been taking Lithium for his manic reactions and continued to take it along with the Prozac his doctor had recently prescribed. In the inquest a jury ruled that the drugs "may have been a contributing factor" in this case.

Joseph Wesbecker's experience with Prozac began to arouse public awareness to the seriousness of the adverse reactions connected to this drug. Tragically, Wesbecker's reaction, nor any warning since then has been loud enough or clear enough to awaken us all to the painful reality of the potential very serious dangers of the Specific Serotonin Reuptake Inhibitors.

On March 6, 1992, Jim and Carri Pizzuto's only child, Marc, 22, brought that awareness home for them by putting a gun to his head and pulling the trigger. Jim has spent every minute since then asking himself over and over and over again why he did not listen to every word of the television program he saw on Prozac several months earlier. Or why he did not heed the warnings given. How he wishes now that the program would have been more bold and straightforward rather than being so "politically polite" in presenting both sides of the issue. Why didn't the program reach out and grab him, shaking into him the fear he now has of the drug? Why didn't it make him realize then the impact those warnings could have made in his own life within a few short months? Why didn't it make him realize the reality of the danger lying in wait for his own loved ones? Why did it have to be Marc who taught him that lesson in a way that will be imbedded deeply and painfully within his soul forever?

Now the questions never end for Jim and Carri, nor for Marc's friends and family. Now with an intensified interest they closely listen to every news report of violent or bizarre behavior or violent suicides and murders and wonder if anyone knew enough to ask if Prozac was involved. They worry about those left behind with all the same questions - those who have fewer or no answers about this drug than they had - answers which would help them begin to understand the tragedies with which they are left to cope.

Marc Pizzuto had deeply touched the lives of many in his short 22 years. Throughout his childhood, he was loving, energetic, confident and contented. His parents saw no signs of depression except for brief periods during his last two winters, when he complained of symptoms resembling Seasonal Affective Disorder (SAD). A doctor at his Maryland University health center prescribed Prozac. Five weeks later Marc was missing classes (something he had never done before), sleeping excessively, and the following week he was dead. Jim describes his son as "the most remarkable and gifted person I have ever known". He felt it a privilege to have been Marc's father. Even though he has every reason to be prejudiced in his opinion of his son, Jim Pizzuto does not stand alone. Marc was loved and admired by all he met. One of Marc's classmates in his Conflict Partnership class shared his feelings about Marc with their professor, "We always got into long discussions after class, and I never could keep up with Marc's depth of thought. I admired the way Marc seemed so fascinated with every aspect of life. He was the kind of person I wanted to be."

Their professor, Colman McCarthy, is also a writer for *THE WASHINGTON POST*. He described Marc as "a young fellow who glowed with life and had ample self confidence to handle the routine academic ups-and-downs that periodically come to every college student...He had qualities that would hearten any teacher: a reflective mind, an appetite for the give-and-take delights of classroom discussion and a writing style that was sensory in tone because he avoided the stiffness of term-paper prose in favor of letting his feelings flow. Marc, in the General Honors program, (He kept a 3.8 average and was on an partial academic scholarship.) had the rarest of undergraduate gifts - intellectual openness. He savored exploring new ideas and seeing where they would take him. He spoke of becoming a professor."

Marc wrote two papers for Mr. McCarthy's class: "THE UTILITY OF A NONVIOLENT LIFESTYLE" and "CONFLICT PARTNERSHIP - A REMARKABLE NEW APPROACH TO MANAGING CONFLICT." In the second paper Marc wrote: "I am rather fortunate. I feel my parents have taught me many of the techniques found in *CONFLICT PARTNERSHIP,* techniques that are indeed effective. Unknowingly, they have taught me by their example as well as through their interaction with me. Yet I am now more aware of the nature of conflict after reading this book, and I believe I am better equipped to handle future conflicts with greater skill."

Marc's statement should help us to understand why all who knew him wonder why he handled his last conflict in a manner so totally contrary to every non-violent example he had set for 22 years. They wonder why this solution was so adverse to those principles he had always lived with so much conviction. Everyone wonders, that is everyone who does not yet understand the violent compulsive behaviors which can be chemically induced through the altering of brain function.

Jim reflects upon his son's life: "He was blessed with an abundance of natural qualities - exceptional good looks, a strong tall six foot stature, confident blue-grey eyes, casual sandy colored hair and an unforgettable smile. He was charming and witty, thoughtful and considerate. He was especially blessed with a wonderful mind and a genuine concern for others. He was the center of our world and all that parents could hope for...Marc was determined in his convictions but always considerate and open to new ideas. He was genuinely concerned with the lives of people, the people close to him and the people of the world...He belonged to environmental and nature clubs and world conflict resolution groups. He thought and spoke creatively about world issues. His potential was infinite. He made good judgments in all aspects of life. He developed his mind with dedicated study and learning. He passionately loved reading and after absorbing its wonders he would pleasantly articulate the essence of his newly acquired philosophies. He cared for his health with physical activity and good dieting habits. He enjoyed sports and daily maintained his fitness with exercising and running. He was a non-smoker and ate wholesome, healthy foods. He was a vegetarian. He felt the excessive waste in polluting fertilizers for growing grain to feed beef and the extravagant waste in grain for beef could be put to far more efficient and humane use in feeding the starving peoples of the world. Furthermore, he was opposed to the way that animals are confined and raised in feeding pens, and did not want to contribute to the animals' abuse by the meat industry. Marc cast his vote by living his principles - unfailingly, those principles were sound and just."

Marc had been a foreign exchange student which allowed him an opportunity to develop deep and enduring friendships with families and students in other countries around the world. All mourn the loss of their friend and the lost promises of the future. Marc was especially fluent in French, but spoke other languages as well. His English skills were impeccable. He loved and studied extensively European and Asian history and cultures. He loved learning and often expressed his conviction that learning is pure joy. He was actively involved in reducing world conflict through better understanding.

In Marc's memory, his fellow students and friends at the University Career Development Center, where he worked, planted a Yoshino cherry tree in the center of a prominent square on the university grounds. It's a peaceful place with benches, green grass, tall trees and stately buildings. Along a shaded path, on a brick wall, near the tree they placed a bronze plaque inscribed with a quotation from one of Marc's papers, "THE BEST EDUCATION IS THE ONE THAT INSTILLS THE LOVE OF LEARNING." The cherry tree symbolizes the keen interest Marc possessed for Japanese culture, also, it will bloom each spring and mature into a grand symbol of Marc's fascination for learning.

Jim ends his description of his son with: "Marc's positive spirit and thoughtful consideration was felt by everyone who knew him and remembered by anyone that met him even for a few brief moments. His innate qualities made us love him, his remarkable intelligence, his expressions, his sincerity. He touched us deep in our hearts and made us love him so very much...We were encouraged by his example, his values and philosophies. Even as Marc's father, I frequently sought and benefited greatly from his clear thinking and sound judgment. Through his infancy, and as he grew, he was the greatest joy possible in life for his mother and me. His excellence gave our life great meaning. I was constantly amazed and inspired by his brilliance. That this brilliant mind would in the end conclude that suicide was somehow a solution..."

Is Prozac the catalyst producing in these people an obsessive violent need to kill and be killed ? Are these patients being chemically induced to take their own lives and the lives of those around them? There as yet is no one agency tracking the connection between Prozac and suicide, or Prozac and violent crime. How many deaths have there already been of which we are unaware because of this? How many more deaths do we need to witness? How much more terror to the victims and to the perpetrator himself? How many more wonderfully creative individuals - the greatest gifts to our world - can we afford to lose before we learn the answer to that question? How many more Marc Pizzutos will have the answer to these questions arrive too late for them?

INTRODUCTION

LEGAL VS. ILLEGAL DRUGS
A BROKEN RECORD OF HISTORY REPEATING ITSELF
...OVER...AND OVER...AND OVER AGAIN

We really do not even begin to comprehend how powerfully we can be affected by chemicals. Our "just say no to drugs" campaign scratches the surface but does not dare go too far. If it did it would insult one of the most financially and politically powerful industries in the world: the pharmaceuticals. At this point in time there has been sufficient medical research completed to help us understand what the highly addictive mind/mood altering drugs are doing to us and why they cause such violent and bizarre out-of-character behavior. These drugs, legal as well as illegal, have flooded the market over the last thirty to forty years and yet with each new generation we seem to have to learn our lesson all over again. The use of legal psychoactive prescription drugs has become very widespread because of extremely vigorous marketing campaigns by the pharmaceutical companies. During 1991 it is estimated that approximately *five billion dollars* was spent by the pharmaceutical industry on advertizing alone to encourage us all to use these chemical agents in spite of the massive amounts of medical documentation and governmental investigation indicating the serious and very dangerous side effects they possess, in addition to their devastating addictive potential.

In 1979 the book *TRANQUILIZING OF AMERICA* warned us of things to come in the use of psychotropic drugs. They spoke of how each new drug is heralded as safer, faster and more effective and specific than the one before it, while time and experience proved none of this to be true. Phenobarbital was replaced by Miltown, Miltown replaced by Valium and now Valium has been replaced by Xanax. Each proving to be more dangerous and addictive than the one before. The latest information out on Xanax, ten years after our introduction to this drug that was touted as less addictive than Valium, indicates that as many as one third of the patients are unable to withdraw from the drug *(CONSUMER REPORTS,* Jan. 1993). These authors of *TRANQUILIZING OF AMERICA* warned over twenty years ago, "The most recent developments in the field of psychotropic drugs suggest that science and medicine are on the verge of discovering a way to alter our moods, quiet our anxiety, and increase our intelligence without harmful side effects. Soon it might be possible to pinpoint and isolate the chemical switches in the brain that control mood and intelligence without affecting other parts of the central nervous system. *There is, however, growing evidence that such a chemical world is not likely to be a safe one."* (p. 310)

We now live in that chemical world they spoke of and attempted to warn us about over a decade ago, a chemical world filled with violence. Is there a connection? Throughout this text we will discuss how the chemical changes brought about by these drugs interfere with various brain functions. This disruption in brain function can cause either drastic or gradual changes in the thought processes altering both mood and behavior. One of the most important and serious of the side effects, which is often passed off as only minor, is that these drugs can produce severe disruption of sleep patterns. This disruption in sleep can result in sleep debt which forces the patient into the hallucinogenic dream state during wakefulness. The most recent sleep research is beginning to help us understand more fully how these drugs keep the patient alternating through varying levels of consciousness, including a potentially dangerous sleepwalk state.

Many of these drugs, because of their stimulant profile, can at first deceive the patient and those around them into thinking the patient is improving and performing at a higher level. Although this forcing of the brain into performing beyond its present capacity can produce desired results at first, the results are not lasting. After the drug-induced boost or higher level of performance is achieved, the patient is left in worse condition than before drug treatment through the rebound effects of these drugs. Sleeping aids upon discontinuation leave the patient with equal or even greater insomnia called "rebound insomnia." The anti-anxiety medications upon discontinuation leave the patient with equal or even greater anxiety called "rebound anxiety." The anti-depressants upon discontinuation leave the patient with equal or even greater depression called "rebound depression," etc., etc.

Whether these drugs be legal or illegal at this stage of our ever changing patterns of social acceptance or rejection is of no importance in the context of why they have these effects upon us or how they actually do affect us. We have no time to lose in educating not only the general public, but medical professionals, judges, lawyers, etc. Drugs have too far reaching an impact upon every aspect of our lives and our society. Our ignorance of them and their effects upon us has placed us on the brink of complete destruction - a physical destruction from within ourselves, which in turn affects our families and our society.

The authors of *TRANQUILLIZING OF AMERICA* further comment on our custom of keeping our aspirin, cold remedies, Valium and Ritalin in the medicine chest, our vodka in the liquor cabinet, our beer in the fridge, and our cocaine in a plastic bag hidden in a shoe as we attempt to separate the drugs we use for medicinal or recreational purposes. *"There is, in short, a separation, albeit sometimes blurred, between the drugs we take for medical reasons and those we take for social or recreational purposes. But with the development and widespread use of psychoactive medications for mood and mind control, the separation between the drugs we take to alleviate disease and those we take simply because we want to feel better or different is growing increasingly thin. The experimental drugs for medical use now on the laboratory drawing boards [this was written in the early eighties] might eliminate the separation entirely..."* (p. 314) As we go on to learn the action of the latest of the new psychoactive drugs upon the brain - those drugs which were then on the laboratory drawing boards -in comparison to the now illegal drugs, you will see that the separation between these drugs has become far, far less than "thin."

The question does not seem to be as much "where do we draw the line?" as it is "when do we draw the line?" in removing a drug from the "legal" status and placing it in an "illegal" status. Ethically and morally who has the right to determine just how many people have to die before the step is taken to change a drug from being legal to illegal? The conflicts of interest within the FDA has produced an outcry from many a consumer protection group over the last decade or two as the pharmaceuticals and FDA officials have formed closer and closer ties. It has been documented in many a volume that many FDA officials have worked very hard not to cross the pharmaceuticals so that they would be insured of a good position within one of these companies when they left their FDA posts. This is a practice which is not only unethical, but should be declared illegal.

Most of us are aware of the problems arising from our medical use of the amphetamines, cocaine, heroin, etc. for various ailments in the past. Now let us examine more closely the history of the psychoactive drugs and their beginnings. It may be as much of a surprise to you as it was to me. Those who saw the movie AWAKENINGS with Robin Williams - a movie adapted from Dr. Oliver Sacks' book and his real life experience, will recall the discussion between the doctor and his superior about the ethics of using the drug El Dopa to attempt to bring patients out of their catatonic state. The superior warned, *"Freud believed in miracles, prescribing cocaine like it was candy. And we all believed in the miracle of cortisone until our patients went psychotic on it!"*

Freud, the father of psychiatry, was thrilled with his discovery of cocaine and himself became addicted. His example paved the way for many psychiatrists after him who used themselves as subjects to determine the effects of the mind-altering drugs. How they felt they could use mind-altering drugs which would affect their judgement, even to the extent of producing hallucinations, and still be capable of gaining any perspective into how the drug was affecting them seems far beyond logical reasoning, but this self-experimentation became the common practice. Just how common it is today would be interesting to know. Much has been written and reported as of late about the use of these drugs among physicians. NBC news devoted a special news feature to this subject in September of 1993.

Freud, as most who are addicted to a drug will do, highly recommended the use of cocaine. A close friend of his, Ernst Fleischl von Marxow, a pathologist, had become addicted to morphine after surgery. Freud attempted a cure by recommending that he use cocaine. The drug-induced euphoria did help him with the morphine withdrawal. Cocaine produces a prompt yet brief euphoria followed by a sudden "crashing" into a depression, requiring continued use and higher and higher doses to produce the continued euphoria. Unfortunately because of his use of cocaine in stronger and stronger doses, von Marxow became completely psychotic. His was one of the earliest recorded cases of cocaine-induced psychosis - one of our first glimpses into the creation of insanity through the use of drugs.

The effects of cocaine upon the brain are long term. As we will discuss in detail later, it can cause panic attacks and other problems years later because of its long term effects upon the brain. It creates learning and memory difficulties. Yet cocaine was once used as a cure for depression, especially the depression associated with mania in bipolar disorders. In light of the fact that cocaine is a stimulant and stimulants cause mania, the use of the drug for manic depression seems quite illogical. The National Institute on Drug Abuse (NIDA) estimates that approximately six million Americans regularly use cocaine. Many athletes are tempted to use cocaine because of its a\lity to enhance performance, yet the effects are short term and the cost is great. William Gildea, a sportswriter for *THE WASHINGTON POST*, described the use of cocaine by some athletes as "a nightmare of physical suffering, depression and paranoia, craving cocaine more than life itself."

Cocaine creeps up on you, and it won't let go. "It can make a person feel awake and alert and produce a brief state of exhilaration, or pleasurable excitement. But these feelings are short-lived, as the effects of cocaine wear off rapidly. To maintain a cocaine 'high,' the user must repeatedly ingest the drug, and cocaine is highly addictive. Some people can become cocaine addicts after only a few days of repeated use. Others take longer to get hooked, but prolonged use causes addiction eventually." (*DRUGS AND SPORTS,* p.57) Frequent cocaine use is demonstrated by episodes of shaking and sweating, restlessness, anxiety, insomnia and becoming easily angered. Often users do not realize they're hooked until after loosing their careers and families.

Steroids have serious and powerful psychiatric side effects. The statement from the movie AWAKENINGS also mentioned the strong support of the medical community for the use of cortisone before they discovered that it also chemically induced psychosis in their patients. Cortisone is a steroid. It may help us to understand the psychiatric side effects produced by steroids if we know that adrenalin (epinephrine) hormones or steroids, such as cortisone, are chemically related to amphetamines, commonly known as "speed." The body produces its own cortisone which we call cortisol. How many of us are aware of the hazardous psychiatric effects brought on by steroids? Patients often experience mood swings. Within seconds they can go from feeling happy to feeling angry or depressed. Steroids definitely have psychological or emotional effects on the people who use them. The steroids can drive a patient completely insane - to the point of experiencing full blown psychosis. ***Studies show changes in brain wave activity in steroid users. These changes are similar to those observed in brain waves of a person who uses stimulants or antidepressants.*** Some of the changes brought on by steroids are "an increase of mental alertness, elevation of mood, improvement of memory and concentration, and reduction of sensations of fatigue, all of which can be partly related to the 'stimulatory' effects of anabolic-androgenic steroids on the central nervous system. Of course the long term effects are the same as they are with stimulants, namely a drastic decrease in all of the above causing depression, loss of memory and concentration fatigue, decrease in alertness to the extent of full blown psychosis. Itil, et al. (1974) found that ***electroencephalographic profiles [EEG - brain waves] resulting from varying dosages of anabolic-androgenic steroids were very similar to those seen with such psychostimulants as dextroamphetamine and the tricyclic antidepressants.*** Others (Broverman, Klaiber, Kobayashi, & Vogel, 1968; Klaiber, Broverman, & Kobayashi, 1967; Stenn, Klaiber, Vogel, & Broverman, 1972) have concluded that the adrenergic-like effects of testosterone on brain function are a result of an elevation of the brain's norepinephrine level, which might result from the inhibition of monoamine oxidase activity in the brain. Further speculation indicates that the 'heightened' state of behavior may well be due to an increased level of norepinephrine in the brain." *(ANABOLIC STEROIDS IN SPORT AND EXERCISE,* p. 163)

Although it has become unacceptable or unethical for athletes, and professional athletes have outlawed the use of steroids, society still experiences many problems from the use of these drugs among athletes. "Sometimes the steroid-induced hostility of athletes spills over into the nonathletic world and affects innocent people. For example, several police officers who used steroids while weight lifting off duty were suspended or fired from their jobs. The steroids made the officers' behavior so aggressive that the men verbally or physically abused citizens they were supposed to be helping. In one incident, a female shopkeeper complained to an officer about the police using her phone too much. The man flew into a rage, pulled out his gun, and shot the woman. She is now in a wheelchair and paralyzed for life." (*DRUGS AND SPORTS,* p. 24-25) In San Diego, California in mid October of 1993, James Buquet entered a health spa shooting wildly and cursing. He was described by one witness as a "crazy psycho" after killing several people and then shooting himself. After an investigation it was discovered that he was using steroids. It is not surprising to learn that Hitler gave his troops steroids as a means to increase aggression.

(An excellent movie called BIGGER THAN LIFE with James Mason is a true life experience of a mild mannered male schoolteacher who becomes completely psychotic and attempts to kill his family after being prescribed cortisone. This is a movie which should be viewed by anyone using any mind-altering drug. Their families should watch it too. I highly recommend it.)

Dr. John Ziegler, who brought steroids to the US after seeing them used among Russian athletes, allied himself with Ciba Pharmaceutical to give study subjects what he considered low dosages (5 mg) of testosterone extract. He, like Freud, administered steroids to himself to observe their effects. But, "...it wasn't long before victory-conscious U.S. athletes were indulging themselves by taking tremendous dosages of steroids that resulted in some severe physical problems. Shocked by the Frankenstein' monster he had built and unleashed, Dr. Ziegler discontinued his experimentation." (*STEROIDS,* p. 28-29) He regretted what he had done so strongly that could he have turned back the clock, he probably would have destroyed his 'miracle drug.' Unfortunately, like all those drugs used experimentally before them, the steroids were here to stay. By the 1950's, steroids were seen as wonder drugs that could fatten cattle quickly to bring a higher price at the marketplace. And although we now know that they are often the cause of cancer because of their very damaging effects upon the immune system, they were originally thought to be a long-awaited cure for cancer.

The steroids fall into two classes: the corticosteroids, such as prednisone and cortisone and the anabolic steroids which have become so popular among athletics for muscle building. Both types cause very dangerous psychiatric side effects which can result in violence. This situation becomes extremely alarming when we realize that an estimated 500,000 young athletes are using the anabolic steroids. The physical side effects alone should be enough to frighten any young developing human being from using these drugs. Although the steroids are used among athletes to increase muscle mass, the muscles developed during the use of the drug disappear upon discontinuation of use. Young men become more feminine and young women become more masculine. Some young men have even had to have a mastectomy to remove unwanted breasts after the use of steroids, a terrible price to pay for larger and stronger muscles which last only for a short time. The steroids also produce heart, liver and kidney damage. They attack every body system as they weaken and destroy the immune system. The psychiatric side effects can result in out of control and out of character behavior, rages causing both injury and death to innocent bystanders, and full psychosis.

In spite of the very serious potential hazards, many use these drugs regularly for many reasons. Prednisone and cortisone are commonly used for many ailments, asthma inhalants, pain from injuries or arthritis, etc. Actually birth control pills are the most widely used of the steroid drugs. Oral contraceptives were first introduced in the early 1960's; today, most birth-control pills are combinations of synthetic steroids. They can produce serious interactions when combined with nicotine. Women report psychiatric side effects from the use of contraceptives as well. Women should be cautioned or warned of these possibilities when they are prescribed these commonly used types of drugs so that they can watch for any of these adverse reactions and alert their physician if a problem arises. Few understand that many of the symptoms of PMS are being induced by these drugs. Cancer expert Dr. Charles Simone adamately declares the cancer risk in conjuction with hormones, "In hormonal use (including both birth control and post menopausal drugs), the risks *far outweigh* the benefits."

Adolescence is when the hormones begin to rush in the body and emotions can be very unsettling and steroids used in this age group can cause many problems. When adding steroids to the body, the patient suddenly has to cope with a flood of hormones that it cannot handle. Steroids cause other effects upon the mind such as trouble getting to sleep, terrible nightmares when they do sleep, some users hear voices, others experience a constant, nagging feeling that people are out to get them or paranoia, others experience feelings of great importance or superiority, and research and anecdotal information suggested some time ago that schizophrenia and manic depression are associated with steroid use. One man, convinced that his mind was controlling a television program he was viewing, flew into a rage when the story did not end the way he wanted it to. Clinical reports suggest that affective and psychotic syndromes, some violent, have been found to be associated with the use of steroids (Annitto & Layman, 1980; Barker, 1987; Choi et al., 1989; Conacher & Workman, 1989; Freinhar & Alvarez, 1985; Katz & Pope, 1990; Leckman & Scahill, 1990; Moore, 1988;

Pope & Katz, 1987, 1988, 1990). Some cases have been reported in which the defendants claimed that psychological and behavioral effects of steroids induced the commission of criminal acts (Conacher & Workman, 1989; 'Doctor,' 1988; 'Ex-player's odd behavior,' 1988; 'The Insanity,' 1988, 'Killing try,' 1988; Lubell, 1989; Maryland v. Michael D. Williams, 1986; Moss, 1988). It is now well understood that excess steroids can produce emotional instability, ranging from euphoria to suicidal despondency (Hall, 1980). Documentation of mental disorders in association with steroids has existed since the early 1950's (Borman & Schmallenberg, 1951; Brody, 1952; Byyny, 1976; Clark, Bauer, & Cobb, 1952; d'Orban, 1989; Glaser, 1953; Rome & Braceland, 1952; Train & Winkler, 1962, Alcena & Alexopoulos, 1985; Fricchione, Ayyala, & Holmes, 1989: Kaufmann, Kahaner, Peselow, & Gershon, 1982; Lewis & Smith, 1983; Ling, Perry, & Tsuang, 1981).

Steroid users often report severe depression in withdrawal. Some people become suicidal as well. Patients report, "They make me more impatient. I'd get angry very easily, especially when I was driving my car. If I had to stop for a red light, I'd get very upset. I felt rushed, always in a hurry, kind of 'on edge' all the time. I also had trouble sleeping at night. My blood pressure went way up, too. I started to lose my hair. And I got some fatty tumors on my body. Steroids made me feel that I could do anything." Increase in muscle strength and power can, in part, be accounted for by neurotransmitter levels (Hakkinen & Komi, 1983; Moritani & deVries, 1979). Research also shows that steroids may in some way modify neural and neuromuscular functions, which supports the belief that elevated norepinephrine or reduced monoamine levels play an important part in the production of increases in muscle power (Alen, Hakkinen, & Komi, 1984; Brooks, 1980; Hakkinen & Alen, 1986; Wilson, 1988). (It is important to note that although the person may feel he is omnipotent, the actual muscle strength is not always there and serious damage may result from this overexertion.) In the following chapter we will discuss the body's hormonal system, why this side effect is present in conjunction with steroid use and why this information is so significant in understanding the role of the SSRIs and why they produce these same types of side effects.

PCP was once thought to be "safe?" Another example of how we are placing ourselves on the brink of destruction by our open arms attitude to all of these psychoactive drugs is the case of PCP. Few are aware that phencyclidine, better known to us as PCP or "Angel Dust" was introduced both as an analgesic (a painkiller) and a dissociative anesthetic. A dissociative anesthetic puts the patient in a dissociative state - a state out of touch with reality and incapable of feeling pain though performing as one who deceptively appears conscious - very similar

24

to a sleepwalk state. PCP was developed and patented in 1957 by Parke, Davis & Company Pharmaceutical. They marketed it under the product name "Serynl" (derived from serenity). Although our experience with PCP has proven otherwise, *according to __medical studies__ the drug was originally considered to have a large margin of safety in humans!* (Domino 1964) By 1967 the problems became apparent even to Parke, Davis who pulled the drug from the market. Not until 1978 was PCP classed as a schedule three drug (having no therapeutic use) - twenty years after Parke, Davis obtained their patent and fourteen years after the study just mentioned which declared it to have a large margin of safety. It reportedly took about *seventeen years* for physicians to understand the dangerous potential of PCP.

Addressing the serious problems presented by this lag time between a drug's discovery and subsequent change in classification, Dr. Ronald K. Siegal wrote, "The time is 1959. Research Laboratories of Parke, Davis and Company in Detroit have just 'discovered' phencyclidine. That announcement added one more drug to the rapidly growing list of psychoactive compounds, both natural and synthetic, which affect behavior...It is now 1978. *With such an evolutionary, albeit natural, lag between the emergence of a new drug and its scientific investigation*, it is not surprising that today, a generation after phencyclidine's discovery, those people born when the drug was first developed are using and exploring its psychoactive properties *whose scientific investigations still lag behind." (PCP PHENCYCLIDINE ABUSE: AN APPRAISAL*, p. 119)

Twenty years after its introduction, Dr. Edward F.Domino, who discovered PCP for Parke, Davis & Company made this statement, "In 1964, when we reviewed the neurobiology of phencyclidine (Domino 1964) it impressed us that the development of a new drug provides the pharmacologist and clinician with a number of surprises. That conclusion is even more true today. Who would, in their wildest imagination, predict that a dissociative anesthetic, which produced a high incidence of anesthetic emergence phenomena and was a drug which mimicked the primary symptoms of schizophrenia by distorting body image, would become the number one drug of abuse in the United States in 1978? Yet that is what the drug culture of our country has accomplished with phencyclidine. Surely a schizophrenomimetic drug in low dosage, and anesthetic and a convulsant in large doses, would not seem to be reinforcing - yet it apparently is to many people who now call it by many different names, including PCP, synthetic THC, angel dust, hog, crystal, animal tranquilizer, horse tranquilizer, peace pill, PeaCe Pill, crystal joint, CJ, KJ, sheet, and rocket fuel. People who abuse phencyclidine have been called parsley monsters when the drug is applied to parsley and smoked. Those who are 'high' on phencyclidine are said to be 'crystallized.' The drug is taken by inhalation, orally, intranasally (snorted), and intravenously. *Knowing what we now know, would any of us who were involved with the early pharmacological birth and development of phencyclidine have ventured further? What have we wrought?"* (*PCP PHENCYCLIDINE ABUSE: AN APPRAISAL*, p. 19)

What impact has just this one mistake by the pharmaceuticals cost society? Even though Parke Davis & Co. removed the drug from the market for human use in 1965, PCP or "Angel Dust" has for years now been a major drug of abuse in the United States. Drug and law enforcement officers dread having to deal with anyone on PCP. Of all the illegal drugs PCP's effects qualify it as one of the very most dangerous. The drug produces almost super human strength in the users and because they feel no pain, it is next to impossible to stop them short of killing them - they just keep fighting. Police have reported incidences where those on PCP have even stripped the flesh from their hands by pulling them through locked hand cuffs.

One 38 year old man who had been smoking marijuana laced with PCP experienced a terrible psychotic reaction. He became very aggressive, attacked a stranger with a razor and decapitated his dog. The interesting thing to note was how long the depression and impaired thinking persisted after discontinuation of PCP use and how much trouble this man had realizing that the delusions he experienced were actually delusions and not reality - a demonstration of the vividness of the dream state in a drug induced psychosis. [The strong inhibition of REM is extremely significant in the production of the hallucinogenic state as you will see in studying the information on sleep disorders in the chapter entitled SLEEP DISORDERS, SEROTONIN, AND THE SSRIs.]

PCP induced psychosis in a "normal human subject" - a case report. In order to see just how much of an impact PCP can have upon innocent victims let's relate a story reviewed in the *READER'S DIGEST*:

These mind-altering effects of the drugs set the stage for a science fiction horror movie. Such was the terrifying experience of Lt. Peter Chmelir as he picked up his luggage after a flight to Florida on June 9, 1978, the same year PCP was classified as a Schedule 3 drug. As he grabbed one of his bags from the luggage carousel he noticed it was coated with a pungent smelling chemical. For a spilt second he considered reporting it, but remembered his friend waiting on him and rushed out. His own personal chemical spill over the next six months turned his life into a hellish nightmare that nearly cost him his life and his career.

After only a few blocks in the car with the bag Chmelir's head began to ache. When he arrived in his room at the base he rinsed the clothes out that had been in that bag. The next morning he bought some detergent and washed the clothes twice. That took care of most of the smell. Late the next morning he put on a pair of underwear from the bag, dressed, went to lunch and then sunbathed for a while. He began to feel lightheaded but dismissed it. He then put on a fresh pair of underwear from the same bag and went to supper. He began to notice a burning sensation in his groin and then began to feel drunk. He made it to his room and after a shower the burning stopped, but he could not concentrate. He was unable to focus on a single thought, lost his peripheral vision. It became tunnel vision and was all out of focus. He asked to be taken to the hospital, even thinking to take a pair of underwear with him for the doctor to examine the chemical. Because of his disorientation his story about the chemical was dismissed. The doctor sent him back to the base assuming it was an allergic reaction and that he should report to the dispensary in the morning. Chmelir awoke at 3 a.m. to terrorizing fear. He was sure he was dying. He called the fire department and by the time they arrived he was hallucinating.

There is very little recall of that Monday, the third day following his flight. He was told he spent the day lashing out, moaning and sobbing. He was tormented by unlabeled fears and distorted horrors. Late Tuesday afternoon his wife returned from a trip and received a call about her husband's condition. She was told he was doing better and would be discharged the following day. Although his head was foggy that Wednesday, his emotions were stable and his control had returned.

Thursday he had a doctor's appointment. In the middle of it he began to feel lightheaded again, emotional control disappeared as he sobbed and babbled off into full psychosis. The diagnosis, "schizophrenia". His wife was flown from California to Florida to be with him. She was shocked by his condition. He could not walk and did not even recognize her. On June 21 she accompanied him to a medical center in California. Although heavily sedated, he became aggressive, hostile and insulting. He had become someone she did not know. He became rational when he arrived in California, but feared he would most likely spend the rest of his life in a mental hospital. Actually his condition improved rapidly and plans were made to release him within a week.

Five days later he dressed in his civilian clothes and went out to eat with his brother. Before they made it to the restaurant Peter became frantic, insisting they would not be able to find their way back to the hospital and his speech began to slur. He spent the night screaming beneath his hospital bed. Then he became physically frozen in a catatonic state. His wife was not permitted to see him. She was taken aside and told that they had discovered PCP in Peter's urine. Doctors still discounted the chemical on Peter's bag. That happened three weeks earlier, how could it possibly be affecting him now? They suspected he must be getting the drug whenever he left the hospital. When confronted, Peter denied ever using the drug. When it was still in his urine ten days later a search was made of his hospital ward. His wife began to research PCP. She found that drug and law enforcement officials are instructed to be very cautious in their handling of PCP because it penetrates the skin on contact and intoxication can also be brought on by inhaling the fumes.

By July 21 Peter was able to return home. All were encouraged by his progress, but the following day while attending a movie with his wife, he grabbed her hand tightly and said he needed to go home. She looked to see his eyes rolling back into his head. At home she undressed him and locked him in the bedroom. The following morning she took him to the hospital went home and collapsed in tears across their bed. Suddenly she felt a warm, burning sensation on her face. Her head felt light. She looked down to see that she was lying across the pants Peter had been wearing. As she held the pants up to the light stains appeared. When she turned them inside out she found them covered with countless tiny crystals. She remembered that police had found that they had to be extra careful about handling PCP because they felt reactions just from touching the drug. Excited about her discovery, she called the doctor Peter had been seeing and told him what had happened to her. He told her she had no training, to stop meddling and he would no longer take her calls!

At the hospital Peter was accused of being a PCP addict and proceedings were made for a medical discharge for him with misconduct. On August 16 he was released from the hospital. Several days later his wife sent a sample of clothing and the zipper from his bag to a poison lab. Two days later the results came, the zipper alone contained two grams of PCP - enough to induce full psychosis for an entire town. He now had his answer to many questions about his experience, but it still took him an additional four months to clear his record with the military. One incident cost him such incredible trauma for a year out of his life, not to mention the lingering effects he must have suffered for years after this.

LSD - All is fair in love and war. The discovery of LSD began widespread scientific attention to the conscious-altering properties of psychoactive drugs. Sandoz Pharmaceuticals discovered LSD in 1943 and began to market it in 1947 under the product name Delysid. Sandoz suggested both experimental and analytical applications in research. In other words they actually advocated the chemical induction of a model psychoses in a normal human subject with LSD. They suggested chemically inducing psychoses in normal human beings. The hope was that this would help them discover the organic causes of mental disease. The ethical and moral question is "Where were they to find the 'normal human subject' in which to induce an LSD psychotic reaction?" Who would volunteer? With Sandoz' recommendation to psychiatrists, LSD was used to create a typical schizophrenic reaction in patients with the hope of discovering more about this mental disorder through the LSD induced psychosis. This attitude seems to persist among those looking for answers to how schizophrenia is produced. The psychedelics have continued to be a boon for psychiatric and brain research. In 1986 Dr. Solomon Snyder of Johns Hopkins University, wrote *"...a class of compounds with no demonstrated therapeutic use, a history of extensive abuse, and the ability to provoke psychosis. **Yet many brain researchers value the psychedelic agents above any of the other psychoactive drugs.** These scientists are immensely interested in understanding why the changes wrought by LSD, mescaline, and psilocybin seem to affect the very core of the user's consciousness...the research into psychedelic drugs has already enriched our understanding of how the brain regulates behavior."* (DRUGS AND THE BRAIN, p. 179, 205) Have these scientists been so intensely interested in learning the effects of these drugs that they have become overanxious in using them on an unsuspecting general public?

If there is at the present concern over the disclosure of government experiments with radiation, it should be of great interest to learn of our government's extensive involvement in LSD and other psychosis producing drug experimentation. At Dachau during World War II, the Nazis had experimented with mescaline, in search of a drug that would, according to a intelligence report by the U.S. Navel Technical Mission, "eliminate the will of the person." In 1947, the same year that Switzerland's Sandoz introduced Delysid (LSD), the United States organized the Central Intelligence Agency (CIA). They too had a great interest in drugs for chemical warfare and mind-control in particular. After several years of using scopolamine and liquid marijuana they began searching for additional, even stronger mind-altering drugs and turned to LSD. Their goal was to find a chemical which would: #1 cause a disruption in memory, #2 discredit individuals by producing aberrant behavior, #3 alter sexual patterns, #4 elicit information from the person, #5 open one's mind to suggestion for mind control, and #6 create addiction and dependence. *(STORMING HEAVEN, LSD AND THE AMERICAN DREAM)* (If the reader will turn to the chapter entitled PATIENT REPORTS they will find those on Prozac reporting all six of these results as reactions to the drug.)

The CIA had a real heyday with LSD research. In 1953, as they turned a hopeful eye to LSD, their secret project, focusing on chemical warfare and mind control, MK-ULTRA, was born - a project which would not be known to the public for many years to come. They were initially funded $300,000 for investigation of several drugs from cocaine to nicotine. The Agency considered LSD to be of such promise that in November, 1953 they sent two men with a black bag containing $240,000 (80% of their funds) in cash to Switzerland to buy up Sandoz's entire supply of LSD. They were authorized to purchase an unbelievable amount of 10 kilos - 100 million doses. Much to their surprise they discovered that Sandoz's total output of LSD since its discovery in 1943 was only forty grams, not quite two ounces. After negotiations Sandoz agreed to supply the CIA with 100 grams of LSD every week and also to notify them of anyone else who was ordering the drug.

The CIA then turned to Eli Lilly, the makers of Prozac, who had previously introduced Heroin and Methadone in their products list, as a domestic source for LSD. They proposed that Lilly develop a synthetic LSD since the natural source of LSD, ergot fungus, was difficult to cultivate. A company memo dated October 26, 1954 by Eli Lilly to then CIA head Allen Dulles announced that they had been able to bypass the need for ergot fungus in processing the drug and had come up with an LSD made solely from synthetic sources. They went on to suggest that with this breakthrough in mass production that "in a matter of months LSD would be available in tonnage quantities." Lilly also went on to state that they were continuing their research to develop a "covert use" of LSD. *(ACID DREAMS)* The following December *TIME* magazine reported that *LSD "may actually help psychiatrists clear up mental illness."* It was also promoted as a cure for alcoholism and as an "aid in facilitating psychoanalysis". In fact, the LSD advertising campaign now has an *all too familiar ring* as we recognize many of the same claims Lilly has been making for Prozac over the last six years. The *MERCK DIRECTORY* lists Lilly as obtaining two patents on LSD just two months after the *TIME* article hit the press. Lilly offered to supply unlimited amounts of LSD to the CIA and as the memo to Agency head, Allen Dulles, pointed out, this "meant that LSD could finally be taken seriously as a chemical warfare agent."

Next the CIA turned to the psychological community, particularly those who were already investigating LSD's relation to mental illness, to help them with their research. "Most were eager to help, provided the Agency picked up the tab. They had few moral qualms: if the CIA wanted to finance basic research in an area ignored by traditional organizations like the National Institute of Mental Health, where was the problem?" *(STORMING HEAVEN, LSD AND THE*

AMERICAN DREAM, p. 81) Their fronts were the Josiah Macy Foundation and the Geschickter Fund for Medical Research. They paid out as much as $40,000 per year for research at Mass. Mental Health. Harold Abramson in New York received $85,000 for his research project. Others included Carl Pfieffer at the University of Illinois, and Harold Hodge at the University of Rochester. As reported by Dr. Robert F. Ulrich and Dr. Bernard M. Patten at the Annual Meeting of the American Academy of Neurology (1990), in Miami, Florida, the men hired to carry out this "morally questionable research" were given government grants to do so - our tax dollars at work.

The CIA had trouble obtaining subjects for their research so they turned to George Hunter White. He referred to the drug as "Stormy" to describe the unpredictably variable effects of LSD. During the day White was busily engaged tracking down drug pushers, yet as the sun went down he became the pusher. White employed prostitutes for a series of experiments from coast to coast. April 13, 1953, a brothel operation, dubbed "Midnight Climax", was born. They disguised their "laboratory" as a bordello where the unsuspecting "clients" were brought in, secretly dosed with LSD and then their behavior was observed behind a two-way mirror. Just as the Nazi doctors in Dachau preyed on the helpless, the CIA searched for subjects who were unable to resist. They used prisoners, mental patients, sexual deviants, the terminally ill, foreigners and ethnic minorities. The Addiction Research Center of the US Public Health Service Hospital in Lexington, Kentucky was a place for heroin addicts to kick their habit. It was also one of fifteen penal and mental institutions the CIA used as a supply of guinea pigs for its covert drug research. *They worked hand in hand with the National Institutes of Mental Health (NIMH).* "When the CIA came across a new drug (usually supplied by American pharmaceutical firms) that needed testing, they frequently sent it over to their chief doctor at Lexington, where an ample supply of captive guinea pigs was readily available." *(ACID DREAMS*, p,24)

It has since been disclosed that by the mid 60's 1500 unsuspecting military personnel were also used as guinea pigs in LSD research. Some have filed suits against the government for damages. Edgewood Arsenal, headquarters of the Army Chemical Corps., had for twenty years employed Nazi scientists on their staff. These scientists had been brought to the US after World War II through a program designed to utilize the skills of German researchers and technicians called Project Paperclip. They had employed at least eight Nazi scientists who were involved in administering psychoactive chemicals to soldiers. "No avenue of experimentation was ignored and no population ruled out as being unfit to act as experimental guinea pigs. Men, women, children, prisoners, mental patients, criminal sexual-psychopaths, schizophrenics, the elderly, and even terminally ill cancer patients were all used to perfect for the CIA the techniques of total control of the mind." *(THE MIND MANIPULATORS,* p. 151)

"Within the CIA itself, Gottlieb [the agent in charge of chemical experimentation], White and his associates were taking LSD regularly, tripping at the office, at Agency parties, measuring their mental equilibrium against those of their colleagues. Turn your back in the morning and some wiseacre would slip a few micrograms into your coffee. It was a game played with the most exalted of weapons, the mind, and sometimes embarrassing things happened. Case-hardened spooks would break down crying or go all gooey about the 'brotherhood of man'. Once or twice things went really awry, with paranoid agents escaping into the bustle of downtown Washington, their anxious colleagues in hot pursuit. After one spectacular chase the quarry was finally run to ground in Virginia, where they found him crouched under a fountain, babbling about those 'terrible monster(s) with fantastic eyes' that had pursued him across Washington. Indeed every car he met had sent a jolt of terror through his body." *(STORMING HEAVEN - LSD AND THE AMERICAN DREAM,* p. 82)

Although records indicate that as early as 1953 the ridiculously dangerous drug-induced antics of the CIA turned deadly, they did not cease their LSD "research" until 1958. The deadly 1953 incident was the case of Dr. Frank Olsen, an army doctor who specialized in designing chemical warfare projects like lipstick that would kill the minute it touched the skin, deadly deodorants, etc. It was decided that he would make a good candidate for LSD experimentation. Two days after unknowingly ingesting LSD at a MK-ULTRA party where he drank punch which had been secretly spiked with the drug, he believed he was going insane and committed suicide by jumping to his death from a New York hotel window. It was not until years later that the truth came out and in 1979, twenty-six years after his death, his widow was finally awarded $750,000 in connection with her husband's death by the U.S. government. So with our money these men were paid their salaries, they used our money to pay for the LSD and the "research," they used us as uninformed guinea pigs and then they had us pay for the damages. They certainly knew how to add insult to injury.

Even though secret operations ended in 1958, the CIA made it clear that they would continue to keep a close eye on contemporary research by the pharmaceutical companies as they proceeded with their research for a sort of behavior-changing drug - one to fit their specifications for mind control which might be marketed for use in psychoanalysis. Apparently they retained a hope that the pharmaceutical companies might yet find a drug to fit their specifications through research in psychiatric drug treatments. Their suggestion that they would keep a close eye on the progress of the commercial interests should have been quite an incentive for any aggressive profit seeking company. How many of the psychoactive drugs presently on the market are there as a result of this hope of landing a government contract? Knowing the history of these drugs makes it difficult, if not just plain insane, to trust them.

When the CIA's Inspector General analyzed the ethics of MK-ULTRA in 1963 with such morally questionable projects as Midnight Climax, he was more concerned with the public finding out about the project rather than the fact that citizens were being subjected unknowingly to a test of behavior altering drugs! He stated that he feared that public knowledge of this information would ruin the reputations of not only the Agency and their agents, but also put the reputations of the professional researchers in jeopardy. He apparently did not realized that the activities of those individuals had already ruined their reputations and his concern was an afterthought. In light of this information about the CIA and its repulsive beginnings is it any wonder that President Kennedy had called for the dismantling of the CIA just before his assassination?

To demonstrate the controversy surrounding the use of LSD in this country, at the same time that the *NEW ENGLAND JOURNAL OF MEDICINE* called for an end to all research with LSD, what should have been the most unlikely organization of all, the National Institute of Mental Health was funding 33 LSD projects at the cost of $1.7 million in tax dollars. How long was it before the general public woke up to the psychedelic nightmare they had begun to experience with LSD? By mid 1966 there where three Congressional subcommittees conducting hearings on LSD, the Juvenile Delinquency Subcommittee of the Senate Judiciary Committee; the Subcommittee on Intergovernmental Relations of the House Government Operations Committee, and the Subcommittee on Executive Reorganization of the Senate Subcommittee on Government Operations. In October of 1966 possession of LSD became illegal in every state in this country.

"Crazy faith in better living through chemistry" A large portion of this information on the CIA and LSD was reported at the Annual Meeting of the American Academy of Neurology in 1990 by Drs. Robert F Ulrich and Bernard M. Patten in a presentation entitled, *"The Rise, Decline, and Fall of LSD."* LSD's developer was Albert Hofmann. Drs. Ulrich and Patten related that, "Hofmann, himself suspects that the materialistic American life-style and resultant feelings of alienation from nature and lack of a meaningful philosophy of life drew people" to LSD. He *"favored the potential uses of LSD; stating that*

33

if people learned to use the drug more wisely under the proper conditions, in medicinal practice, and in association with meditation, it could become a 'wonder child'." (Keep in mind that this is a drug known to twist every perception we possess as humans and was first marketed to chemically induce psychosis.) These two doctors reacted to Hofmann's opinion by stating, *"We now know that will never happen. LSD was part of an era of crazy faith in better living through chemistry."*

Only three years after this presentation was made to the nation's neurologists, this "crazy faith in better living through chemistry" they expected to never happen again is exactly what Dr. Peter Kramer's new book, *LISTENING TO PROZAC, A Psychiatrist Explores Antidepressant Drugs and the Remaking of the Self*, is rehashing for us. It would be interesting to learn how Drs. Ulrich and Patten feel about Dr. Kramer's suggestion that we create a better living through the chemistry of Lilly's latest "wonder drug," Prozac. In fact it would be interesting to know if Dr. Kramer himself realizes that he is proposing once again Hoffman's philosophies. As we proceed further and take a closer look at the similarities in action which these two drugs, Prozac and LSD, have within the brain, you will see why it is so curious that such similar arguments have been raised to justify the use of these two Lilly progenies.

Although Congress attempted to stop the spread of LSD after the CIA experimented with it, now, exactly fifty years after the discovery of LSD, the drug is making a comeback. It's use is skyrocketing among young people. Among young adults, about one of 10 has experimented with LSD. According to Dr. Henry Abraham, director of psychiatric research at St. Elizabeth's Hospital in Boston, "Use of LSD is really like playing Russian roulette with chemicals," Abraham said. "You can spin the chamber and maybe five times you get away with it. Maybe the sixth time you blow your brains out. Instead of bullets, they are using drugs. God bless 'em."

What debt we owe to those who introduced us to the wonders of LSD. The pharmaceuticals have given us one dangerous and highly addictive psychoactive prescription drug after another: heroin, methadone, cocaine, LSD, the amphetamines and methamphetamines, steroids, PCP, Qualudes, Extasy, etc., etc., etc. The list goes on and on and has not stopped yet. Once these drugs have been released to the public for medicinal purposes, how do we ever control their use? Education as to their effects appears to be our only hope. If we can understand what we are doing to ourselves and the cost involved to each of us personally and then to society as a whole, perhaps we will see the insanity behind our reaching out so rapidly and with such trust, devouring each new drug as fast as they offer one more. This memory of past mistakes with these previous drugs, which time and experience have proven to be extremely dangerous, should warn us of impending problems in the future and instill a far more cautious approach to our use of prescription drugs, especially new ones. Learning from past mistakes is one of our most important reasons for the keeping of records and studying history, because learning from the mistakes of others is far less painful than learning from one's own mistakes.

Yet have we really learned anything from these devastatingly disastrous mistakes in our past with such seriously mind-altering, highly addictive drugs - drugs which in the beginning were thought to be "safe"? How long can it take us to learn that once out there it takes lots of time and red tape to remove them from the market? And even after they are removed, stopping their illegal use once a large population has become addicted to them is next to impossible. Although these drugs have caused some of the most terribly violent and destructive behavior known to man, it does not appear to be the case that we have learned our lesson on drugs and their effects as yet. We jump to try all the new ones as they are candy coated and dangled in front of us on our television sets, in magazines, in newspapers, etc., etc., yes, even by the doctors we are trusting with our lives.

After first being used in medical practice in India in 1950, methaqualone came to the United States in 1965. It was marketed as a sleeping pill and daytime sedative under the brand name Quaalude. Once again scientists believed that this drug's chemical differences from barbiturates would prevent the addiction and dependence problems patients had encountered with other sedatives. And once again federal regulators saw no need for strict control of the drug. By the 70's, Quaalude was being widely abused on college campuses, and in 1981 alone, methaqualone was implicated in an estimated 20% of traffic deaths in some areas of the United States. Tolerance to methaqualone develops rapidly, leading users to crave higher doses, thus producing potential overdoses.

Congress attempted to curb the tide of psychoactive drugs. Senator Thomas Dodd, Democrat from Connecticut, had enough vision to attempt to curb this drug situation with his "Psychotoxic Drug Control" bill in the mid 60's. At the time he was serving as the chairman of the Senate Subcommittee to Investigate Juvenile Delinquency and had become concerned about drug trafficking - especially prescription drugs being diverted into the illegal market. Perhaps his bill was inspired earlier when in 1963, President Kennedy's Advisory Commission on Narcotic and Drug Abuse recommended that all drugs "having a potential for psychotic and anti-social behavior [specifically including the tranquilizers, which medical authorities testified in reality make patients more anxious than before] be deemed by law dangerous drugs subject to strict federal controls".

In another senate subcommittee Dr. Donald Louria gave a warning of the impact that a mother's use of psychiatric drugs has upon their children: *"...if the mother is a daily tranquilizer user, then the child is three and a half times as likely to use opiates (such as heroin), five times as likely to use stimulants or LSD, seven times as likely to use tranquilizers as an appropriate control group whose mothers were not daily tranquilizer users."*

Senator Thomas Dodd's Psychotoxic Drug Control bill included President Kennedy's Advisory Commission's recommendation. It passed the Senate in 1964, but died in the House. It would have automatically deemed dangerous and subject to strict federal control amphetamines and barbiturates and any products containing these substances. It would have then authorized the Secretary of Health, Education and Welfare to strictly regulate any substance found to be *"habit forming because of its medically stimulant effect on the central nervous system; or...any drug which contains any quantity of a substance which the Secretary, after investigation...designates as affecting or altering, to a substantive extent, consciousness, the ability to think, critical judgement, motivation, psychomotor coordination, or sensory perception, and having a potential for abuse when used without medical supervision."*

Senator Dodd made his report to Congress on August 3, 1964. He reported that over the previous five years, the illegal use of the billions of these pills had reached epidemic proportions. The following is a summary of his concerns:

"...I refer to the staggering amounts of psychotoxic drugs that are diverted every year into illegal channels, millions of which end up in the hands of our Nation's youths...I reported to the Senate on August 24, 1961, that in the year 1960, drug companies in this country produced 5 3/4 billion capsules of barbiturates and 4 billion tablets of amphetamine drugs. This is in addition to millions of bootleg drugs that find their way into the black market...during the last five years, the illegal use of the billions of these pills...has reached epidemic proportions. The results of this traffic which have come to our attention, revealed the following picture:

"The illegal use of these drugs is increasing at a fantastic rate among juveniles and young adults.

"The use of these drugs has a direct causal relationship to increased crimes of violence.

"The use of these drugs is replacing, in many cases, the use of the 'hard' narcotics, such as opium, heroin, and cocaine.

"The use of these drugs is more and more prevalent among the so-called white-collar youths who have never had prior delinquency or criminal records.

"The use of these drugs is increasingly identified as causes of sexual crimes.

After voicing these concerns he concluded in this meeting and subsequent meetings with this summary, "Mr. Chairman, I feel this bill has had as much study, analysis, and consideration at this point as any piece of legislation I have ever been associated with...Since May 23, 1961, when I first introduced this bill, it has been subjected to the scrutiny of the President's Commission of Narcotic and Drug Abuse; the Department of Health, Education, and Welfare; Treasury; Justice; and State; the law enforcement agencies in New York City and the State of California, where this problem is greatest; the Association of Juvenile Court Judges; the International Juvenile Police Officers Association; the Pharmaceutical Manufacturers Association; and the distinguished representatives of a number of religious faiths. All of these groups, without exception, have approved of or endorsed this bill over the last 3 1/2 years.

"...It was publicly and repeatedly supported by the late President Kennedy. It has the support of every group that knows anything about this problem. It has been backed by every witness who testified before the Juvenile Delinquency Subcommittee, including three drug company presidents...Mr. Chairman, I do not know anyone who is against it."

A glimpse at politics in medicine in America. He quickly learned that one organization had just voiced their opposition - the American Medical Association. (Keep in mind that these drugs were heavily advertized in AMA publications and the revenue from this advertising was a major financial resource for them.) They called for *education* rather than *legislation.* Senator Dodd responded that this course of action would be "to say nothing, in my opinion, and I cannot really find words strong enough to express my disapproval of that course of conduct. *The house is on fire, and we do not need a lesson in how to prevent the starting of fires. What we need now is to put the fire out and go on with our fire prevention work.* " *(BY PRESCRIPTION ONLY,* p. 89-91, 198-199)

And so our battle continues with one mind-altering prescription drug after another adversely affecting our lives and proving to be more dangerous and addictive that the last. Children and their parents seem to be awakening to the dangers of Ritalin, the popular methamphetamine [exactly the type of drug Senator Dodd and President Kennedy were so concerned about] used for hyperactivity in children. Dr. Peter Kramer points out that many people feel more alert and productive on amphetamines, although it is only short term. He then adds this qualification, "But amphetamines are addictive and cause paranoia - they are drugs of abuse - and for these reasons we allow them to be prescribed for very narrow medical indications, chiefly ADHD." (*LISTENING TO PROZAC*, p. 245) ADHD is Attention-Deficit Hyperactive Disorder, the label we use for a child who is unable to pay attention in our all too often inadequate and boring school system of today. Hypoglycemia, heavy metal poisoning, such as lead poisoning, or allergies have all been found to be biological causes for ADHD. Giving a child a stimulant for ADHD brought on by any of these biological disorders does not make any sense, as the stimulant would only worsen the condition in the long run even if temporary results were achieved. The amphetamines given for ADHD are "drugs of abuse," "addictive" and "cause paranoia" and we are giving them to kids?! Incredibly bright on someone's part! What on earth are we doing to our children? What kind of future does this offer them when they are being conditioned to an addictive mind-altering drug at such an early age? The Canadian magazine *WESTERN REPORT* in an article entitled "Silent Scourge - How two obscure prescription drugs cause most of our urban crime" (February 2, 1987) credited Ritalin, this highly addictive psychiatric drug, a form of "speed" and a class #2 narcotic, and the painkiller, Talwin, as being responsible for 70 percent of Canada's urban crime.

Ninety-five percent of hyperactives are male. If male brain function is compared to the female brain function, we find one reason for this high incidence rate of ADHD in young males. Neurologist Richard Restak explains, "The male brain learns by manipulating its environment, yet the typical student is forced to sit still for long hours in the classroom. The male brain is primarily visual, while classroom instruction demands attentive listening. Boys are clumsy in fine hand co-ordination, yet are forced at an early age to express themselves in writing. Finally, there is little opportunity in most schools, other than during recess periods, for gross motor movements or rapid muscular responses. In essence, the classrooms in most of our nation's primary grades are geared to skills that come naturally to girls but develop very slowly in boys. The results shouldn't be surprising: a 'learning disabled' child who is frequently 'hyperactive.'" (*THE BRAIN: THE LAST FRONTIER*, p. 205)

Even the drug which maimed and deformed thousands of children through their mothers' use of the drug, Thalidomide, a sleeping pill, was promoted as safe during pregnancy. This was being done even though the manufacturer, Merrill, had reports coming in from around the world of deformities being produced in the babies born to mothers who had used the drug. So many lives were affected by this drug which is still marketed in third world countries and is being considered for use now for AIDS patients in spite of what we should have learned from our previous experience with it.

Clearly doctors should show *extreme caution* in their prescribing of these mind-mood-behavior-altering chemicals, especially the newer ones like Halcion, Xanex, Prozac, Zoloft, Paxil, Luvox, Effexor, Anafranil, etc., where our knowledge of the drugs are still sketchy. And patients should show *extreme caution* in using these drugs, many of which we have found to be extremely addictive even after being used in low doses for short periods. Time and experience are beginning to prove these new drugs to be just as addictive and deadly, if not more so, than those drugs which have gone on before them.

Because the large majority of the drugs involved in our "Just Say No To Drugs" campaign were "gifts" from the pharmaceutical companies it seems only right that they be the ones to fund our drug war. Why should we use our tax dollars to clean up their mistakes? They are the ones who made the huge profits from them. Let them cover the massive expense involved in policing, rehabilitating, jailing and imprisoning, etc., which we now cover for them. This innovative implementation of recompense might bring a very rapid solution to our drug problem world wide. If the pharmaceutical companies really were held accountable for their actions by having to pay the damages in pain and suffering and death caused by their drugs, they may be more cautious about the drugs they put on the market. This manner of payment for their actions would seem far more appropriate and ethical, rather than the current practice of using our legal system to hide behind, tying up the courts as a stalling technique to keep these deadly drugs on the market longer in order to accumulate additional profits. When they are forced to recall the drug, they are allowed to say "whoops, goofed again" as they file bankruptcy or pay minuscule fines and walk away leaving a trail of victims behind them. These are victims which we then take care of for the rest of their lives with our tax dollars. They additionally leave behind them a trail of new drug addicts, unsuspecting patients who now are unable to break the endless chain of one mind-altering drug after another. We will with our tax dollars fight for years to help them overcome their addiction or dependence and put their lives back together so that they can become productive members of society again. Or as the brain damage from the drugs they cannot be withdrawn from progresses, we will pay to have them committed to mental institutions or nursing homes. It is long past time for these companies who have become extremely wealthy at our expense to start paying their own way and accounting for their mistakes. There is no doubt that if this were the case we would see far fewer of these deadly mind-altering, behavior-altering, addictive drugs on the market.

CHAPTER 1

BLISS IN A BOTTLE
...OR JUST OUR LATEST
RUDE AWAKENING TO THE DANGERS
OF MIND ALTERING DRUGS?

"Never before Prozac has a medication been so misrepresented by so many people for so long in the absence of adequate data." .....Dr. Mantosh Dewan and Dr. Prakash Masand, Department of Psychiatry, State University of New York, JOURNAL OF FAMILY PRACTICE, Vol. 33, No. 3, 1991

A far too common occurrence in psychiatry is the replacement of older drugs with newer ones that "might" be safer and more effective but often prove to be the opposite. Arthur J. Snider, who was at the time science editor of the *CHICAGO DAILY NEWS* said in October 1963, "My concern is that *the record would show that 90% of the stories we have written about new drugs have gone down the drain as failures."* As you will discover as you read the chapter on legal drugs vs. illegal drugs, history has continued to repeat itself over and over again. The latest statement to demonstrate these continuing promises with the strong possibility of the proverbial "whoops, goofed again" clause comes from the February 7, 1994 issue of *NEWSWEEK,* "...drug makers are now developing compounds that promise faster action against depression and higher success rates...because their long-term effects are largely unknown some experts worry that millions of people are basically serving as test subjects. Many medications, including Valium and thalidomide, have shown their true hazards only after coming into broad use." (p.41, 42)

The director of the Psychopharmacology Service Center for the National Institute of Mental Health, Dr. Jonathan Cole, reported on the antidepressants in the *JOURNAL OF THE AMERICAN MEDICAL ASSOCIATION*, November 2, 1964, "Their place in the physician's armamentarium is still far from clear, although many clinicians feel that the drugs are useful and effective. However, controlled clinical trials of these agents have not always led to unequivocally positive findings. Even when such findings have been favorable to the drug under study, the differences between the efficacy of the drug and a placebo have not been as great as one might wish, or as one might have anticipated *after reading published reports of uncontrolled studies."*

He went on to say that the question with MAOIs "is whether their therapeutic efficacy is sufficient to offset the potential risk of their causing severe reactions. Even those...that have no apparent tendency to cause liver or brain damage have, nevertheless, the innate ability to potentiate the effects of a wide variety of other pharmacological and toxic agents, including sedatives, stimulants, ephedrine, histamine, epinephrine, and bee venom..."

FDA failures produce hundreds of deaths around the world. An example of what Dr. Cole was referring to is the MAOI Parnate. Parnate was introduced in March of 1961 by the makers of the latest SSRI, Paxil, and within a three year period had been the subject of 190 medical articles worldwide. Psychiatrist Arthur Egelman, who was the FDA medical officer responsible for the antidepressant Parnate dissented May 21, 1964 in a memorandum to allowing Smith Kline & French [Beacham] to remarket Parnate after it had been temporarily pulled from the market. He stated, *"There is no question that this is a dangerous drug. Attempts to surround its use with a thicket of contraindications, warnings, and precautions are unwieldy and impossible to apply. In addition, this does not tell the physician that even if he should avoid all these pitfalls his patient may die from the drug anyway...Its supposed rapid action in the treatment of depression is felt to be due to its amphetamine-like effect. It should be underscored that this is NOT an antidepressant action. If it were we should use the amphetamines as antidepressants. I deeply regret the prolongation of human suffering and the sacrifice in human life which will follow the resumption of marketing of this relatively ineffective drug."* He subsequently resigned.

Six years after the FDA approval of the drug it was disclosed that only four controlled medical studies had been completed for the drug and that none of them were completed *before* the FDA approved Parnate for marketing. It was found to produce death from a dangerously rapid rise in blood pressure. This was originally thought to be experienced by only .01% of users, but in 1967 the incidence rate shown in scientific trials was *at least 100 to 2700 times greater.*

Another drug, Sparine (promazine hydrochloride), was a potent tranquilizer manfactured by Wyeth Laboratories. who was pushing for its release before testing was completed. Dr. Barbara Moulton was the FDA physician in charge of the application for the approval of the drug. She too resigned from her post as an FDA medical officer because of what she witnessed in the politics behind this particular drug, stating that because of the FDA's failures "hundreds of people, not merely in this country, suffer daily, and many die..."

We have been warned about the dangers of overuse, such as in using the antidepressants for mild depression. Dr. Cole went on to warn us that, *"Since many of these drugs are, if not potentially dangerous, at least quite potent* *pharmacological agents, there is justifiable concern about their overuse for the treatment of mild depression. "*

Speaking of Miltown, Equanil, Librium and Valium he said, "The extent of use of these drugs was staggering, thanks in good part to massive sustained advertising campaigns that provided a major revenue source for publications such as the *JOURNAL OF THE AMERICAN MEDICAL ASSOCIATION, MEDICAL TRIBUNE,* and *MEDICAL WORLD NEWS. " (BY PRESCRIPTION ONLY,* p. 186-188, 213b, 213e)

This practice of massive advertising campaigns for drugs in order to convince us and our doctors that we "need" various drugs and specifying which drugs we do need should be a great concern for us. *CONSUMER REPORTS* discussed this issue at length in two articles which ran concurrently in the February and March 1992 issues entitled *"Pushing Drugs to Doctors"* and *"Miracle Drugs or Media Drugs?"* These articles are a "must read" for anyone who is interested in learning more about the politics behind convincing us we need so many drugs to deal with problems in life. They estimate a figure of 5 billion dollars was spent in 1991 for this type of advertising and add, "Though doctors insist their scientific training, high intelligence, and sophistication enable them to resist manipulation, the truth is that skillful marketers can influence M.D.s just as easily as they can sway the rest of us..." The pharmaceutical companies spend more on this advertising than they spend in research and development of products.

The authors of *FORTY-SOMETHING FOREVER* report this as well, "The pharmaceutical industry, which influences med school curriculum (by providing the research funds to support university labs), would rather young docs learn to depend on drugs than natural cures. Once graduated, most doctors receive ongoing medical education via the drug detailmen who visit their offices periodically to provide literature and inform them of medical advances - (translated into English that means an update on their firm's newest FDA-approved drugs) - or if they are avid followers of their medical journals, they'll read 'advertorials' - research reports favoring the very drugs promoted in the periodical's ads." (p. 304)

Dr. Dale Console once pointed out that if a car does not have an engine, no amount of advertizing could make us believe it did. Nor would it take the consumer a decade to determine that all he had under the hood was an advertizing agent rather than a motor. Yet for years after the antidepressants made their debut there has been uncertainty among many distinguished scientists as to just what is under the bottle top.

Our latest search for bliss in a bottle has led us to the Specific Serotonin Reuptake Inhibitors (SSRIs), with Prozac leading the parade and Zoloft, Paxil, Lovan and Luvox trailing close behind. Are they going to prove to be bliss in a bottle or just our latest rude awakening to the dangers of mind altering drugs? Since Prozac is the most rapidly accepted psychotropic drug ever and has been out long enough to have a track record, we will discuss it in particular, realizing that this information will help us to project the future of Prozac's analogues - Zoloft, Paxil, Lovan, Luvox, etc. As these analogues begin to be used with more regularity we will have more experience to draw upon. As all of them are designed to raise the level of a brain chemical called serotonin, learning the ramifications of this procedure will be our main focus, enabling the reader to understand what *any* drug designed to have this effect upon serotonin should produce.

Whether you personally are using one of these drugs or not, everyone must be made aware of the cost we will pay as we pick up the pieces of the SSRI aftermath, not just the cost to individual families, but the cost to society as a whole. At some point, most people will either be prescribed or have close association with someone who is prescribed neuroleptics, antidepressants, or other psychoactive drugs. Prozac is the most popular antidepressant on the market today as it is handed out like candy for depression, yeast infections, post-surgical pain, P.M.S., Chronic Fatigue Syndrome, flu, acne, listlessness, hormonal imbalances, hypoglycemia, etc.

Ignorance is bliss and our bottle of bliss runneth over. Drs. Dewan and Masand told us at the beginning of this chapter that we have never known of another drug before Prozac that has been so misrepresented by so many for so long in the absence of adequate data. When considering our past track record of the tragic results brought on by our ignorance of these types of drugs, the realization our ignorance of this new group should make us realize we had better become informed about them as rapidly as possible. Your doctor or therapist may have bought into the enthusiastic promotional literature from the companies that manufacture such drugs, and may be unaware of or downplay their risks while touting their benefits. Specialists have trouble keeping up with research and for non-specialists it is next to impossible. In spite of this 63% of antidepressants are prescribed by non-specialists. According to a study in the July 1993 issue of *ARCHIVES OF GENERAL PSYCHIATRY* non-therapists spend an average of *only three minutes* discussing the patient's case. It only takes a minute to write out a prescription for a drug where searching for an underlying disease could take days, weeks, even months to discover. In many cases, the risks and side effects of these drugs, which are being prescribed far too rapidly and irresponsibly, are serious and lifelong, and affect half or more of the people using them over prolonged periods of time.

People and their families who are candidates for such drugs are usually desperate and debilitated, and are not in a position to fully investigate the efficacy and safety of recommended drugs during their crisis, especially the newer drugs with so little information being available on them. You owe it to yourself and your loved ones to take advantage of educating yourself to the myriad of problems now arising from the use of Prozac and this whole new class of antidepressants.

The purpose of this book is to inform the consumer first of all of the latest medical reports out on Prozac and the other SSRIs and of what patients are reporting from their own experience after using them. These are drugs which were rushed through the FDA approval process based on only five and six week studies. Since the consumer becomes a "guinea pig" after the first six weeks of use, he needs to be made aware of what others in this "real life" laboratory test are experiencing. And he needs to know what the latest medical data is indicating, so that he can evaluate his own situation. It is also written as a reminder, since most of us seem to have little memory or even any knowledge of the fact, that almost every one of the so called "street drugs", which have been the focus of our "Just Say No To Drugs" campaign, were in their beginnings "gifts" of the pharmaceutical firms. Many were hailed as "medical miracles" before their dependence or addiction and deadly behavior altering side effects became obvious, transforming them into "controlled" substances, i.e., Heroin, Cocaine, LSD, PCP, amphetamines, methamphetamines, etc. Additionally it is written to inform the reader of the latest research on sleep disorders and how this research applies to our topic. Psychoactive drugs, both legal and illegal, repress REM sleep and disrupt normal sleep patterns which can cause bizarre psychotic reactions or dissociative states known to us as: delusion, hallucination, mania, akathisia, panic attack, depersonalization, paranoia, etc. and in the extreme, the potentially violent REM Sleep Behavior Disorder - a sleepwalk nightmare where the patient acts out violent dreams while sleepwalking.

It is also written with the hope of bringing understanding and healing to so many patients and their families who have been adversely affected by these new drugs, the hope of restoring a sense of dignity to those individuals and their families who have had it robbed from them by the use of these mind-altering prescription drugs...those who in following doctors orders have had their lives altered forever...*that this information in bringing awareness will help erase the shame and lift their pain through understanding, so that they and their families can once again hold their heads high and know how to put their lives back together again.*

It is a very unfortunate situation that the large majority of not only the general public, but the medical community as well, understand so little about drug reactions, drug interactions and allergic reactions to drugs. This is even more true *when it comes to the mind altering drugs.* Even though doctors are the ones who recommend these drugs, they generally receive little education on drugs in medical school and what is learned after that is often picked up from a pharmaceutical sales rep. Many doctors admit that their drug information is gained from the newspaper. We would hope that a specialist, such as a psychiatrist, who is focusing on a limited number of specific types of drugs, would have a better working knowledge of them, but unfortunately even that isn't necessarily so. A pharmacist or one who specializes in drug abuse tend to be the most knowledgeable. Since 80% of Prozac is prescribed by general practitioners this lack of information, *especially on behalf of doctors*, spells trouble with a capital **T** for all of us. We need to understand far more about this subject than we have in the past. Our society is inundated with drugs. When do we begin to learn from our mistakes? How bad does it have to get before we wake up? The problem is so massive that drug interactions make up 40% of all accidental poisonings and in 1979 the World Health Organization documented this to be the cause of one forth of the deaths within hospitals. It is estimated that 125,000 deaths will be attributed to prescription drug reactions this year.

We are all aware that people can have various reactions to drugs...hyperventilation, rashes, hives - many adverse reactions, even cardiac arrest, seizures, stroke and death. It seems that we tend to grasp far more clearly the physical effects produced by drugs, but the amazingly powerful emotional, mental and behavioral reactions to these drugs escape us. These reactions can be so bizarre that they can make us question reality itself. *When it comes to the "mind-altering" or psychoactive drugs, how many of us actually understand that the primary reactions to these are **typically mental and emotional** reactions brought on by interference with thought process and brain function? This malfunction produced by the drug reaction in turn affects the patient's responses, judgement, behavior, cognitive reasoning, decision-making abilities, etc., etc., etc. - virtually any area of mental or emotional response.* Mental and emotional areas are those areas targeted by these drugs and are, therefore, those areas which become affected by the psychoactive drugs. Even in our court system there is a great lack of awareness concerning this issue in spite of the fact that psychoactive prescription drugs have been around for decades.

As pointed out by *WOMAN'S DAY* in an article entitled, *"IS YOUR MEDICINE*

MAKING YOU CRAZY?" (8/11/92), even drugs given for high blood pressure, heart disease, asthma, insomnia, contraception, arthritis, epilepsy, ulcers, inflammation, glaucoma and colds can produce *psychiatric* side effects. Many act like mild amphetamines, making people feel hyper or restless. They can produce depression, disorientation, delirium, hallucinations, agitation, anxiety, confusion, paranoia, insomnia, mood changes and memory loss. Of course the incidence and intensity of these psychiatric reactions should prove to be higher with the drugs classified as mind-altering: painkillers, antianxiety drugs, sedatives, anesthetics, tranquilizers, the antidepressants, antihistamines, and the many other psychoactive drugs.

The possibility of drugs prescribed for physical complaints being the cause of various psychiatric reactions is very real. The possiblities are depression, confusion, memory loss, anxiety, agitation, irritability, hallucinations, paranoia, mania, delirium, etc. It is therefore, extremely important for caution to be taken by both the physician and the patient to first rule out this as a possible cause of these symptoms. The psychiatric drugs are far too often prescribed for these reactions to various other drugs with no investigation into a drug reaction being the possible cause for these symptoms. Giving a patient an additional drug to treat a reaction brought on by another drug would only mask and complicate the underlying disease process and put the patient at greater risk to experience even more serious drug reactions by adding one drug on top of another.

How often are patients being prescribed Prozac or other powerful antidepressants for the symptoms being produced by the drugs they were given for other complaints? How many physicians take the time to find out which medications, including the over-the-counter medications, their patients are using that might be causing depression, anxiety, restlessness, etc. *before* they prescribe a psychiatric drug? How many patients realize the importance of providing their doctors with information about other medications they are using? How many realize that even mixing the over-the-counter medications with prescription drugs could cost them their lives? Dr. Jack Gorman, director of psychological studies at Columbia University's College of Physicians and Surgeons, made this statement to the writer of the *WOMEN'S DAY* article, *"Even medications that don't usually cause problems, such as antibiotics, can produce psychiatric side effects in some individuals. **Whenever you notice a change always ask, 'Could a drug be causing this?'"***

The article went on to mention many drugs with cause these effects. An example of some of the drugs that can cause psychiatric side effects and a few of their reactions are: Antianxiety drugs like the benzodiazephines (Valium, Librium,

47

Xanex, etc.) cause depression, disorientation, delirium; Anticonvulsants like Dilantin, Tegretol, Klonopin cause depression, disorientation, delirium, hallucinations, etc.; antidepressants like the SSRIs, Wellbutrin, MAO inhibitors, imipramine, Elavil, Lithium, etc. cause agitation, restlessness, anxiety, etc.; Antihistamines (many cold remedies and sleeping pills like Benadryl) cause disorientation, delirium, hallucinations in high doses, depression, etc.; Antihypertensives like Reserpine, Aldomet, Guanethidine, Catapres, Inderal, etc. cause depression, delirium, etc.; Anti-inflammatories like Indocin, Naprosyn, etc. cause depression, confusion, paranoia, delirium, hallucinations, etc. and the corticosteroids cause depression, anxiety, delirium, paranoia, mania, etc.; Antimicrobials like Acyclovir (Zovirax), Ampkotericin B, Flagyl, Keflin cause confusion, delirium, paranoia, etc.; Asthma medications like Theophylline, aminophylline, etc. cause anxiety, insomnia, etc.; Decongestants like Pseudoephedrine, etc. cause anxiety, restlessness, insomnia, etc.; Estrogens like oral contraceptives or estrogen replacement cause mood changes, depression, etc.; Glaucoma meds like AK-Zol, Dazamide, Diamox, etc. cause depression, disorientation, etc.; Heart medications like Digitalis, etc. cause depression, anxiety, disorientation, delirium, etc.; Painkillers like Xylocaine, etc. cause depression, delirium; Opiates like meperidine, Percodan, etc. cause agitation, delirium, etc.; Salicyclates (aspirin) cause agitation, confusion, hallucinations, delirium, etc.; Parkinson's medications like Cogentin, Akineton, amantadine, etc. cause depression, delirium, hallucinations, nightmares, etc.; Sleeping pills like Compoz, Excedrin-P.M., Sleep-Eze3, Sominex, etc. cause disorientation, delirium, etc.; Dalmane causes depression, confusion, delirium, etc.; Halcion causes memory loss, disorientation, delirium, agitation, etc.; Stimulants like amphetamines cause anxiety, paranoia, mania, depression, etc.; Ritalin causes hallucinations, etc.; Ulcer medications like Tagamet cause disorientation, delirium, hallucinations, etc.

Depending upon the patient's sensitivity to the particular drug, these effects can range from mild to severe. All of this definitely gives rise to the question, "Just how many of our "diseases" are drug-induced or are reactions to other drugs, which are subsequently treated with additional drugs to treat the psychiatric reactions?" We do not yet seem to be accustomed to the fact that *a drug can chemically alter one's behavior and emotional and mental reactions by chemically altering their minds.* The large majority of us apparently do not yet fully comprehend the term "mind-altering". Few of us have read medical reports such as those mentioned in this text and especially those in Appendix B which repeat over and over again that *reactions such as violence, suicidal ideation, hostility and obsessive-compulsive behaviors are being "chemically induced/ drug induced".* The fact that these types of psychiatric reactions are brought on by a drug reaction is discussed openly and repeatedly throughout technical medical literature.

Dr. James W. Long in his discussion of Prozac in *THE ESSENTIAL GUIDE TO PRESCRIPTION DRUGS 1992* explains, *"A review of relevant literature on this subject reveals that the **development or intensification of suicidal thoughts during treatment (regardless of the severity of depression) has been documented repeatedly for many antidepressant drugs in wide use.** It is apparent that suicidal thinking may emerge during treatment with any antidepressant."* And Fava and Rosenbaum state in a letter to the *JOURNAL OF CLINICAL PSYCHIATRY*, in November 1991 that "...emergence of suicidal ideation or behavior has been observed with many antidepressant pharmacotherapies."

When we are under the influence of a drug, who is in control, us or the drug? We are the ones in control of our own lives and our behavior. We are the ones who make our choices in life, right? As a general rule this is true, but how can this apply when we unknowingly choose to use a mind-altering drug which interferes with our behavioral responses? How many would assume that a patient has *"chosen"* how they are reacting to their medication if they had an allergic reaction to a certain antibiotic? Is he to be *condemned* for breaking out in a rash or hives? Or how many would say of someone who was given a drink that was "spiked" with alcohol, without his knowledge, that he should have had control over how he reacted to that "mind-altering" substance? Because no one had informed him that his drink contained a mind-altering substance, would he be expected to drive as if the alcohol did not affect him or perform other functions as well as he did before he ingested the alcohol? Would he be the one responsible for allowing the alcohol to affect his ability to perform? Does it become the *fault* of the individual for reacting in exactly the way this substance affects anyone? This is, of course an absolutely *ridiculous* assumption. Someone given an extremely deadly chemical does not *decide* that he is going to die as a result of ingesting that chemical. Control is exercised in making the choice to use or not use a substance. We do not have control over how a substance affects us, just as we have no control over various drug reactions. *Drugs control us, we do not control them. The only method available to us for controlling how drugs affect us is by us choosing not to use them.* Any child involved in their school's "Just Say No To Drugs" campaign can tell us that. The only choice we make is in whether or not we take the drugs, we have no choice in how we react to them. Yet, with a mind-altering substance, such as Prozac or the other psychoactive drugs, this is exactly the totally ridiculous view being taken by much of the public, by many in the legal system, and by physicians (who should certainly be aware of these reactions and know better). *Prozac and the other SSRIs were designed to chemically alter the brain and thereby affect one's thoughts, mood and behavior.* Even though these drugs were intended to stop depression and prevent suicide, a drug can often have a paradoxical or opposite reaction from what it was theorized to do. When Prozac or the other SSRIs do create a paradoxical reaction and the patients report that it is *adversely* affecting their mood and behavior, why would we condemn the patient for having reactions to the drug? *There is absolutely no logic behind this reasoning.*

A patient's responsibility lies in being informed about a drug and what it does. Yet, if patients are deprived of that information, how can they be held accountable for the results? In a case such as this the patient becomes accountable or responsible for one thing only - using a product, in good faith, according to the knowledge provided to him by those he has trusted with that responsibility - his physician and his pharmacist, the manufacturer of the drug and the Food and Drug Administration (FDA).

In the case of this new class of drugs, the SSRIs, I believe that those who are responsible for providing drug information have failed in their responsibility to the patient. In this light the patient becomes just as much an innocent victim as those who are affected by his altered behavior. The patient, in order to avoid becoming an innocent victim because of this lack of information, had better accept the responsibility for himself to become informed. However, in our complicated drug testing and approval process, obtaining such information can be very difficult. For instance, when Prozac was introduced to the market almost six years ago it had not been tested for possible withdrawal effects. Now the patients who have been forced into discovering this on their own are reporting a very high rate of serious withdrawal and dependency. Sexual problems were not reported in the beginning and now the most recent studies show that at least a third of the patients report these side effects. Little, if any, warning was given about Prozac's interactions with other drugs. Now we know that it magnifies the level and the effects of many other drugs by ten times or more causing life threatening toxic reactions. Suicidal ideation was not listed as a side effect to in the original studies and had to be added to the warnings on the drug two and a half years after its introduction. In fact Prozac and all the other SSRIs obtained FDA approval on studies which spanned a mere *five or six weeks*. It is amazing that these drugs can produce so many horrifying adverse reactions as are listed in the package insert within the first 5 or 6 weeks. During that short testing period for Prozac 15% of the patients had to end their participation in the study because of adverse side effects. After those initial five and six week periods of use the patient becomes a guinea pig. Many physicians will admit that if you are among the first to use a new drug you are actually participating in the testing process for that drug.

Dr. Irving Stone in his book released in 1975, *"THE HEALING MIND,"* p. 17 & 18 stated, "The oath of Hippocrates requires that I administer no poisons to my patients even if I am requested to do so. The ancient teacher also advised his students that the first law of healing was, 'Above all, don't make things worse'. In a report from the World Health Organization, we are advised that *one of every four people who die in hospitals is killed by the drugs he or she is prescribed. It is believed that this is the result of the physicians being unfamiliar with the dangers of the new drugs which they freely prescribe.* The 'pill for every ill' approach to disease has backfired. We are killing as many people or more with the "cure" as does the unchecked disease."

Is Prozac proving to be one of the cures which is killing as many or even more as the disease for which it is prescribed? Is it really the "wonder drug" it has been promoted to be or is it the Thalidomide of the 90's, the "Mother's Little Helper of the 90's, the LSD of the 90's, or even worse? Thalidomide, another psychoactive drug - a sleeping pill, was the cause of over 5000 cases of babies born with missing limbs to mothers who used the drug before it was banned back in the 50's. Since more women than men are being prescribed Prozac the question has been asked, "Is Prozac another Miltown or Librium, the 'mother's little helper' from which we expect too much and about which we know too little?" (*LISTENING TO PROZAC*, p. xvii) And the reason we must pose the question about Prozac being the LSD of the 90's is at the very least threefold. Number one, it is patented and manufactured by the same pharmaceutical company who gave us LSD, Eli Lilly. Number two, the advertizing campaign and promotional push for the two drugs has been extremely similar. Number three, the target in the brain for both Prozac and LSD is the neurotransmitter, serotonin and both act as enhancers of serotonin, that is they both raise the level of serotonin (we will discuss this similar action in detail in the chapter SEROTONIN DOUBLETALK).

Almost overnight Prozac has become the biggest money maker ever for Eli Lilly - without a doubt it is their "golden goose". While we reach out in desperation for a "quick fix" for depression, etc., exercising our faith in a marvelous marketing campaign designed to make us believe that Prozac would be the answer for "all that ails us," Prozac has exploded in profits for Lilly - bringing in over $100 million every month. And Lilly hopes to see even more profit by gaining approval for Prozac's use in treatment for obesity with a capsule three times the average dose and a name change to "Lovan." (We should note here that the latest studies out on the effectiveness and safety of Lovan are indicating that it will not be approved. [*Business Week,* June 22, 1992] But Lilly doses not give up easily and unfortunately, as you will learn in the chapter LILLY AND POLITICS, efficacy and safety are not always as motivating as politics and profit in reaching these decisions.)

Prozac was the first in this new class of anti-depressants, the SSRIs, and costs many times more than the drugs used previously for depression. This whole new group of medications work directly on the brain to raise levels of the neurotransmitter, serotonin, a brain chemical that is believed to affect depression. The fact that this is such a new approach in treatment should call for caution in the beginning rather than the belief that this would be a *"wonder drug" or a "cure all",* with so little caution being demonstrated in administration, dosage, monitoring, observance for withdrawal symptoms, etc. Patients everywhere are being sold on Prozac as an answer to any problem. It has become very fashionable or faddish and is commonly referred to as the "Yuppie Upper" or "Puppie Upper." Since being introduced to the market on December 29, 1987, by Eli Lilly, an Indianapolis-based pharmaceutical company, Prozac has had a dazzling career, claiming star status after Lilly's skillful sales promotion, including cover stories in *NEWSWEEK* and *NEW YORK*, which promoted it as the "wonder drug" of the 90's, just as Lilly's LSD had been promoted as the "wonder drug" of the 50's and 60's in the magazine articles then. People were walking into doctors offices asking for Prozac after the initial barrage of media attention. Doctors stated that they had never seen anything like it. The *SALT LAKE DESERET NEWS* reported a local health official as stating that the use of Prozac is so prevalent in his local area that it should be declared one of the four food groups. A Salt Lake County Drug and Alcohol Abuse official, when asked if they had any statistics on the use of the drug locally replied, "Sure, you can't sling a dead cat here without hitting someone on Prozac." There are entire families being placed on the drug, even children as young as three years of age! Concerned family members report that the drug is being passed around at their family reunions like chewing gum. A councelor, who is a personal friend, came home one evening to find a six month supply of Prozac in a paper bag on his porch with a note that read, "You seem a little down. I'm sure this will help." At this point it would not surprise anyone to hear that Baskin Robbins is announcing that "Prozac" is their newest flavor. It has been promoted for use in almost every ailment known to man. From PMS to premature ejaculation, even as a cure for whatever it is that keeps a patient from not dating early enough in life, we are being led to believe that Prozac is the answer. Promoters have "pushed every button" known to humanity: unhappiness, obesity, sexual dysfunction, shyness... about the only thing we have not heard it will cure is poverty, but the reports are bordering on that now.

PROZAC: PANACEA OR PANDORA?

If you are not using the drug yourself, you most likely know at least one, but more likely several, who are using Prozac for a wide variety of complaints ranging from listlessness to the flu, headaches and hormonal imbalances brought on by the initial stages of pregnancy to yeast infections and Lyme's disease, and now shyness. And if it isn't bad enough that medical doctors are handing these drugs out so freely, the pharmaceutical companies have been making a concentrated effort to encourage non-medical practitioners such as psychologists and social workers to recommend these types of drugs to their clients. We have already begun to see the results of their campaign in the form of Dr. Jim Goodwin. Dr. Goodwin is a psychologist from Winatchee, Washington who is being dubbed in the press as the Pied Piper of Prozac because he has 100% of his patients on either Prozac or the newest SSRI, Paxil. He is a practioner who is using the drug himself and has for four years now.

A young mother, two blocks from my home, was just prescribed Prozac for the flu. The niece of a close friend, another young mother, was just given Prozac by an eye, ear, nose and throat specialist for dizziness. The wanted her to use it for two weeks and come back if the dizziness continued and *then* he would do the medical tests to determine what should have been the first concern - an inner ear infection. Luckily both young women knew enough to throw their prescriptions away and find a new doctor. In relating her Prozac experience to her boss, the second young mother found that her boss had an even more bizarre Prozac experience. She went in to see her physician about acne on her back. She too was given Prozac for her ailment. She obediently used her Prozac prescription for a short time. When asked by her co-workers whether or not the Prozac helped her acne, she replied, "Sure, after two weeks on Prozac I could have given a damn whether I had acne or not!" Another close friend who thought she may be expecting her first child searched out an older OBGYN in hopes that the doctor would be more conservative. She explained to him that although this would be her first child, and had no experience to draw upon, she was sure that she must be expecting because she had recently become quite weepy and moody for no apparent reason. She felt these symptoms were an obvious sign that her hormones were changing because of the pregnancy. The doctor returned with the results of her tests and the good news that she was indeed expecting her first child. He warned her about using any drugs, including aspirin, then wrote out a prescription for Prozac for the moodiness and weeping. She knew enough about Prozac to be absolutely appalled at his suggestion and found another doctor.

This practice of handing out such a powerful mind-altering substance like it is candy is great cause for alarm. Such widespread use would indicate that everyone everywhere should be concerned enough to become better informed.. This is a drug which alters the mind, thoughts and actions of the patients, thereby affecting not only the patient, but anyone who interacts in any way with that individual patient. For this reason the public should be made aware of how Prozac works in the body and upon the mind. They should be aware of the allegations being made nationwide of extremely violent behavior and suicide as side effects of Prozac. They should be made aware of the massive amount of medical literature which demonstrates the potential violence that is possible with this drug and the other psychoactive drugs. They should also be aware of the allegations surrounding insufficient testing by the manufacturer. They should be concerned about the potential long-term disabling effects upon the patients. They should be concerned about what effect this drug could have upon the brain function of the children being born to those presently using Prozac - what effects it may be having upon the developing nervous system affecting brain function and development, as well as, the child's behavior patterns for years to come after in-utero exposure. We are the ones who end up picking up the tab for the costs involved when a drug causes death, disability or criminal behavior. It costs us in higher taxes, higher insurance rates, additional law enforcement, prisons and jails, an increased number of disability benefits for botched suicide attempts or for the families left behind, or for long-term debilitating physical side effects, etc., etc. If Prozac is causing such violently destructive thoughts leading to murder, as so many patients are reporting, we also stand the chance of losing our lives or the life of a loved one as an innocent bystander through another's drug-induced behavior.

Although Prozac was reported to have fewer side effects than most antidepressants, and this was the basis for the aggressive marketing that has pushed Prozac to the top of the charts, the FDA lists approximately 575 side effects. Additionally, Lilly admitted to the FDA on April 20, 1990 that they did not include "suicidal thoughts" as an adverse event and therefore, did not look for that as a side effect in their clinical trials on Prozac. They also directed those conducting studies not to "include signs and symptoms of depression continuing since admission to study." The Review and Evaluation of Efficacy Data pointed out that this would have altered the evaluation for the efficacy of Prozac, "Not surprisingly, many antidepressants (and anxiolytic) agents do produce adverse effects which are known to be symptoms of depression, (e.g., insomnia, nausea, anxiety, tension, restlessness) leading to a possible under-representation of these effects." Not including these reactions would have lowered the actual figures for adverse reactions.

Other critical information was withheld. Recently released FDA records have revealed that Prozac was shown to include potential risks of "*intensification of the vegetative signs and symptoms of depression...* " They also disclosed that Lilly was aware of and had reported to the FDA just two months before Prozac's approval 27 deaths in a document entitled "Deaths Reported During or After Fluoxetine Treatment." Dr. Hummel, one of the administrators at Utah State Mental Hospital, has expressed that he has also noticed that in some patients it appears that Prozac is multiplying the depressive state. After seeing a very serious adverse reaction in someone close to him, he has questions about why no one seems overly concerned about what is happening with Prozac. He uses the drug in only 5% of his patients because he does not see that it is any more effective than other antidepressants, and, in order to be used safely, it requires extremely close monitoring in order to be used safely.

As of October, 1993, 28,623 complaints of adverse side effects had been filed with the FDA, including 1,885 suicide attempts and 1349 deaths. Elavil, another anti-depressant has received 2,000 complaints in 20 years on the market. Prozac had accumulated almost three times that number just in the first two years. Valium, the most prescribed drug on the market from about 1972 to 1982, in 22 years received less than 7000 complaints and faced a very vocal public and medical outcry against it's excessive use when it was discovered that it was extremely addictive and produced terrible withdrawal symptoms. Prozac has been out only six years and the most severe emotional side effects did not even come to public or professional attention until February 1990 and yet there are 28,623 complaints registered, a figure higher than any other drug in the history of the FDA. The general rule of thumb for estimating the impact of these reports made to the FDA is that they represent anywhere from one to ten percent of the actual figures. In the Journal of the American Medical Association David Kessler, FDA Commissioner, indicated that the higher figure of 100 times what is reported are the actual figures according to one study, "Only about 1 percent of serious events are reported to the FDA..." *Working with a 1 to 10% rate would indicate staggering figures ranging from 286,230 to 2,862,300 actual adverse reactions, 18,850 to 188,500 actual suicide attempts and 13,490 to 134,900 actual deaths associated with Prozac! These figures are unheard of in the history of the FDA - never have they seen anything that compares.* Jane Heimlich, in *HEALTH AND HEALING*, states "Prozac has the distinction of having the most ADRs [adverse drug reactions] of any drug in history..." (See chapter entitled LILLY & POLITICS for additional statistics from various medical sources which indicate *even higher figures* for these serious reactions. Fava and Rosenbaum report in a study entitled "Suicidality and Fluoxetine: Is There a Relationship?" that only half of the physicians they contacted completed and returned their questionnaire on Prozac and suicide. They felt that "Data may have been missed if clinicians were reluctant to report a negative adverse effect such as suicidal ideation due to their prescribing...")

Lilly had embarked upon just as an aggressive marketing campaign five short years previous to the approval of Prozac with their arthritis "cure" Oraflex. April 20, 1982 Eli Lilly announced FDA approval of Oraflex, "a new direction in antiarthritic therapy". The press release was glowing. It stressed the safety of the drug, pointed out that it had been well accepted in England and was available in several other countries. Of course the advertizing was the same old story that Oraflex, just as they have told us about Prozac, was also better than the other medications then available. The marketing campaign was so successful that after the first 21 days on the market 64,000 prescriptions were filled for the drug at a price of $1,300,000. Approximately two months later nearly 500,000 people had tried Oraflex. That is when things began falling apart for Lilly and their newest wonder drug, Oraflex. British doctors began reporting very serious side effects, such as perforated ulcers, liver damage, kidney damage and gastrointestinal bleeding and death associated with Oraflex. By August 4, 1982 England outlawed the drug and the following day, succumbing to FDA pressure, Lilly removed Oraflex from the market in the United States. Only three months on the market had produced 43 deaths. In England where the drug had been available for almost two years the death rate had reached 96. "Sixty Minutes" reported, *"...what the American public didn't know while it was being bombarded with praise for Oraflex was that there were some dark secrets in the drug's recent past. That while some were hailing it as a wonder drug in the United States, there were people overseas who were cursing it. "* Disturbing as it may be there were Lilly executives who knew about the serious adverse reactions to Oraflex and were aware of at least 29 deaths *before* the drug gained marketing approval in the United States. Lilly maintained that they did nothing illegal or unethical by not divulging this information. But they plead guilty to criminal charges on August 22, 1985 and were fined a mere $20,000 (the maximum fine) for withholding the information. The $20,000 to Eli Lilly should have been nothing to them at all when you consider that they bring in over $100 million every month on Prozac alone. This seems a very small payment when it involves the loss of 139 human lives.

Joe Graedon, in his book *THE NEW PEOPLE'S PHARMACY,* reported Lilly's ethics during the Oraflex situation. "The company has steadfastly insisted that no reporting to the FDA was necessary because the deaths that occurred in Europe were to be 'expected' from drugs like Oraflex. Because I was shocked when I learned that Lilly 'expected' so many people to die, I got in touch with an FDA official to get the agency's opinion. When I told him that Lilly still maintained that its drug was no different from any of the other arthritis agents, he was caught off guard. He responded that 'between you and me, it takes a lot of balls to say that.' Another argument that the Indianapolis pharmaceutical manufacturer had used in its defense was that officials didn't have to report overseas deaths because they were the responsibility of a foreign subsidiary. And that, furthermore, United States regulations don't require notifying the FDA of deaths of non-American patients under some conditions. A different FDA spokesman had an equally candid reply to this tack: 'Horseshit!'"

As it all came out in the end Lilly was withholding information about British cases from the United States while they withheld information on the US cases from the British. With this information on US cases the British government drug authorities would likely have banned Oraflex sooner than they did. This withholding of pertinent information about their drugs by Eli Lilly is presently the subject of an ongoing federal grand jury investigation. In December 1992 Lilly's quarterly report to stockholders reported, "A federal grand jury in Baltimore, Maryland is conducting an inquiry into the company's compliance with the Federal Drug Administrations' regulatory requirements affecting the company's pharmaceutical manufacturing operations." The *INVESTOR'S BUSINESS DAILY* reported, "The FDA said there were objectionable conditions in nearly every area of Lilly's Indianapolis capsule and tablet plant...*In nearly every system examined, the available data were found to be incomplete or inaccurately summarized...*"

Morton Mintz a reporter for the Washington Post, and a Niemann Fellow who won the Raymond Clapper award for reporting the thalidomide tragedy describes his book, *BY PRESCRIPTION ONLY*, a book which could have been the warning to prevent all the tragedies we have seen with drugs since 1967, "Here we shall see that there have been instances when our excessive trust in certain Corporate Consciences has been rewarded with inadequately and even fraudulently tested drugs, with useless drugs and inferior versions of good drugs, with protraction of illness, and with waste of our money. In order that sales may begin and continue, regardless of whether we are healed and spared pain, evidence of serious and even lethal effects has been withheld from the responsible government agency and concealed from the medical profession and the public." (p. xiv)

After the Oraflex fiasco, we all should have been ready for the deja-vu scenario presented to us in the form of Prozac. In light of the overwhelming avalanche of adverse reaction reports filed with the FDA and horror stories of death and terror beyond anything Hollywood could have dreamed up, Lilly continues to defend this new drug as well. Once again they stress that we should just "expect" these reactions with this type of medication. With Prozac they have given us a slightly different slant to their defense. This time we should "expect" the deaths to be brought on by the disease itself - depression, not their newest wonder drug.

Dr. Paul Leber, director of the FDA's neuropharmacological drugs product unit, was quoted in the July 3 , 1990, issue of *NEWSDAY* as referring to Prozac as "a very hot item", adding, "People are thrilled about the drug, maybe wrongly." Dr. Peter Kramer says, "People to whom medication has been prescribed often express concern over unknown side effects, and this concern is understandable. There are instances in which taking medication has had *terrible unanticipated consequences ...medications do not always behave as we expect them to."* (*LISTENING TO PROZAC*, p. 125)

Approximately sixty lawsuits had been filed before the first edition of this book went to press in September 1991. By March 1992 that figure had jumped to 125. Lilly's stockholder report for December 1992 lists a figure of 170 pending suits. How many more are in process we do not know. We do know that the problem is so massive that the American Trial Lawyers Association set aside an entire division to deal specifically with Prozac litigation several years ago. Appeals to Congress for a Congressional investigation have also been filed. Survivors of Prozac have circulated petitions to request that Congress step in and investigate Prozac, asking that it be removed from the market, if not permanently, at least temporarily, until further testing can be done.

In March, 1991, a Houston attorney, Paul L. Smith made a statement in *THE TEXAS LAWYER*. "In my opinion we are just scratching the surface of what a potentially dangerous drug this is." After it was reported that his firm specialized in Prozac suicide litigation his office was flooded with calls, not only from people who had lost a loved one, but also from those who were offering to serve as witnesses because they themselves had bad experiences on the drug. Hon. Leonard Finz, an attorney also handling many Prozac cases and himself an ex-New York Supreme Court Justice, warns, "There are literally thousands of people out there who are having uncontrollable rages and not understanding why. We're sitting on top of an explosive nightmare!" And attorney Kelly Thompson stated the spring of 1991 on CNN'S LARRY KING LIVE, "I say to anybody in America who has a loved one who has committed suicide, 'Get a blood test and let's find out what's in them.' We are guinea pigs for new drugs. We should have a data bank so we could find out what is going on. This drug [Prozac] was put on the market in record time. It has escalated to the number one drug. They [Eli Lilly Pharmaceutical] give trips to Hawaii for prescribing it! The people when they retire from the FDA go to work for these big drug companies. I think we need to watch it closely! Either there's a lot of extreme incidental incidences occurring all over this country or something could be there!"

Ralph Nader's consumer protection group, The Public Citizen, requested early in 1991 that the warnings connecting Prozac with suicide and violence be made more visible by placing them right on the product label. Their medical experts felt that this was called for in the light of the large number of adverse reaction reports made to the FDA and the abrupt discontinuation of a case study on Prozac where five out of eight patients experienced "de-novo [feelings not experienced previously] emergence of intense violent suicidal and/or homicidal ideation." [The reader should be made aware at this point that the FDA hearings called for by Nader began with five out of the ten FDA voting panel members disclosing their financial ties to various drug companies - a direct conflict of interest. A more detailed account on this issue can be found in the chapter entitled, LILLY & POLITICS. It remains a mystery, an embarrassment and cause for investigation as to why these panel members were allowed to vote after such disclosures.]

One young woman, who was a bitter victim of Prozac, made the statement that it would do no good to fight to warn others about the dangers of this drug because no one would listen until enough people were affected - then, and only then, would something be done. She had a sister who had lost her life in a Prozac suicide and another sister whose life was also left shattered by the use of the drug, while she personally was still in a body cast one year after she attempted to take her own life in a car accident while on Prozac. In my experience, her case, where multiple victims are involved, is not an isolated one but a common one. At least one half of the reports I have received have involved *multiple victims of adverse reactions,* not just one. We need to ask ourselves, "Just how bad does it have to get and how many need to be affected by Prozac before we do something about this drug and its analogues, Zoloft, Paxil, Luvox, Lovan - the other SSRIs?"

Maria Malakoff and her husband Gary were both pharmacists in Florida until Prozac changed their family forever. After a few months of Prozac use Maria impulsively attempted suicide, realized it was a reaction to Prozac and discontinued her use of the drug. She tried to warn her husband of the danger she felt he was facing by his continued use of Prozac. He assured her the drug was doing him good. Gary continued to assure his wife until he stopped his use of Prozac forever by putting a gun to his mouth and pulling the trigger in front of Maria and their four children. Maria and Gary's pharmacy was the first pharmacy to remove Prozac from the shelves. Now through her pain and anguish Maria sends a warning to all of us, **"The day is not far off that every family in this country will be affected in some way by Prozac!"**

CHAPTER 2

UNDERSTANDING DEPRESSION, MANIA, ETC.

The 90's have been designated by the U.S. government as the "Decade of the Brain". This miraculous three pound thinking organ is what makes us human. It produces feelings - feelings of pleasure or pain, happiness or sadness, love or hate, inner peace or turmoil, pride in our actions or remorse because of them, joy or sorrow, hope or despair, etc. With our brain we command the actions of our bodies, i.e., movement of legs, arms, fingers, toes, etc. With our brains we read, reason, form and express ideas, calculate, create, etc. With it we gather sights, sounds, odors, words, thoughts, etc. and record them for future reference. The various functions of the brain are endless. Marvelously and mysteriously the brain accomplishes all of these in the twinkling of an eye. Every ten seconds it can absorb 10 million bits of information - 4 million from the eyes, 5 million from the skin, and 1 million from hearing, smell and taste. It is difficult to comprehend the complexity or the amazing sensitivity of these processes.

The brain is a collection of 100 billion neurons (nerve cells) and a trillion support cells and is protected by more bone mass than any other organ. The neurons are so minute that they are only 1/100th the size of this period. The tentacles which come off the neurons, dendrites, have a space between them which is a millionth of an inch. This tiny space is a synapse. The neurons communicate with one another by sending messages through electrical discharges across these synapses. In order for that electrical message to cross a synapse chemicals called neurotransmitters must travel across this space to trigger a chemical reaction on the other side. Too much or not enough of one transmitter or another (there are approximately 75 known neurotransmitters) can profoundly affect muscle strength, mood, thinking, behavior, memory, etc. Many hormones are also classed as neurotransmitters. Epinephrine (adrenalin), norepinephrine (noradrenalin), angiotensin, and CCK are all classed both as neurotransmitters and as hormones. The effects of hormones and neurotransmitters on behavior overlap greatly. Actually there is little difference between them. There is a difference in how the hormones and the neurotransmitters are released, with the neurotransmitters being released near a targeted cell and the hormones being carried by the blood to the target, but even this distinction is blurry. So as we venture further into the subject of neurotransmitters, keep this very close relationship between the neurotransmitters and hormones in mind. In fact more and more scientists are classifying the brain itself as a hormone secreting gland.

So what is depression? Generally depression is divided into three types: Unipolar (profound low moods), Bipolar (a combination of depression and mania, "manic-depression" - swings from high to low and back again which can be a one time experience or chronic) or Dysthymic Depression (chronic feelings of depression with feelings of normal moods for periods of time). It should soon become apparent to you as we go on that these are all just varying degrees of the same disorder. We do know that depression is generally triggered by a traumatic event or a buildup of a series of stressors (emotional, physical, chemical, etc.) or traumatic situations throughout life. This goes on until a point is reached where the ability to cope becomes impossible. Usually the more rapid the onset of symptoms and more clear the event which precipitated the depression, the easier it is to treat and the shorter the time required for recovery. Those who develop long term depression tend to be those who experience overwhelming stress or a *constant* barrage of traumatic experiences with no break or little opportunity to recover from each episode, thus allowing a festering of the problem within.

The key is in having an opportunity to recover from the stimuli or stressor. With the opportunity to recover from each stimuli or stressor the patient does not reach a feeling of overwhelm. Depression is often described in terms of "overwhelm." Exhaustion can easily be substituted for the term overwhelm - exhaustion brought on by a constant barrage of stressors with no opportunity to rest and recover from each and every stressor. Whether the cause of the stress be physical, emotional, spiritual, chemical, psychological, financial, etc., this feeling of overwhelm is caused by stress to the point of exhaustion. The problem arises when we reach our own specific limit of energy available to us to handle a problem. If we have sufficient energy and have not yet exhausted our supply, we will find ourselves capable of handling the problem. If our energy levels are depleted we will experience "overwhelm" or "exhaustion" or "depression," depending upon which term you choose to use. The degree to which we experience this feeling of overwhelm will be determined by the degree to which those supplies are depleted coupled with the rapidity with which we correct the problem. No matter what type of stressful or traumatic situation we face, if we have the energy, the time and opportunity to recover and the knowledge it takes to solve the problem, it will not overwhelm us - it will not cause depression.

Elevated body steroids and enlarged adrenals are evidence of both stress and depression. Dr. Kramer mentions that, "A host of observations associate depression with abnormalities in stress hormones. Many depressed patients, if given a substance that ordinarily causes the body to decrease its output of cortisol, fail to suppress - that is, the system is so revved up that it no longer responds to ordinary forms of regulation. Cortisol levels (the amount of hormone in the blood) are high in many acutely depressed adults. Autopsies often show the adrenal gland to be enlarged in adults who have died by suicide. The gland is also enlarged, according to imaging studies, in about a third of depressed patients. *Put briefly, elevated, nonsuppressible cortisol levels can be a marker of depression. Elevated cortisol may even account for certain symptoms of depression. "(LISTENING TO PROZAC*, p. 115)

So why would excess in the adrenalin hormone, cortisol, be a biological indicator of depression? It is via our endocrine glands and nervous system that we process stress. The glandular system keys us up for action in order to produce peak accomplishments in critical situations it keys us up through the body's steroids. After the initial excitement, it has long been known that a depressive state follows. Both actions are critical and valuable to the individual. It is simple to understand and see the value of being keyed up for top performance in a crisis - it is a life saving measure. But we haven't seemed to realize yet that it is equally important to go into the secondary phase of being keyed down - the depression phase which forces us to rest and replenish ourselves from the keyed up phase which has used up much of our energy reserves. This process prevents us from carrying on for extended periods at top speed, resulting in "burn out" or what is being referred to as "overwhelm" or "depression."

We all have inherited constitutions or biologic conditioned responses to stress. It is critical to know that each of us have inherited, as well as, acquired conditioned responses to stressors. So *how* we respond to stress is not always up to us, but depends upon the strength of our glandular system. "Let me add now that the choice is not entirely ours. Even the optimum tempo at which we are to consume life is largely inherited from our predecessors...The features of a species reflect the cumulative memories of past generations; individuality results from the gradual engraving upon this inherited background of personal memories (including 'biochemical memories') as they are acquired during a single life-span. In the course of the development of a species, every member of each successive generation must relive - as an embryo before entering this world - the entire history of its ancestors..." (*THE STRESS OF LIFE*, p 419, 434). Although we inherit much of this ability or inability to handle stress from our predecessors, with concentrated effort we can change much of that. We must keep in mind that not only do we inherit from our parents and ancestors our ability or inability to handle stress, but we pass that ability or inability down to our offspring. As we learn various ways of minimizing stress in our own lives and building a stronger glandular system in ourselves to withstand stress, we are conditioning our future children with an advantage in handling the stressors they will face in their lives by passing on to them a stronger glandular and nervous system.

The body's steroids are like amphetamine (speed) and can produce the same effects. Steroids change the way the brain and the body work and excess steroids can be very harmful to both. The brain controls the glands, which release these chemicals we call hormones or steroids. It tells them when to release a hormone and how much of each hormone to release. The body knows how much sleep it needs and how much food it needs. The body also knows how many hormones it needs for healthy growth, balanced metabolism, etc. The abnormal excesses of steroids only confuses the body. The brain keeps a very careful measurement of these chemicals. It makes sure that the body has the right amount of each. When we disrupt this balance we cause a multitude of adverse conditions in the body and the mind.

The steroids are a crucial part of the body's defense system. After an injury, they assist in providing the body with the energy needed to defend itself from damage and to keep the blood pressure at the necessary level. *"Keep in mind that the hormones are meant to alarm you and key you up for peak accomplishments. They tend to combat sleep and to promote alertness during short periods of exertion; they are not meant to be used all day long. If too much of these hormones is circulating in your blood, they will keep you awake, just as a tablet of amphetamine would.* (Incidentally, amphetamine is chemically related to adrenaline.) Your insomnia has a chemical basis, which cannot easily be talked away after it has developed; and at night in bed it is too late to prevent it from progressing." (*THE STRESS OF LIFE,* p 424) Insomnia itself is a powerful stressor as the body pumps adrenalins in order to keep you going in an exhausted condition. Forcing yourself through a usual day's work while you are sleepy can produce another sleepless night because of the excess adrenalin pumping through your system. This cyclic development is difficult to break. The best remedy is to make up the sleep debt as soon as possible to reduce the amount of stress accumulation or excess adrenalins.

Drugs which force the body to raise its own level of steroids also produce this amphetamine effect. They may make you feel alert and bounding with energy. Yet, when the effects wear off, you feel down and depressed. This is called "rebound depression." And because these drugs force the body and the mind to continue on in a depressed or exhausted state, the rebound depression is worse than the original depression. Those stimulants which we consider mild stimulants (nicotine, coffee, chocolate, caffeinated drinks - *any stressor in our life has a stimulant effect upon us through our adrenalin responce*) do this as well, setting us up for the "need" for stronger and stronger stimulants the next time we crash from the present high. Some stimulants can make pain easier to bear, and they cause a surge in confidence. The amphetamine like adrenalin rush makes us feel "high." Often, these people believe they are doing better, when in fact their performance is worse. Amphetamines or adrenalin rushes can also make people feel more aggressive than usual. Elevating the steroid level in any way, via chemicals (mild or strong) or various stressors which will cause the body to go into a stress response. It does so by elevating its own adrenalin levels in preparation for what it reads as an excessive need. This will often result in deep depression after the excess adrenalin produces a high which can vary from a euphoric or hypomanic episode to a manic or psychotic episode.

Acute stress vs. chronic stress. The effects of brief stressful periods, lasting from a few seconds to a few hours which calls for vigorous action is considered a state of acute stress. The effects of acute stress are minimal because we have the opportunity to recover between stressors. We can encounter another kind of stress which is chronic stress. This is produced by problems that seem to go on forever, problems that we can do little or nothing about - sudden death of a loved one, a lingering court battle, undiagnosed illness, poverty, business failure, *prolonged use of stimulants of any kind* (including the common stimulants like nicotine or caffeine consumed daily in sodas, coffee, chocolate, etc.), etc. The body's response to chronic stressors differs from its response to temporary emergencies or the acute type stressors where one can nullify the effects through taking the time to recover from the stressor. With chronic stress the stress response becomes conditioned or gets into a groove of over-reacting as if each mild stimulus or stressor is instead a major one. This biological conditioned response begins to make mountains out of molehills and keys us up too much with each new crisis. Mild stressful situations then begin to cause the same internal crisis situation as serious stressful situations should. The body automatically responds to what it now reads as an even greater cause for alarm and begins pumping excess adrenalins to key us up and prepare us for what it perceives as a crisis. This unnatural overreaction is the end result of being subjected to chronic stress. And the excess of adrenalins begin to produce the same reactions as if you were using amphetamines, ie., elevation of mood then depression of mood, increased alertness ten decreaed alertness, reduction of fatigue followed by crushing fatigue, improvement of memory and concentration followed by an inability to concentrate or remember, increase in both energy and insomnia followed exhaustion and sleepiness, and so on.

Our internal regulator of this adrenalin response is the hypothalamus gland. Steroid secretions from the adrenal glands, ovaries, and testes are controlled by the hypothalamus in the brain. The hypothalamus regulates the amounts of hormones released from the pituitary gland. These pituitary hormones, such as gonadotropins (sex hormones) and ACTH - adrenocorticotropic hormones (stress hormones), are all proteins. They cause the steroid-producing centers (adrenal glands, ovaries, and testes) to produce steroids, which then influence the brain and many different organs of the body. Stress excites or stimulates both the axis composed of the hypothalamus, pituitary gland and adrenal cortex, and the sympathetic nervous system. Prolonged stimulation of the hypothalamus/pituitary/adrenal axis causes the effects of this axis to become more prominent than the sympathetic nervous system. This can retard growth and development. This effect upon retardation of growth also accelerates aging as it inhibits the rebuilding process. The cascade of hormones produced follows this process: the hypothalamus causes the anterior pituitary gland to secrete the hormone ACTH, which in turn activates the adrenal cortex causing it to secrete cortisol and several other stress hormones. The cortisol both elevates blood sugar and enhances metabolism. This increase in fuel supply to the cells gives them the ability to sustain a high level of activity during stress. After this high level of performance the body shuts down in order to use any remaining energy to rebuild supplies for the next crisis. Therefore, an individual with elevated cortisol secretion may be withdrawn and inactive as the body shuts down in order to replenish its reserves - a hypo-adrenergic condition. Basically this process biologically forces us into a much needed vacation. If the body energy reserves are depleted or overdrawn to the extent of having pushed ourselves too far into a state of exhaustion, the cortisol flow is turned back on in response to this additional stressful situation. This begins a vicious cycle which is difficult to break. If the body and mind are allowed to rest the system will normalize and regain its mental and physical energy levels. If the much needed rest is not supplied, a craving for stimulants to force the body even further than it has the ability left to force itself will develop. Unfortunately this chemical stimulation of adrenalins only additionally depletes the mental and physical reserves causing an even greater depression, exhaustion, and depletion of energy levels when the inevitable crash emerges after the chemically induced energy level ("high") wears off. If the body and mind are continually pushed beyond their limits and not allowed the time to rest and rebuild even death can result.

Hormones (steroids) are essential and their balance critical to both mental and physical health. Hormones control the way our cells use the nutrients in our food. They regulate protein and carbohydrate metabolism. They maintain the body's mineral and water balance. A disruption in those hormones can cause severe depletion of essential nutrients. This can lead to more serious mental and physical disorders over time as the depletion becomes greater and greater and cells begin to die from starvation. This is a large part of the reason that another health problem associated with excess steroids is cancer. According to cancer expert Dr. Charles Simone 60% of cancers in women and 40% of cancers in

66

men are nutritionally based. Because the steroids are essential in maintaining blood pressure, any disruption can also cause problems with maintaining that critical balance. If we add steroids to our body it can cause many problems. "People using steroids often lose their memory. They lose their attention span. They can't concentrate for very long. They lose their ability to cope with stress. They also lose their ability to feel pain." (*DRUGS AND SPORTS*, p. 25) The result is the same when the excess in steroids is caused by our body's own over-response in the production of steroids during stressful situations or through the over-response produced by the constant use of daily stimulants, such as caffeine, nicotine, etc., which are included in a multitude of products we now consume on a daily basis.

Protecting the body's stress mechanisms is what is of utmost importance in physical, mental, emotional and spiritual health. Whether the stressor be chemical, physical, mental, emotional or spiritual, the result is the same - it disrupts body and brain chemistry and produces excess steroids to assist in the crisis situation. The consistent exposure to various stress situations will cause the adrenals to begin to over react. This automatic over response to ever milder stimulants produces a wide variety of mental and physical disorders through the excess body steroids. The liver is our main detoxifying plant for these excess steroids and other chemicals. When the liver is busy detoxifying chemicals (including medications) or the cross-linked proteins produced by protein binding drugs, etc., it is using up the supply of enzymes it would generally have used to neutralize any excess body steroids. If we want to avoid a dangerous build up of steroids we must keep our liver functioning properly and make sure it is not overburdened with work.

Abnormal increases in cortisol can be very damaging to the immune system. As cortisol and other hormones shift energy to the processes of increasing blood sugar and metabolism, they shift it away from the manufacture of proteins, including the proteins necessary for the immune system and growth and development. This adverse effect upon growth and development is one of the reasons why stimulant drugs or drugs which increase adrenalin (cortisol) flow should not be used during pregnancy or during childhood or adolescence. Taken before puberty they can, not only retard, but even alter sexual development. Internal growth and development is retarded as well as the outwardly obvious development, such as height. Adolescents experience more severe reactions because of the profound hormonal imbalances they are already experiencing in puberty. In acute stress or short term stress this shift in hormones may not be a serious problem; however, stress (elevated adrenalin levels) that continues chronically for weeks or months weakens the immune system and retard growth and the ability to rebuild tissue. *In other words, chemically inducing an elevated level of cortisol produces chronic stress.* These changes, while helping the body to sustain prolonged activity, do so at the expense of decreased immune system activity and decreased growth and development.

What is the result of constant excess adrenalin production brought on by prolonged stress? The elevation of the body's steroid levels induces a *constant alarm response*. Virtually every organ and chemical constituent of the body is involved in a stress reaction. This constant chemical alarm situation keeps all body systems keyed up. Depending upon the metabolic processes, the level can vary, producing a constant keying up and then shutting down effect or crashing. The crash produces depression. Athletes who push and push themselves in preparation for cometition often experience depression after the competition is over. The suffer a crashing from their own excesses of adrenalin. This constant excess of adrenalin, which pushes the system well beyond its energy reserves as an end result, causes a type of Post Traumatic Stress Syndrome or symptoms similar to Chronic Fatigue Syndrome. When these abnormal excesses of the adrenal steroids are produced by prolonged periods of stress, we find that it becomes very difficult to sleep. Some may become euphoric or carried away by an unreasonable sense of well-being or buoyancy, "not unlike that caused by being very slightly drunk." This euphoric state is often followed by excessive sleepiness or a sense of deep depression, which may even go so far as to produce suicidal tendencies. Profound mental derangements may result, which we must note, disappear when the hormones are allowed to balance and normal sleep patterns are restored. Amazingly, with enough steroids in the blood, whether produced by the body or by an injection of synthetic steroids, the depression phase can actually be followed by complete anesthesia. Dr. Selye warned years ago, "There remained no doubt that hormones can affect consciousness and that...*they act very much like an excess of alcohol, ether, and certain narcotics, which tend to cause excitement followed by depression*...it is instructive to know that stress stimulates our glands to make hormones which can induce a kind of drunkenness. Without knowing this, no one would ever think of checking his conduct as carefully during stress as he does at a cocktail party. Yet he should. The fact is that *a person can be intoxicated with his own stress hormones*...We are on our guard against external toxicants, but hormones are parts of our bodies; it takes more wisdom to recognize and overcome the foe which fights from within. In all our actions throughout the day we must consciously look for signs of being keyed up too much - and we must learn to stop in time. To watch our critical stress level is just as important as to watch our critical quota of cocktails. More so. Intoxication by stress is sometimes unavoidable and usually insidious. You can quit alcohol and, even if you do take some, at least you can

68

count the glasses; but it is impossible to avoid stress as long as you live, and your conscious thoughts often cannot gauge its alarm signals accurately. Curiously, the pituitary is a much better judge of stress than the intellect. Yet, you can learn to recognize the danger signals fairly well if you know what to look for." (*THE STRESS OF LIFE), p. 249, 412, 413)*

Stress is activated by a large variety of things, but with effort we can consciously control our reaction to most of them. Some stressors are general, those affecting the majority of the population in the same way - war, a fire, a chemical spill, a riot, accidents, etc. Others are specific. They are dependent upon an individual's own peculiarities. For example to one who has had a child kidnapped, just their child being out of sight can trigger the same type of stress experienced by the initial kidnapping. For each of us the stressors vary. Beyond serious disease or intensive physical or mental injury, driving in rush hour traffic, hearing our child cry, going into surgery, exposure to a draft, an alarm waking us each morning, a phone ringing in the middle of the night which could signify an emergency situation, or even expressly joyful situations can be enough to activate our body's stress mechanism producing a flow of our own steroids - the adrenalins and the noradrenalins in the brain. Our perception of a potentially stressful situation can make all the difference in how that stressor affects us. If we possess the knowledge to handle a particular crisis situation, we react in a vastly different manner than one who does not have that knowledge. In an accident one who has knowledge of emergency medical techniques will busy themselves assisting victims while those without this knowledge will most likely panic and become hysterical because they lack the wisdom to know *how* to handle that crisis. Our bodies come already programed with our responses to physical and chemical stressors. This is evident by the fact that babies, animals, the severely retarded, etc. - those incapable of being consciously convinced of the harm of a particular chemical, say a deadly poison, will die upon the ingestion of the poison.

We all experience stress as a part of life. As we keep in mind the similarity between hormones and neurotransmitters and the fact that the brain is part of the glandular system, we can see that as stress builds over time it does so within the glandular system of the body. This untreated or unresolved stress takes its toll, not only upon us, but upon our children and their children as well as we pass on acquired inability to handle stress. This weakens us physically, mentally, emotionally, spiritually, etc. for generations to come. In the past the main focus in research was on how our thoughts and emotions affect our bodies. Little was considered in how body processes or changes affect mentality. We have now begun to look at the biological causes for mental conditions. At the center of all of the research is something our lives are filled with anymore - stress.

Stress is generally manifested either by unusual aggressiveness or passive indolence depending upon the present state of one's constitution or inner strength and ability to handle that stress. In general the following are some of the symptoms of stress:

1. Accelerated pulse rate or pounding heart
2. General irritability
3. Depression
4. Hyperexcitation or hyperkinesia (inability to take a physically relaxed position such as sitting quietly or lying down, moving about for no reason)
5. Hair loss
6. Dryness of the throat and mouth
7. Loss of appetite
8. Impulsive behavior or emotional instability
9. Overwhelming urge to cry or run away (indicative of the "fight or flight" associated with adrenalin - epinephrine)
10. Inability to concentrate
11. Flight of thoughts and general disorientation
12. General fatigue
13. Loss of the joy in life
14. General panic, afraid for no reason
15. Emotionally "keyed up"
16. Trembling or nervous ticks
17. Easily startled, "jumpy"
18. Nervous, high-pitched laughter
19. Stuttering or speech difficulties
20. Grinding of the teeth
21. Insomnia
22. Sweating (apparent by close inspection of skin)
23. Frequent need to urinate
24. Indigestion
25. Nausea
26. Diarrhea
27. Migraine headaches
28. Premenstrual tension or missed cycles
29. Neck or back pain
30. Excessive eating
31. Increased smoking

32. Alcohol addiction
33. Drug addiction
34. Increased use of mind-altering drugs
35. Nightmares
36. Neurotic behavior
37. Psychoses
38. Prone to accidents (this is why pilots and air traffic controllers are generally checked for stress and restricted in their use of mind-altering drugs)

The preceding symptoms are the result of hormonal imbalances brought on by various types of stressors. Dr. Hans Selye, one of the great pioneers in the physiology of stress, lists the above symptoms as clear markers of stress. Then he points out that all of these "easily-detectable manifestations of stress are the result of deranged hormone secretion or nervous activity" (*THE STRESS OF LIFE,* p. 173). The more signs or symptoms which are apparent, the more obvious is the seriousness of the condition. These symptoms of stress are the same symptoms given as the symptoms of all the various mental disorders, including depression. Almost everyone of these is used as an excuse to prescribe Prozac or another psychiatric drug. Nevertheless they are also often reported as side-effects of the psychoactive drugs. Let's take a look at why this happens.

Stress is measured medically by testing for elevated levels of the adrenaline (epinephrine), corticoids, or ACTH. Another determining factor is Corticotrophin Releasing Factor (CRF), which is responsible for the release of ACTH and subsequently the adrenal corticoids, cortisol (cortisone), and corticosterone. Another marker for stress is enlargement of the adrenal glands, which is often found in those who have committed suicide. This indicator of stress, the enlargement of the adrenal gland, can be caused by many factors - all those things which cause a chemical stress response process within the body, ie., shock of any kind, pregnancy, insulin treatment, diabetes, low oxygen, overexertion, hyperthyroidism, exposure to cold or shock producing agents, a wide variety of drugs, high protein diets, infections, diets low in magnesium and vitamin B, etc. The body is going to react to anything harmful to it and the wear and tear produces this adrenal enlargement as the end result of its adaption process in filling the excess of demands made upon it for more and more adrenalin hormones.

The medical diagnosis for elevated, nonsuppressible cortisol levels is Cushing's disease. This inability to control the level of cortisol produces obesity (similar to what is seen with someone on steroids such as Prednisone), bone loss, depression, mania, etc. Cushing's is difficult to detect. Even though preliminary test results may not demonstrate evidence of Cushing's, several months down the road the same test will produce a clear diagnosis. So we are talking about varying degrees of this disorder, the milder degrees are not detectable, while the increasing severity becomes easier to detect. As a result, physicians often misdiagnose Cushing's syndrome as depression.

Keep in mind that elevated cortisol levels have been discovered consistently in various mood disorders and have been implicated as the cause of these disorders. Cushing's is the clinical state resulting from the sustained overproduction of cortisol. Cushing's comes on gradually and insidiously and in varying degrees. It can be produced by overactive adrenal glands caused by an adrenal tumor or by pituitary hypersecretion of ACTH or an ACTH producing tumor in another organ such as the pancreas or bronchials. Cushingoid syndrome is the proper term used when Cushing's is chemically induced as a side effect to drugs - the most common offenders are the corticosteroids, ie. cortisone, prednisone, dexamethasone, etc. in either creams or inhalants (such as asthma medications) or by direct ingestion or injection.

The signs and symptoms of Cushing's are: emotional instability - fluctuating from a wide range of euphoria to depression or full psychosis such as mania; insomnia; aggravation or irritability; decreased ability to handle stress; diabetes; decreased glucose tolerance; fasting hyperglycemia; increased urine glucose levels; muscle weakness due to either potassium loss or metabolism of muscle mass; fractures due to decreased bone mineral; retardation of bone growth in children; edema; protruding abdomen; girdle obesity; fluid retention around face and eyes ("moon face" or mongoloid look); slender arms and legs; fat deposits across the shoulders and around the waist; acne, clitoral enlargement, abnormal hair growth and masculinizing features are apparent in women; abnormal mammary glandular function in men which may produce milk; peptic ulcers; capillary weakness due to protein loss; hypertension from sodium and water retention; increased production of androgen steroids; depressed immunologic system; suppressed inflammation response may mask severe infections; poor wound healing; purple striae in skin; tissue wasting; calcium in urine due to bone demineralization; increased potassium excretion; renal disorders; etc. In Cushing's syndrome physicians and family are to remember that emotional lability is produced by this disorder as well as an inability to handle stress. Therefore, it is recommended that situations which upset the patient be recorded and then avoided if at all possible. It is critical that the patient get the physical and mental rest he needs. The patient with Cushing's syndrome requires painstaking assessment and vigorous supportive care. This disorder can lead to a fatal adrenal crisis as the adrenal glands reach the exhaustion point. All of these cautions are good to note with those who have had reactions to the use of the SSRIs as well. When this disorder is chemically induced, the remedy is discontinuation of the offending medication in order to halt the disease process and restore health.

Mania and depression as well, can be intentionally created in a normal healthy subject in a laboratory setting by inducing a series of stimuli be it physical, chemical, emotional or etc. Both mania and depression are progressive and potentially lifelong conditions and can through this process of intentionally introducing a series of stimuli clearly be induced in a normal healthy human being. This process of inducing a series of small stimuli or stressors at first demonstrates no visible symptoms. But the effects of those stressors begin to multiply over time. In response the body becomes accustomed to producing more and more adrenalin in response until it takes only a mild stressor to set off an overabundance of adrenalin release. At this point the previously normal patient can go into a manic reaction which will continue until the excess adrenalin slows and normalizes and the patient crashes into depression and exhaustion from his own body's over reactive stimulant.

Other results of a prolonged or exaggerated stress response are mania, sleep disorders, panic attacks, anxiety, etc., and in the end chronic fatigue. Some of the most common psychiatric and physical diagnosises made after prolonged use of Prozac are bi-polar depression (more commonly referred to as manic-depression), panic or anxiety and Chronic Fatigue Syndrome. Although not generally recognized, these conditions are closely related in their origin. As we proceed into the next chapter and learn the effect of this class of drugs, the SSRIs, upon body steroids, you will see why these disorders can be the direct result of using Prozac, Paxil, Zoloft, Lovan or Luvox or any of the drugs that raise the level of the neurotransmitter, serotonin.

What is manic-depression and why is it that periods of mania are followed by periods of depression and fatigue? First let us examine what is happening throughout the entire body system to cause mania. This is a revving up of all body systems through a series of stimuli or series of stressors. This is most obvious when it is induced via chemical stimuli such as cocaine, alcohol, etc. Most of us are aware of the various drugs which rev the user up through their stimulant effect. Actually stimulants include a whole range of substances from caffeine to cocaine. They make you feel alert and energetic. They can make pain easier to bear, cause an increase in confidence and a "high" feeling. They can also make one feel more aggressive. Even though those using stimulants believe

73

they are doing a better job, it has been demonstrated repeatedly that their performance level is actually worse. Then when the effects wear off, you feel "down" or depressed and fatigued after using up your energy reserves.

The commonly used legal stimulants would be caffeine (found in tea, coffee, aspirin, No-doz, soda, Vivarin, etc.) and nicotine. (If it was shocking to you to learn that nicotine was considered by the CIA for mind control experimentation, you need to know that although we generally think of nicotine as a "mild" stimulant, it is known to be a highly addictive, poisonous chemical which causes addiction after only a few weeks of use. Additionally in 1985 there were 300,000 tobacco-related deaths in U.S. as compared to 643 reported cocaine-related deaths.) Sugar is another one which we do not generally think of as a stimulant, but it is. Meat can possess stimulant properties as well. Besides having a high protein content which can interfere with liver function, it often contains many chemical residues such as antibiotics, steroids, etc. Many over-the-counter preparations contain stimulants. Illegal stimulants are speed (amphetamine and methamphetamine), cocaine, PCP, etc.

These stimulants irritate one or more areas in the body system - pushing all functions beyond their normal capacity. Metabolic rate is speeded up. Because of their effect upon the adrenal glands the user is chemically forced into a "fight or flight" situation. The user braces himself for an emergency. Muscles are keyed up to either fight or flee, respond aggressively or panic. This is how they produce can induce violent behavior. Glandular functions are all forced beyond their capabilities producing increased sexual activity, "racing thoughts", going days with little or no sleep, etc. A few additional areas which become revved up are the social, sexual and financial. Most manics become social butterflies. Many become very sexually active. Most spend large amounts of money whether they have it to spend or not. After the manic phase the individual crashes in most of these areas and finds himself not wanting to be near anyone (part of this reaction is embarrassment because of their impulsive and out of character actions during the manic episode), disinterested in sex or sexually dysfunctional, and financially destitute or in debt or behind bars.

Mania is all too often the side effect produced by antidepressants. Although Kramer admits that keeping patients on antidepressants long-term is becoming a widespread practice as of late, he points out that this is being done "even in the face of evidence that antidepressants can set off episodes of mania". He describes mania as an "extreme and often psychotic state in which the brain is racing...manics often seem sociopathic in their indifference to the consequences of their acts...irritability can be an early sign of mania."

So why is mania often produced by antidepressants? This is because of the "revving up," or amphetamine type reaction these drugs produce. Remember that amphetamine and adrenalin are similar chemical structures. This stimulant effect begins revving up all body systems forcing them beyond their present already depleted capacity clearly manifested by the symptom of depression. This approach of using drugs with a revving up or amphetamine effect can be likened to approaching someone who has just run a marathon and collapsed at the finish line and kicking him until he gets up and runs another marathon, kicking him all the way and never allowing a period of rest. The result of this approach is obvious. It is my opinion that the terms depression, overwhelm and exhaustion are interchangeable. They are the same. Whether the initial stressor was chemical, physical, financial, emotional, spiritual, etc., the end result is the same - excess adrenalin release. This uses up our energy reserves and we drop lower and lower with each additional stressor if we are not allowed the time to heal from the first and second and so on.

Robert M. Post notes that kindling of epilepsy appears very similar to manic depressive illness, in particular rapid-cycling bipolar patients. Remember, mania can be produced by a series of small stimuli which also at first demonstrates no observable reactions.Epilepsy can be induced in this way. Depression can also be induced through the same technique as it follows the period of excitement with each episode becoming more complex than the previous one. (The most prominate feature of kindling is sleep disruption and as we go into the chapter on sleep you will begin to understand that connection to each of these disorders.) Manic depression or bi-polar disorder is often diagnosed after Prozac use in patients I have interviewed. Rapid cycling bipolar disorder can best be described in a patient's words to me about his Prozac experience, *"I was happy one minute, horribly depressed the next minute and very angry the next, with no apparent reason for any of these feelings."* This is a rapid moving from high to low or low to high for no obvious reason. And as Solomon Snyder points out, "...each 'depressive' episode is more complex, both behaviorally and biologically, than the preceding one." *(DRUGS AND THE BRAIN, p. 121)*

Creating these various reactions via stimuli is called kindling. Kindling is the term used to describe this process because the effect is similar to the kindling produced by adding wood shavings to a fire. This is a term generally used in conjunction with seizures. Although the stimulus induced in the brain is not considered a seizure, it produces a seizure-like effect causing an abnormal excitability in the brain so that the brain becomes so sensitive to stimulation after an excess of stimulation that even a cup of coffee, or other milder stimulant, will set this kindling process off, thereby producing the same adverse effect which the primary drug had originally caused. The brain develops a "hair trigger" response. The patient's sensitivity to stress, chemical or otherwise, appears to change so that a very small amount of any type of stimulus can set off a reaction. These reactions may occur frequently and may be produced for months or years after the initial stressor which brought on the first episode. Those who previously had a high tolerance during their drug use also find that this is no longer the case. We are familiar with the latent reactions produced in conjunction with LSD and latent reactions experienced in conjunction with post traumatic stress syndrome. Our body's defense reactions fall into a groove and begin to always respond with the same exaggerated hormonal response, whether it is appropriate to the situation or not. The system becomes acclimated to overreaction. Constant stress, whether drug induced or produced by all the other various causes of stress in our lives, a situation of constantly being on the edge of a crisis, conditions the body to over-respond.

Although often nothing observable becomes apparent to us or a physician with many various initial stressors or stimulants throughout our life, research shows that they are clearly and subtly taking their toll on each of us. Seizures can even be kindled in experimental animals through this method. At first nothing is apparent after applying an electric current, but after a series of intermittent small stimuli, the animal will have a mild seizure. Less and less electricity will be required each time the seizure is replicated. Even intermittent, rather than a constant state of stimulation over time will cause the animal to seize spontaneously, with no electrical stimulus at all. Then the time between the seizures decreases, and they come not only more often but with greater impact or complexity. We know that kindling causes structural changes in nerve pathways with the initial stimulus, before seizures become apparent. This is believed to be caused by a series of chemical reactions. "These substances include hormones that determine whether the cell makes new connections with other neurons or change shape. Kindling rewires the brain...the brain reshapes itself anatomically in response to small noxious stimuli." (*LISTENING TO PROZAC,* p. 112)

So even though we experience stress throughout our life and induce much of it through the use of stimulants which directly produce these constant smaller stimuli within our brains and think they are not affecting us, the body is keeping a very accurate and detailed account. Each time we introduce a stimulant or are subjected to stress it begins to add up - it begins to kindle an overreaction - an overreaction which has been demonstrated to produc depression, mania, and even seizures. In this day and age avoiding all stressors would not be a simple task, but there are many things we can do to avoid stress as well as correct it in our lives. It would be a logical conclusion that in order to avoid this type of reaction in our lives we would want to avoid as many of the smaller stimuli as possible in order to avoid the greater problems as they accumulate. In light of this understanding, if you still feel you cannot avoid these milder chemical stimulants, it would be wise to use them very sparingly.

Kramer notes that those psychiatrists who question the "transformative powers of Prozac" believe that what Prozac does is " makes people silly, impairs their judgement, substitutes false euphoria for mild depression." In other words they believe it is causing a revving up or manic like reaction. Kramer goes on to explain that manics sometimes "enjoy [?] a less extreme state of euphoria and energy, called 'hypomania.'" He then refers to it as a "noteworthy" side effect of Prozac. Hypomania, a mild form of mania, is a mental disorder. It is an abnormal, unhealthy state - a disease state. Why would anyone consider that "noteworthy"?

Mania and hypomania are both types of insanity. There is nothing "noteworthy" about being manic or hypomanic, nor in attempting to chemically induce these conditions. Achieving self-confidence and self-appreciation through one's achievements in life and through developing one's talents is noteworthy and healthy, but being chemically induced to believe that we are better than everyone else or that we are someone we are not, ie., Christ, Napoleon, is exactly what we define as insanity. Even though mania produces an incredible belief in one's self, when there is no connection with reality the individual can accomplish little good. This is a false sense of confidence in a false reality. It is insanity. what is noteworthy about insanity? There are far more safe and productive ways for the brain to take a vacation. That is what dreaming is designed to accomplish. Personally I prefer dreaming while I sleep comfortably in my bed, rather than acting one out in front of the rest of the world.

Kramer explains that he believes hypomania makes the patient more confident and more aggressive. Hypomania is a slightly euphoric state which removes inhibitions and allows for aggressiveness, but by what method? It is achieved by a blunting of alertness and awareness, robbing the patient of a fully conscious state. Assertiveness is exercised by first being fully alert and aware of every aspect of a particular situation and then having the internal fortitude, the courage, to assert oneself. Aggression brought on by hypomania is an entirely different situation producing an illusion of assertiveness and inhibiting the process of individual growth. In a toxic state consciousness is impaired. This impairment leads the patient to struggle to determine what is real and what is a dream. This fits with what is known about the mental state of patients experiencing an acute schizophrenic decompensation. Psychosis enters in as the patient resolves his confusion by adopting his delusions and attending to his hallucinations as if the they were real. It should become apparent as we continue on (especially from the information in the chapter on sleep) that hypomania is a mild dream state in which alertness and awareness are blunted. In this semiconscious state the inhibitions an individual would normally place upon himself in a fully conscious state are removed. Chemically inducing an uninhibited aggressive state is a far cry from a healthy assertive step forward in life.

After prolonged stimulation, eventually all systems, physical, mental and emotional reach a point where they have been pushed to their limit and become totally depleted. At that point everything shuts down (physical, spiritual, mental and emotional) and refuses to go any further in a desperate attempt to save our lives. In other words, the individual "crashes." This is when the depression part of manic-depression enters in. Let me stress once again that in the manic phase *all systems, physical, spiritual, mental and emotional* are forced beyond capacity. Therefore, it must be remembered that in the depression phase it is again all systems that subsequently "crash", become depressed and must be replenished. All the laws of the universe require that those reserves which became depleted from overuse be replenished before the person is restored to a healthy state in each area, physically, spiritually, mentally and emotionally. In other words, it's pay back time. Just how long this "crash" or depressive period lasts depends upon just how far the reserves were depleted or overdrawn and how much these systems are assisted in rebuilding and restoring those depleted reserves. One is so completely exhausted physically, spiritually, mentally and emotionally after the manic "high" or stimulant phase that the patient feels completely unable to go on. Energy reserves have been, not just depleted, but even overdrawn. If glandular dysfunction after the manic episode was not enough to physically induce an emotional depression, all of the other embarrassing repercussions stemming from the out-of-character behavior would be more than enough to cause a depression even in an individual of considerable emotional strength.

Using a drug with a stimulant effect at this point could be compared to forcing a breaker on your electric box to go back on and stay on when it has already, as a safety measure, cut itself off. This obviously poses many serious risks. It is the same with the body and the mind. Stimulants keep turning the body's breakers back on when they should be shut off to allow for rest and a regeneration of energy supplies and the rebuilding of nutrients. *Compensation must be made.* Recuperation from a manic episode can take quite some time. Such a high geared chemical rush causes an incredible low. When you hit such an extreme low in so many areas, it is often difficult to begin the climb back up. This stage of a drug induced manic-depressive state is often labeled Chronic Fatigue Syndrome (CFS). Whether this is a correct diagnosis or not remains to be seen as we understand more about CFS. There are those experts who do believe that CFS is brought on by an accumulation of environmental toxins. If those toxins are not stimulants which would bring on mania, the individual bypasses the manic phase and goes directly to the depressive phase because of the sluggishness caused by the severity of the toxic effect and the individual's ability to fight the effect, CFS is the diagnosis. So depending upon the type of toxin which accumulates in the body, an individual may or may not experience a high before the depressive low recognized as CFS.

If, rather than rebuilding our physical, spiritual, mental and emotional "banks" by providing the required rest, nutrients, love and caring, etc., we attempt to force ourselves out of the depressive state with additional ever stronger stimulants, what will be the result? The new level "high" brought on by the drugs will crash to a new all time "low." All these various systems will reach an even greater depressive state. This method of drug therapy will work - temporarily, but never long term. Our systems can only handle so much of this continued forcing beyond actual energy supplies. This is why patients experience rebound depression with antidepressants which is often worse than the depression they originally took the drugs to cure. This is no cure, only a postponing of the inevitable. How long one wants to stay on this roller coaster is their decision, but is also determined by their capability to endure the effects as they become more and more severe.

There is no wisdom in forcing the body. It will not function as it should and it can cost us dearly. We must not procrastinate living the eternal laws of nature which will bring us the level of performance in life that we desire. The title of an excellent book on organization sums it up for us, *IF YOU HAVEN'T GOT THE TIME TO DO IT RIGHT, WHEN WILL YOU FIND THE TIME TO DO IT OVER?* Or additionally one might ask, "Will you get another chance to do it over?" The depletion is dangerous and damaging and can be life threatening and must be dealt with sooner or later. The longer we wait, the more difficult the rebuilding process will be.

Chemically induced mania should subside after the offending chemical is flushed from the system and the body allowed to rest from the ordeal. When the mania or revving up period and subsequent depression is induced by chemicals, either ingested intentionally or accumulated from environmental pollutants, it should subside after the chemical is flushed from the system, unless permanent damage has been done. Depending upon the cumulative effect of the stimulating

79

chemical, this high/low cycling will continue until the chemical has been flushed completely out of the system. As long as the stimulating chemical is circulating in the system, the manic depressive reactions will continue. The intensity of the highs and lows ease up markedly as the drug is tapered down and discontinued. Then if no additional stimulants are used during this washing out period, the roller coaster ride should be much milder as the patient comes down. (A manic reaction during the withdrawal period from the SSRIs will be a much stronger possibility if the drug is discontinued abruptly or additional drugs are used. Several reports have been made on a reaction in combination with anesthesia during this withdrawal period as well.) How long this period of cleansing the chemical from the body may take is determined by the amount of chemical accumulated; the protein binding aspect, along with other accumulating aspects of the offending chemical; the body's ability to metabolize the residue; and whether or not additional chemicals are being added on top of what the body is already attempting to flush. Once the chemical is washed out and all body systems are replenished, proper functions are restored to a normal level along with the ability to face life and its challenges. Then is health restored.

As we begin to see the effects of these chemicals upon us the vision of their impact becomes staggering. Their is such a widespread use of so many mind-altering chemicals which possess a stimulant effect to the entire system, not only those we use as "medications" by directly ingesting them into our bodies, but those with mind-altering effects which are sprayed as pesticides, used as preservatives, fed to farm animals to increase their weight, sprayed on vegetables and fruit to produce greater harvests, chemicals in our environment which surround us everywhere. Their effects upon our quality of life should alarm us enough to ask if the benefits outweigh the risks we are now finding that they produce, not only in destroying our environment, but in the wholesale destruction of our bodies, emotional stability, our minds - our very souls.

Mania has been found to be associated with Prozac and reported in many studies (Settle 1984; Chouinard 1986; Lensgraf 1990; Nakra 1989; Turner 1985; Jerome 1991; Achamallah 1991; Venkataraman 1992). Many more reports of mania are listed in Appendix B. A couple of cases reported by Venkataraman are quite representative of the rest and would be beneficial to review. One 15-year-old girl after 5 months on 40 mg. of Prozac became increasingly irritable, grandiose, impulsive, distractible, elated with a decrease in sleep, and her judgement became impaired. She began skipping school and attempted to steal her mother's car. Her speech was pressured and mood expansive. A decrease in dose stopped the manic reaction.

The other, a 14-year-old girl after 5 months on Lithium and 20 mg. of Prozac became increasingly agitated, irritable, unstable, with increased motor activity, decreased sleep, and poor concentration. A decrease in dose did not stop the deterioration of her condition in this case. She became progressively impulsive, including sexual promiscuity, truancy, alcohol abuse and running away from home. They state that her "insight and judgement were markedly impaired."

In these two cases the patients were adolecents. This is a time of many hormonal changes brought on by puberty and because of this upheaval of hormones they are far more sensitive to powerful mind altering chemicals, often resulting in serious reactions. To interfere with hormonal balance in this period of a child's life by giving a powerful antidepressant is an excellent means of inducing mania. It continues to amaze me that parents and others around these children are not alert and aware of the progressing manic reaction. They all too often report that they are pleased with the child's "assertiveness and new found confidence." They remain completely unaware that they are describing hypomania, or the beginning stages of mania. I fail to see anything "noteworthy" about the way these two young lives were impaired and families adversely impacted by the hypomanic and manic reactions induced by Prozac. These are real people. These children's lives have been altered in a way that will profoundly affect them throughout their lives. How do you say "Whoops, goofed again" and walk away when this is a human being, a child who had a normal life to look forward to before this? Even if the child lives through this drug induced manic experience, what kind of feedback does it give them about who they are, their own strengths and weaknesses, their own feelings and their own mental stability? Are they capable of discerning what was drug induced as compared to their own actions or choices made by them in a fully conscious state - those actions or choices for which they should assume responcibility as opposed to those which were chemically induced? A manic reaction is a horribly devastating experience as reality sets in and the patient realizes what his out-of-character behavior has been. Hypomania naturally progresses into mania if the chemical stimulation continues. Hypomania is often just the beginning stages of mania. Why would anyone praise Prozac for inducing hypomania? Looking for a chemical to induce hypomania, which will not in the end produce full blown mania, is ridiculous. Now let's go on to learn just how the SSRIs and other antidepressants produce mania in patients.

CHAPTER 3

HOW DO THE SSRI ANTIDEPRESSANTS WORK?

Just how do the SSRIs work and what do they do? The SSRIs presently on the market are Prozac, Zoloft and Paxil. Fluvoxamine or Luvox, is expected to be approved right away by the FDA. All of these drugs are very similar in action with only very slight variations. They were all created to specifically affect the levels of the neurotransmitter, serotonin, in an attempt to chemically raise 5HT serotonin levels. In fact nearly all of the antidepressants raise 5HT serotonin. Either through increasing serotonin output or by increasing post synaptic sensitivity, they all raise 5HT serotonin levels. The SSRIs are touted as the latest "better mousetrap" because they have a much stronger affect upon 5HT serotonin. And although we hear that they are more effective for depression than other antidepressants, there is no medical evidence to suggest this. "Moreover, there is no evidence to suggest that selective serotonergic agents are more effective than other, less selective agents in the treatment of depression" *(SEROTONIN IN MAJOR PSYCHIATRIC DISORDERS*, p 79).

Serotonin is the neurotransmitter believed to affect depression and our moods. It is believed to affect pain, REM sleep, sexual desire, etc. It assists in regulating aggression and violence, impulsive behavior, appetite, the drive to act, anxiety, fearfulness, ability to think clearly before acting, judgement, perception, etc. This neurotransmitter, although it has a strong impact upon brain function, is largely manufactured in the enterochromaffin cells of the intestinal tract. *Serotonin affects nearly every area of brain activity.* Serotonin binding sites are found throughout the brain and most predominantly in the raphe nucleus. Projections from these cells ramify to all brain areas, including the frontal cortex, the striatum, and limbic system, affecting the hypothalamus and hippocampus.

"Prozac comes from a world that most doctors don't understand." If you ask a professional, preferably one who is trained in psychopharmacology, the study of drugs which affect the mind, just how the SSRIs work and what the theory behind the mechanics of Prozac was, they will attempt an explanation which always ends with, "Actually we really don't know what Prozac does or how it works within the brain or how any other antidepressant works in the brain." Because we yet know so very little about the brain, this is all guesswork. Dr. Peter Kramer calls Prozac "a new and relatively untested drug" and adds, "It comes from a world even most doctors do not understand." After admitting that we don't really know just how Prozac does work, the general attempt at an explanation goes like this: "Prozac is

'designed' to prevent the re-uptake of 5HT serotonin by binding to the cell receptors and the pre-synaptic cell membranes that serotonin normally passes through within the brain." This process is believed to block 5HT serotonin so that it cannot pass through into the blood stream where it is quickly inactivated or metabolized. The theory is that this binding effect of Prozac will raise the level of 5HT serotonin by holding it in the brain and not allowing it to be expelled. The levels of this neurotransmitter would then begin to build up within the patient's brain.

Dr. Kramer pointed out that "...most of what interests researchers is not so much cortisol produced by the adrenals as the *substances in the brain that stimulate the adrenals.* There is a cascade of such hormones; one brain center stimulates another, and so on down the line until a hormone is released that causes the adrenals to produce and release cortisol. At the top of the cascade is a substance produced in the brain called corticotropin-releasing factor (CRF). Elevated CRF levels can be measured in the brains of rats subjected to stress - and here is where a more homologous model of stress and depression emerges..." (*LISTENING TO PROZAC*, p. 115). From the time that researchers first looked at steroids as an answer for mental disorders they have felt that the "stress hormone" cortisol would be discovered to be the biochemical link between stress and depression. Dr. Kramer discusses the importance of stress hormone levels (adrenalin, cortisol, etc.) in depression, suicide and violence "...not only depression but also temperament rests on and is sustained by levels of neurotransmitters and stress hormones...Indeed, we should be surprised if a medicine that resets the norepinephrine and serotonin systems does *not* directly alter temperament." (*LISTENING TO PROZAC*, p. 175) Before progressing any further we should note that there is an increasing body of evidence to suggest that any drug which affects serotonin will affect the noradrenergic (norepinephrine) system (Frances et al. 1987; Manier et al. 1987; Potter et al. 1985). From this we can see that the SSRIs, which are designed to specifically affect serotonin, will also affect norepinephrine. We can therefore, be assured that they will alter temperament, including.

The SSRIs' effect of raising 5HT serotonin levels in turn elevates the body's steroid levels. Now that we have discussed the critical role of body steroids and their connection to depression, we need to understand how the SSRI antidepressants enter into the picture. What Dr. Kramer did not go on to explain, after telling us that how depression is determined medically or chemically is by elevated cortisol levels and that researchers have been looking for the chemical trigger that causes excess cortisol, is that when serotonergic agents are used to elevate serotonin levels, that the *elevated serotonin consistently manifests an* *accompanying rise in blood corticosteroid (cortisol, cortisone, etc.) levels*. This is the case whether it be serotonin precursors (those agents the body uses to manufacture serotonin, ie. tryptophan), agonists drugs (which produce a release of serotonin) or SSRIs (which block the reuptake of serotonin). Studies demonstrate that the neurotransmitter serotonin acts as a stimulant of the hypothalmo-pituitary-adrenocortical axis (Fuller 1981), thereby producing excesses of body steroids. Serotonin, if not the specific substance, it is apparently one of those substances in the brain that researchers have been searching for, which clearly stimulates the adrenals.

Elivated levels of CRF, cortisol, ACTH, etc. are evidence of both stress and depression, yet, in animal studies the SSRIs *increase* levels of ACTH, cortisol and prolactin (Stark et al. 1985; Lesieur et al. 1985 & Jones, Hillhouse and Burden in *FRONTIERS IN NEUROENDOCRINOLOGY*, Vol. 4). Studies also demonstrate that serotonin levels correspond with the daily rise and fall pattern of corticosteroid secretion. *In fact **one single dose** of 30mg of Prozac clearly increases cortisol levels by an absolutely amazing 200% (Petraglia et al. 1984)*. If one single dose causes such a significant increase in cortisol, what kind of increase in cortisol levels can be expected when someone is taking Prozac on a daily basis? Prozac has also been demonstrated to increase the release of CRF (Gibbes and Vale 1983), implying that an accompanying increase in ACTH and cortisol levels will follow. As we already knew that excess cortisol is a marker for depression and these studies were published three years or more before Prozac was approved, it remains to be seen why it was ever approved as an antidepressant.

This information about the effect of serotonin on body steroids is extremely significant. Taking Prozac or any drug which elevates serotonin levels, in turn consistently elevates body steroids, thereby producing a nonsuppressible pattern of chemically induced elevated cortisol levels. This increase in body steroids can explain many things: It certainly helps us to see how Prozac and the other SSRIs can get someone who is depressed (overwhelmed or exhausted) up and moving. No wonder patients talk about the drug beginning to "kick in" for them as 5HT serotonin builds. This in turn kicks the adrenalin flow straight from neutral or reverse into high gear. It is by this method that an SSRI can get a depressed patient up and moving. Even though they can get a patient up and moving, from what we have just learned, what should we expect to be the long term effect in using this method? We should expect the SSRIs to produce even more depression, if not while using the drug, certainly after a period of use this increase in depression should be expected. While taking the drug, the constant adrenalin effect of revving up the patient would postpone the inevitable "crash."

Yet, if Prozac is doubling cortisol levels with just one dose, and elevated nonsuppressible cortisol levels are a marker for depression, it should follow that the end result of using Prozac is a drastic *increase* in depression. This also helps us to understand why many patients who have never experienced depression before using Prozac, those who were given the drug for various reasons other than depression, report experiencing depression *after* Prozac use. It explains why so many report a worsening of depression in conjunction with the use of the other SSRIs.

The effect of serotonin in elivating body steroids also gives reason for the "amphetamine effect" felt with the use of Prozac. Cortisol is an adrenalin hormone and adrenalins (epinephrines) are like the body's own version of amphetamines. Adrenaline or epinephrine and amphetamine are chemically related so an increase in adrenalin is similar to a dose of amphetamine. Prozac and the other SSRIs produce this effect by chemically supplementing the body's own adrenalin through forcing the glands via an increase in 5HT serotonin to drastically increase their own production of the glandular version of amphetamine - adrenalin. Prozac or any SSRI should also logically produce the same mental and physical side effects associated with the use of steroids. Once again, the only difference is that these drugs accomplish this by artificially forcing or chemically increasing the body's own steroid production. We should, therefore, expect the serious physical and psychiatric reactions of both the steroids and amphetamines to be associated with the SSRIs. We do know that imipramine, considered a milder enhancer of serotonin than the SSRIs, magnifies the effects of the amphetamines (Carlton, 1961). The most obvious reason for this is that it raises 5HT serotonin which in turn increases the body's own adrenalin (amphetamine). It should follow that any drug which increases serotonin will also magnify the effects of the amphetamines. In fact behavioral syndromes caused by the amphetamines such as side to side head weaving, head tremor, paddling, etc. have been prevented by depleting 5HT serotonin. These behaviors are magnified by the increase of 5HT serotonin and in fact 5HT serotonin is believed to be the means by which the amphetamines induce these behaviors (Solviter et al. 1978). Keep in mind through all of this that experts have clearly cautioned over the years that the amphetamine effect is a detrimental, ineffective and even counterproductive approach to treating depression. This approach cannot be used without the inevitable "crash" which is the depressive state we originally set out to cure with this treatment.

When 5HT serotonin levels are raised there is a rise, not only in cortisol, but also in prolactin. Excess prolactin can cause headaches, diabetes, or gradual loss of vision. In women specifically it can produce amenorrhea (absence of periods), lactation, or infertility. In men it can produce impotence and breast enlargement.

Logically we should expect the similar result of Cushingoid syndrome from the use of the SSRIs. Cushingoid syndrome is a chemically induced non-suppressable increase in body steroid production and the SSRIs chemically induce a hypersecretion of steroids - ACTH, cortisol and adrenalin. Because 5HT serotonin stimulates the hypothalmo-pituitary-adrenocortical axis, any drug which increases 5HT serotonin should produce the same end result of chemically inducing Cushingoid syndrome. All of the antidepressants in general increase serotonin to some extent. This is the logical explaination for their amphetamine type effects. They also in long-term use should produce the same result of chemically inducing Cushing's syndrome. Yet the SSRIs, because of their direct and very potent effect upon serotonin, should understandably produce these effects far more rapidly than the other antidepressants. The new antidepressant just approved by the FDA, Effexor, should produce a double stimulant effect through its indirect effect upon cortisol levels via both elevated serotonin levels plus its direct effect upon noradrenalin or norepinephrine (the adrenaline in the brain and nervous system). It is understandable why it is being called "Prozac with a kick." The patient ought to feel as though he has been kicked when the inevitable crash occurs with this new drug.

Although enabling the depressed patient to get back on his feet, through a drastic rise in adrenalin, it is clear that these drugs are intensifying the symptoms of both depression and stress. As we just mentioned, not only depression, but also stress is measured by excesses in cortisol. A magnification of the patients' original level of stress is produced by these chemicals through the activating of the adrenergic system. Remember that Dr. Selye warned that the body falls into a groove of having an exaggerated response to stressors. This is a kindling process. When a drug stimulates the adrenals the patient is robbed of his internal glandular control. The adrenals begin to rush at the slightest provocation causing: mania, depression, akathisia type reactions (inability to rest or relax, anger, irritability, violence, etc.), hallucinations, electrical surges throughout the body, etc. - all of the symptoms we listed previously which are considered manifestations of stress. Our bodies normally control excess steroid levels through inactivation in the liver and/or through the release of the hormone or neurotransmitter, acetylcholine. As the liver becomes impaired through the use of drugs, which are very toxic to this vital organ, or as the brain and nervous system no longer possess the ability to produce acetylcholine, the body loses its ability to control its steroid levels any longer.

The first psychotherapeutic medication was Chlorpromazine (Thorazine) an antihistamine. The antihistamines are also known to bring on an adrenalin or epinephrine rush, including the fight or flight response. In fact the amphetamines (known by the street term as "speed") were first developed and marketed for the treatment of asthma. Anyone who has had either a history of street drug use or antihistamine use are prime candidates for a rapid reaction to the SSRIs or any of the other drugs that either stimulate the adrenals or suppress the cholinergic system, or even more so to a drug which does both. The anticholinergic effects of some drugs impair the ability to produce choline which helps to neutralize excess adrenaline. This inability to produce acetylcholine is the disorder found in Alzheimer's disease. Patient reports on Prozac indicate that both systems, the adrenergic and cholinergic, are being affected.

Why raise serotonin when it in turn raises steroid levels and produces a wide variety of mental and physical disorders? We already know that the most critical sign of stress is elevated cortisol levels and that elevated serotonin levels produce this excess cortisol. Therefore, one thing we can do to avoid this excess stress - stress which can cause intoxication - intoxication even to the point of anesthesia, besides a wide variety of fatal physical ailments, is to avoid drugs which elevate 5HT serotonin levels. Knowing what we do about the connection between elevated serotonin levels and their production of a stress response with accompanying elevated steroid levels should make any of us extremely concerned about using drugs which are intended to elevate or enhance serotonin levels. Those drugs being used medically to raise serotonin levels are the SSRIs - Prozac (Fluoxetine), Zoloft (Sertraline), Paxil (Paroxetine), Lovan (Fluoxetine), Luvox (Fluvoxamine), etc., the new Effexor (Venlafaxine), Deseryl (Trazodone), Anafranil (Clomipramine), Lithium, BuSpar (Buspirone), Gepirone (congener of buspirone), Ipsapirone (congener of buspirone), Eltoprazine, MAOIs, serotonin agonists and precursors, the tricyclic antidepressants, etc. ECT (electric shock treatment) as well raises serotonin.

Animal studies demonstrate that in the initial administration Prozac actually causes the brain to shut down it's own production of serotonin, thereby causing a paradoxical effect or opposite effect on the level of serotonin. We have no research to verify just how long this shutting down of serotonin production continues. A decrease in the brain's serotonin levels would indicate the necessity for extreme caution. Lower levels could make drastic changes in a patient's behavior, leading to the reports similar to what we have been receiving from the medical community on Prozac over the last several years. (Check medical references in Appendix B.) Dr. Peter Breggin stated in the April, 1991, issue of Insight Magazine that, "This [shutting down of the serotonin production] should have set off red flags at Eli Lilly."

To further complicate the paradoxical effect of the SSRIs actually *lowering* serotonin levels, we do not know through double blind clinical studies how, as the brain works to protect itself from either the drastic depletion or enhancement of serotonin levels, this could be creating a constant upheaval in the serotonin level. This rebound action could cause the level to fluctuate up and down bringing on a "roller coaster" effect as the brain fights to protect its neurochemical balance and the the drug continues to produce its iffect of disrupting the balance. Important to keep in mind is the fact that whether the level is going up or down, any disruption, whether it be a raising or lowering , of *any neurotransmitter* can cause drastic changes in brain function, behavior, mood, memory, sleep patterns, cognitive reasoning abilities, etc. The neurobalance of the brain is very delicate and sensitive and repercussions form a disruption of that balance are extensive. Many are long lasting and perhaps irreversible. in the metabolism or turnover of serotonin within the brain can have very drastic repercussions. "The nervous system is complex and full of redundant pathways, so we should not imagine that a given behavior depends on a single neurotransmitter. Still, a given type of synapse seems to be more important for some functions than for others. Consequently, *an excess or deficit of activity at a particular type of synapse may produce altered behavior, even abnormal behavior.* " (*BIOLOGICAL PSYCHOLOGY,* p. 81)

Our diet directly affects serotonin levels. The studies which indicate that diet may affect violent behavior, such as; Mawson & Jacobs, 1978, have led to additional studies on how the diet affects serotonin levels. The brain's neurotransmitters are manufactured from the foods we eat. As much as all of us may be getting tired of hearing about what we are doing to ourselves by not being responsible about our diets, we obviously *desperately need* to hear it again. We need to hear it again because now we are beginning to understand that it is affecting our mental health. Physical disease and death can be very difficult situations to handle in life, but mental disease and insanity is something most of us absolutely dread. Who wants to take a chance on losing control of our own thoughts, mood and behavior. Control of our diets can provide the mental control we all desire. Diet does directly affect thought, mood and behavior by either providing the nutrients for the production of essential neurotransmitters or providing blockages to nutrients by way of additives, pesticides, artificial sweeteners, preservatives and other chemicals. *This includes many medications, which can interfere with both the production and utilization of neurotransmitters* (R.J. Wurtman, 1982, 1983; Wurtman J.J., 1985; Wurtman, Hefti, & Melamed, 1981). It is unbelievable that few doctors ask a patient for a history of medications the patient has been using may have brought on the depression they are experiencing. They need to start realizing that drugs do interfere with neurotransmitter synthesis and utilization and allow their patients a period of time to recover from the previous drug's effects before prescribing something for depression.

L-tryptophan is the natural precursor of serotonin. It is an amino acid which is converted to serotonin once it enters the brain. It has been found that foods low in tryptophan decrease serotonin synthesis (Lytle, Messing, Fisher, & Phebus, 1975). In light of these studies it would be wise for those with symptoms indicating low serotonin levels or those who wish to avoid low serotonin levels to increase their intake of foods that contain higher levels of tryptophan which are the carbohydrates and avoid foods low in tryptophan and those foods which compete with tryptophan for entry into the brain which are the heavy proteins.

There are those foods which inhibit serotonin production by blocking the entry of tryptophan into the brain. These foods which inhibit tryptophan are the high protein foods - those of which our society has had a large overdose during the last several decades. Over the years researchers have found that increasingly lower amounts of protein are what is more beneficial to us, not the high protein recommendations of the past. A meal high in protein will cause lower amounts of tryptophan to reach the brain as the other proteins compete with tryptophan for entry into the brain. Carbohydrates increase the flow of insulin. Insulin in turn removes the other proteins from the blood which compete with tryptophan for entry into the brain. In this way carbohydrates increase serotonin production.

Dr. James Wasco, medical writer for *WOMEN'S DAY,* warns that we are far too quick in our use of "medication" for emotional problems. He adds that the danger in this pill popping quick fix solution is that it "all too often" results in addiction or dependence as larger and larger doses are required to get the desired effect. Changing one's diet to provide the brain with the proper fuel to balance its own levels of serotonin should be a logical first step to a solution to a solution for depression before ever considering using drugs which can produce extremely serious side effects. Over the last several years we have learned that cutting back on our protein intake, especially meats, will lower our risk of high cholesterol, heart disease, cancer, etc. Now we see it can also help to keep our brains functioning properly, especially when it comes to the production of serotonin.

The standard rule of thumb for good health, physical as well as mental, is to eat more fruits, vegetables and grains and less fat. Avoid nicotine, caffeine, and other stimulants. Make sure the proper quantity and quality of rest and relaxation are obtained. Retiring to bed at an early hour adds more to good mental health than most would imagine. Exercise vigorously several times each week. Whatever you do, do most of what you do in moderation. In face of the risk of loss of control over our mental health and behavior, we must be willing to learn these simple lessons. What means might nature use to warn us even more strongly that these basic laws of health are the foundation of our well being as individuals, families, cities and nations? Nature has a way of rudely awakening us when we ignore such basic lessons in life - in this way it prevents us from harming ourselves and jeopardizing our lives.

NutraSweet can lower serotonin levels. The amino-acid tyrosine reduces the amount of tryptophan which crosses the blood-brain barrier for use in the manufacture of serotonin. Foods high in phenylalanine (such as NutraSweet) can pose a serious problem because phenylalanine actually blocks the entry of tryptophan into the brain, thereby also inhibiting the synthesis or manufacture of serotonin. This is not the only disruption in the neurotransmitter activity caused by phenylalanine. Since it is a precursor of dopamine, norepinephrine and epinephrine (the brain and nervous system adrenalin), it can also increase the levels of these neurotransmitters while lowering the level of serotonin. This is an excellent formula for producing agitation and irritability and violence. After ten years on the market, one of NutraSweet's most recent advertisements makes the claim that it has been "put in everything" and now it is available by the spoonful. This increasing use of NutraSweet could certainly have set many people up for problems involving low levels of serotonin. This information certainly raises questions in my mind as to how and why NutraSweet was ever approved by the FDA. It is rare for me to interview someone who is using Prozac who is not drinking at least a gallon or generally two to three gallons per day of diet soda sweetened with NutraSweet! The patients have noted that they were both amazed and confused by their extremely high consumption of these diet drinks. This craving for drinks with a substance which lowers brain serotonin is, to me, a strong indication that the brain is desperately attempting to balance its levels of serotonin as Prozac triggers a drastic fluctuating of the balance of this neurotransmitter.

The brain is such a delicate and extremely complicated structure about which we know so very little. Why would we even dare to take a chance on disrupting the balance of any of the neurotransmitters? The slightest changes can have remarkable consequences in thought patterns, coping abilities, behaviors, memory, mood, cognitive reasoning ability, sleep patterns, etc., etc., etc.

Does Prozac accumulate over time? (Be sure to read the latest research on this issue by Dr. Craig Karson in the following chapter.) Prozac, just as all the other

90

serotonergic drugs, is a highly protein binding drug (94.5%), in theory blocking primarily serotonin in the brain for extended periods. But it also binds to other proteins or toxins in the blood, making them too large to be broken down and expelled readily by the body. The Physicians Desk Reference (PDR) states that Prozac binds to "human serum proteins, including albumin and glycoprotein. The interaction between fluoxetine and other highly protein-bound drugs has not been fully evaluated but may be important [see Precautions]." (PDR 1990, p.905) Warnings to prescribing physicians about Zoloft elaborate a little more on the relevance of this highly protein binding aspect, "Because sertraline [Zoloft] is tightly bound to plasma protein, the administration of Zoloft (sertraline hydrochloride) to a patient taking another drug which is tightly bound to protein (e.g., warfarin, digitoxin) may cause a shift in plasma concentrations potentially resulting in an adverse effect." Keep in mind that a large number of drugs developed over the last few decades are very highly protein bound. For instance, approximate protein binding percentages for Valium is 98%, Halcion 80%, Xanex 82%, Zoloft 98%, Paxil 98%, etc. This binding to body proteins and other drugs would causes excess stress to be placed on the organs and glands involved in metabolizing and elimination processes, i.e.. the liver, pancreas, kidneys, lymph glands, etc. Those patients having extremely adverse effects immediately tend to be those who are mixing Prozac with other drugs, those with pancreatic, liver and kidney weaknesses, those in a weakened physical condition, or those with a past history of diseases affecting those organs, including a past history of excessive alcohol usage or drug abuse, or years of constant prescription drug use, especially psychoactive drugs or drugs which induce psychiatric side effects.

Eli Lilly states in their clinical pharmacology warnings on the product that "Fluoxetine [Prozac] is extensively metabolized in the liver...As might be predicted from it's primary source of metabolism, liver impairment can affect the elimination of fluoxetine...This suggests that the use of fluoxetine in patients with liver disease must be approached with caution. If fluoxetine is administered to patients with liver disease, a lower or less frequent dose should be used." With this in mind, it is a frightening observation that one of the more frequent complaints of adverse reactions made to the FDA about Prozac is "impaired liver function". The signs which indicate impaired liver function, those which should be watched for in order to prevent even more servere malfunction are: nausea, vomiting and abdominal pain. The liver is considered one of the most important, if not the most important, chemical laboratories of the body. One might view the body's energy level from the position of its capability to remove the chemical scars of life. Removing chemical scars is the function of the liver. This implies that our energy level is based upon the capacity of our liver to function properly.

Every biologic process leads to chemical changes, thus requiring proper liver function in order to process these chemical byproducts. These products should be soluble or subject to destruction and elimination, thus enabling us to restore and rebuild without accumulation of toxins. When the process of elimination is rapid, and recovery complete, our tissues undergo little change and we remain *healthy and young*. There is however, a percentage of all biologic reaction products that are insoluble, or less rapidly removable than their rate of production. Cross-linked proteins, chemicals, calcium deposits, and many other products of biologic activity would be included in this category. This accumulation of debris also interferes with the liver's ability to manufacture vital hormones and enzymes, the ability to neutralize additional poisons, control the body's own steroid production, which, in turn, affects the immune system, blood pressure and heart function, brain, kidney, pancreas,etc. function - all vital organs are affected causing serious damage to the entire system, a shortening of life and destruction of health. *"Mere excessive accumulation suffices to block the machinery. It could induce the changes we consider characteristic of aging by the mere presence of ever larger amounts of inert waste products and the consequent inability to produce indispensable vital ingredients at the proper rate." (THE STRESS OF LIFE, p. 431)*

This concern of liver impairment is one that has been expressed over and over again in conjunction with the use of the antidepressants and many other medications. *If a patient is taking a drug which impairs the organ essential in controlling the amount of medication the body retains in the blood, how safe is the drug?* Once liver function is impaired, any chemical can rapidly accumulate within the body to toxic levels, producing adverse reactions and even death.

The pharmaceutical product warnings on Prozac as of May 1990 mention the possibility of this drug precipitating hyperglycemia (diabetes), hypoglycemia and pancreatitis. The adverse effects upon the pancreas appears to be causing an imbalance in the blood sugar levels which in turn causes a compulsive desire for excesses in alcohol (See information on the Prozac - alcohol connection in the next chapter.), processed sugars and other stimulants (i.e. cola drinks, nicotine, other drugs, etc.). We have just explained that all of these can additionally impair liver function, increase the chances of drug interaction, and these can cause the pancreas to be pushed into over-reaction because of the additional stimulation. The body's desperate attempt to increase the blood sugar by these means would impair liver function which would in turn then raise the level of Prozac in the system to dangerously higher levels. Thus the vicious cycle of this drug would become self-propelling and self-defeating. The undue stress placed upon the pancreas, even to the point of pushing the once healthy pancreas into

92

malfunction, would cause the excessive craving for stimulants which would then further impair liver function. Combine this with the high incidence reports to the FDA of liver impairment as a reaction to Prozac and we should question anyone's ability, no matter how healthy, to withstand the effects of this drug over a prolonged period of use. *The length of time involved before the adverse side effects, both emotional and physical, begin to appear would only demonstrate the strength of the patient's own constitution to withstand those effects.*

The PDR states, *"The effectiveness of Prozac in long-term use, that is for more than 5 to 6 weeks, has not been systematically evaluated in controlled trials.* Therefore, the physician who elects to use Prozac for extended periods should periodically re-evaluate the long-term usefulness of the drug for the individual patient." The vast majority of patients on Prozac have been on the drug for far more than 5 or 6 weeks and few have been "periodically re-evaluated." Most doctors assume there is no need to do so, either because the sales pitch they received may have conveniently excluded warnings of possible side effects in the attempt to sell this product, or because the typical heavy work load the doctor faces gives him little or no time to investigate the tremendous volume of new drugs on the market. Also, the importance of consistent re-evaluation has apparently not been stressed to the prescribing physician by the pharmaceutical reps, because close monitoring of Prozac is very rare. In fact, it is amazing to see how often the suggestion is made that a patient may need to stay on Prozac indefinitely - even for life. Doctors receive very little training in medical school on drugs. It would make far more sense for doctors to diagnose and pharmacists to prescribe the drugs since they know so much more about them.

Unfortunately it appears there are too many irresponsible health professionals who are not concerned enough about their patients and the adverse effects they are experiencing with Prozac. Much of this stems from their lack of education when it comes to drugs and drug reactions. David Rothman in the February 14, 1994 issue of *THE NEW REPUBLIC* reviews *LISTENING TO PROZAC* and addresses this issue. "To the extent that Kramer is typical of his generation of physicians, it is plain that trusting the medical profession to be strict gatekeepers before therapies, new or otherwise, is foolhardy. Anybody who expects physicians to save us from ourselves, or form the worst imaginable abuses of twenty-first-century medical interventions, whether they involve genetic engineering, pharmacological interventions or surgical procedures, had better start searching for alternatives." It is definitely the attitude of far too many within the medical community, after being persuaded by pharmaceutical reps that Prozac has few side effects that, "This is a wonderful new drug with no side effects. Here, try it. You will feel great." Then they burst into song, "Happy trails to you...Until we meet again. Happy trails to you...Keep smiling until then." The patient rarely even gets the "call me in the morning" on this one! That may seem slightly theatrical, but it is all too real. The doctor *all too often* says, "Here is your prescription for the next year. Unless *YOU* notice any problems, we will see you then." In this way he puts the responsibility on the patient and removes it from himself. If the drug did not alter the mind and impair ones' judgement, the doctor might rationally expect the patient to notice problems which are developing, but few ex-Prozac patients will claim to have been capable of judging whether or not they were having problems with this drug. If they did suspect it was affecting them adversely, they were afraid to tell their doctor because they felt they would not receive the assistance needed to discontinue the use of Prozac or to face the terrible withdrawal. And they often state that they were afraid the doctor would accuse them of having "pre-existing emotional problems," rather than recognizing that these problems are being chemically induced by Prozac. They often cite this as one of their fears even if the drug was initially prescribed for a *physical*, rather than a mental or emotional ailment.

Why is Lilly having problems gaining FDA approval of Prozac for weight loss and is Prozac safe in weight loss? Eli Lilly has been working on obtaining FDA approval for the use of Prozac, with a brand name change to Lovan, as a treatment for obesity - which is often caused by blood sugar imbalances, as demonstrated through obsessive appetite cravings. Therefore, if Prozac is approved as a weight loss remedy we may see a nightmare beyond our wildest imaginations. Another contributing factor to that nightmare would be the extremely high dosage, 60 mg. (three times the dose the majority of Prozac patients are using presently) that must be used to affect a loss in weight.

Even though Prozac has not been approved for use in obesity, there are weight loss programs that recommend it and doctors who suggest that weight loss is a possible beneficial side effect. It is important to understand how this is achieved. First it is generally understood that Prozac will rev up the metabolism, causing it to work beyond normal capacity in the way amphetamines rev up the metabolism. Many patients report the "crashing" of the metabolism after discontinuing use of the drug. This causes an inability to digest food properly thus producing much gas and weight gain. Research suggests that the other method of producing weight loss is through poisoning. When an individual becomes extremely toxic from high amounts of poisons lodging throughout his body, he instinctively goes into a fasting state or semi-fasting state in order to begin flushing out those poisons. This is a life saving instinctive reaction. Eli

Lilly uses serotonin double talk to justify the method Prozac employs to effect weight loss. However, when a *highly accumulative* drug needs to be increased to *three times the average dose* in order to be effective, it should be obvious that the patient is losing weight by going into an anorexic state as a reaction to being *poisoned*. In fact 9% of patients using Prozac reportedly develop this serious eating disorder of anorexia.

Toxicity brought on by large amounts of poison lodging throughout the tissues of the body will force a patient into a fasting state in order to flush those poisons out and save the patient's life. Certainly there are better ways to accomplish weight loss. In the July 3, 1990, issue of the *LONG ISLAND NEWSDAY* this is made very clear by Dr. Merton Kahne, a professor of social psychiatry at MIT. Kahne is involved in clinical trials comparing fluoxetine [Prozac] and another serotonin stimulating drug called dexfenfluramine in overweight but otherwise healthy people. As one who has tested Prozac for efficacy in weight loss, Dr. Kahne's opinion is, *"My general impression is that the anorexic effects are dose-related and that it is risky to prescribe Prozac given the current state of knowledge...*It is likely to turn out that at the lower doses, you may only get a slight weight loss. *To get a more significant effect, you may have to overdose the person...Using Prozac to treat weight problems is like 'shooting a mouse with an atom bomb."*

In the June 22, 1992, issue of *BUSINESSWEEK*, an article entitled, "Prozac is Making Lilly a Little Edgy," discussed Prozac being used for weight loss and marketed as Lovan. It predicts little hope in light of recent studies for the drug being approved. Their prediction seems logical when one finds "increased appetite" listed in Lilly's literature as a side-effect. Yet there are those who continue to promote Prozac's use for weight loss.

These adverse paradoxical reactions are responses due to toxicity. People who reach these toxic levels of concentration of Prozac in their systems are those who suffer adverse paradoxical reactions. Those suffering severe adverse reactions are now dead, either due to violent acts taken against themselves or they have suffered fatal physical reactions; or they are being prosecuted for violent actions they took against others; or they have survived with their lives shattered - mentally, physically, emotionally, and financially. Those who continue to live in this so called "Prozac Hell" are the saddest victims of all. These people describe themselves as: extremely irritable; experiencing overwhelming rages with an intensity they have never felt before which forced them do things they "didn't want to do"; focusing this rage on someone they have cared about, even to the point of stalking them; having violent suicidal or homicidal thoughts;

95

having no feelings of guilt or sense of conscience; experiencing addiction or dependence; having panic and anxiety attacks; feeling "possessed"; developing an "I'll show you!" attitude toward everyone around them; having no memory of who they are; having their memories become so jumbled and confused that they are producing "false memories" of an innocent loved one abusing them; putting on the appearance of being normal while inside having horribly bizarre thoughts; experiencing obsessive compulsive behaviors such as sex, spending, shop-lifting, embezzling, etc.; loss of ability to read, learn or retain information; having extreme difficulty with concentration; having no ability to feel love or concern for those close to them; having impaired judgement (forming a thought sequence to arrive at a decision becomes a monumental task); they feel completely out of control and often develop an overwhelming fear of being controlled by others. (See how patients describe their experiences in the chapter PATIENT REPORTS.)

Admitting such obvious "out of character" behavior for these victims is a devastating thought. They fear that they will be labeled "crazy" because they realize the things they have done are insane. They have never experienced anything like it before and are overwhelmingly shocked and embarrassed and, frankly, very puzzled by their own behavior.

Dr. Breggin explains the toxic reaction to Prozac in an article from THE RIGHTS TENET: Winter/Spring, 1992 issue:

THE PROZAC TOXICITY SYNDROME

"Reports by Prozac survivors present a consistent pattern of compulsively driven thoughts and activities, especially suicidal and violent behavior. Typically the behavior is 'out of character' for these individuals who become hostile, paranoid, euphoric, energized, hyperactive, undisciplined, unable to sleep, subjectively grandiose and omnipotent, and insensitive to the effects of their behavior on themselves or others. Racing thoughts of 'a mind that won't stop going' are typical. Periods of 'crashing' and depression are common. Short-term memory and attention span are almost always impaired. Much more rarely patients become frankly confused and disoriented. Cognitive and emotional difficulties often persist after stopping the drug. Addiction and withdrawal symptoms are common, including severe depression and a worsening of suicidal or violent impulses.

During the drug reaction, individuals do not realize that they are behaving abnormally, but later they may be appalled by their actions. Afterward, they frequently cannot clearly recall their actions. "

This toxic reaction is an emotional nightmare - a mental and emotional "living hell". The symptoms are emotional in appearance, stemming from a chemically induced brain disorder. The toxic reaction is not showing up as a physical malady, but in thinking processes and behavior. Patients do not realize how they are acting while under the influence of the drug. In my opinion the patients who suffer an obvious physical reaction forcing them to go off the drug before they suffer the Prozac Toxicity Syndrome which profoundly affects their mental state, are the "lucky" ones.

The patients' unfamiliar emotions and unacceptable actions, for which they assume they are forced accept responsibility, along with the utter confusion, bring on such feelings of humiliation and inadequacy and loss of self-respect, that the patient becomes even more depressed about their situation in life. He or she continues to take the medication or even allows an increase in dosage, thinking that he must *really need* this anti-depressant. This is the most heart-rending side of Prozac - that the patient, who is uninformed of the side effects, really is led to believe that all these feelings and events are indications of flaws in his own character and not reactions to the drug. The problem is in the human, certainly not our latest cure all. As Michael O'Brien of the Citizen's Commission on Human Rights has so aptly stated, "Prozac is a boon to psychiatrists. It brings in business! A person with a simple problem now becomes a mental patient with serious problems."

Those patients who are being convinced that they are not actually suffering a chemically induced psychotic reaction, but really are going crazy generally become long term mental patients. They suffer years of additional psychoactive drug therapy with each new drug multiplying the toxic effects of the first. Then comes the electric shock treatments, antipsychotic agents, antiseizure medications and/or hospitalization. Attorneys are asking what they should do with the flood of people coming to them. They say the patients are afraid to go back to their doctors because the doctor will either raise their dose, thinking they need more of the drug in their systems in order for it to be "effective" or that the doctor will label them "crazy" or "suicidal" and lock them in an institution.

Although the major lack of awareness tends to center around the emotional side effects of Prozac, there are also serious physical side-effects as well. Generally these physical side-effects are more easily recognized as reactions to Prozac than are the emotional because of our many methods of detecting the physical effects. Unfortunately so many doctors are so completely unaware of these physical reactions to the drug that they, after diagnosing the physical condition, don't even see the connection to Prozac. These doctors then, without discontinuing the use of Prozac, prescribe additional medication for the drug-induced symptoms brought on by Prozac. All of this just further complicates the patient's condition and greatly increases his chances of additional adverse drug reactions or interactions through the addition of more drugs.

Dr. Peter Kramer speaks of additional physical side effects, "Prozac not uncommonly causes nausea, loss of appetite, nervousness, insomnia, drowsiness, fatigue, sweating, rash, dizziness, and headache. More rarely, *it has been associated with damage of one sort or another to almost every body system and organ* - from arrhythmia of the heart to inflammation of the liver to dysfunction of the thyroid gland." *(LISTENING TO PROZAC,* p.311) Some patients report their nausea reaching a point where they began throwing up blood. Terrible burning pains in several organs are reported regularly by ex-Prozac patients - the pancreas, gall bladder, kidneys, stomach, spleen, etc. Several of them have lost at least one of these organs. Unfortunately the surgical wounds do not always heal properly because of the poor wound healing that is produced by the excess adrenalin flow and the patient has to endure repeated surgeries. The pain is almost always reported as "burning". Occasionally it will be a stabbing pain in the same organs. Often urine is reported as "burning". One patient reported such a severe burning from her urine that cold compresses after urination became necessary. Doctors rarely find the cause of the burning in their various modes of testing.

Why do doctors seem to have such a need to defend drugs? Does it somehow validate the worth of their profession because if we didn't need drugs, perhaps we would no longer need them to supply those drugs? Many doctors are telling their patients, who have developed complaints such as seizures, hypoglycemia, diabetes, cancer, pancreatitis, rashes, bronchitis, kidney problems, blood platelet disorders, liver abnormalities, etc., that their use of Prozac had no connection - *even though there are medical evidences linking all these as possible side-effects of the drug.* [Warnings about these possible adverse reactions are listed in the Prozac package insert and multitudes of adverse reaction reports made to the FDA.]

Why would a doctor not immediately discontinue use of a medication when these serious drug reactions occur in their patients? It is a puzzle why doctors feel such a need to defend drugs. Their responsibility is to have their patient's interest at heart, not a drug companies' interests. Our past mistakes with drugs should have taught them more. Are doctors either so busy that they can no longer take the time to read the information on the new drugs they are giving their patients or are there so many drugs on the market now that no one could possibly ever be able to keep up with the volume? Or are too many of them using mind-altering drugs themselves and having trouble thinking clearly?

Contrary to the belief of many patients and doctors, *a physician is human with human weaknesses and with just as much potential as any one else to make mistakes.* Unfortunately any mistake he makes may cost a life, cause permanent disability or brain damage, etc. Why do we place that much responsibility on a fellow human? Patients and doctors alike should learn more about the body and how it functions, what substances we are ingesting and how those substances affect our bodies and our minds. We *must* take the responsibility to think for ourselves and stop expecting others to do it for us. How bad do things have to get before we wake up and take back the responsibly which is rightfully ours? No one has more insight into what is happening within our own bodies than we do. Health is the most important of our responsibilities, because if we do not have it we cannot function as we should to perform any of our other responsibilities in life.

Another serious potential problem involving the physical side effects of Prozac is that the drug is very often prescribed as a painkiller because of its anesthetic type effect. It is given for headaches, chronic pain, post surgical pain, etc. Some patients even report that they have cut themselves just to see if they are still capable of feeling pain. (Rarely do patients mention feeling pain when they report mutilating their bodies.) Therefore, as the patient is using a painkiller on a regular basis, he remains unaware of ongoing or developing physical conditions because his internal alarm system - pain, is blocked.

Many patients, as they are finally beginning to come off the drug after prolonged periods of Prozac use, are finding they have developed several physical ailments, some very serious, during their use of Prozac. They have many unexplained aches and pains that were not there before or that have become far more intense since the use of Prozac. All of these they have remained unaware of during the use of the drug because they could not *feel* the developing disease process through the increasing intensity of the pain.

With more and more long-term use of Prozac, patients are continuing to report additional problem areas in physical side effects that need to be evaluated. The *PHYSICIAN'S DESK REFERENCE FAMILY GUIDE TO PRESCRIPTION DRUGS* lists the following side effects: heart attack, impotence, hair loss, cataracts, kidney disorders, hepatitis, arthritis, breast cysts, breast pain, convulsions, coma, migraine headache, bronchitis, pneumonia, deafness, duodenal ulcer, stomach ulcer, gallstones, pelvic pain, inability to control bowel movements, painful sexual intercourse for women, urinary tract disorders, eye bleeding, spitting blood and vomiting blood.

As Prozac is the common denominator in all these reports and many of the complaints are identical, there is strong indication that many of these were brought on by use of the drug. The large majority of these complaints correspond to the side effects produced by steroids or amphetamines. Blood pressure and cholesterol levels are rising drastically. Severe memory loss, hair loss, sleep disorders, headaches, joint pain, muscle contractions, sweating, nausea, severe abdominal pain (often a burning pain), kidney pain and kidney failure, burning urination, hypoglycemia, diabetes, abnormal liver function, development of various allergies, rashes, development of Chronic Fatigue Syndrome symptoms, chronic digestive problems including poor metabolism, indigestion, gas and diarrhea, ulcers, blurred vision, electric surges shooting throughout the head and body (similar to what is known as "post drug syndrome"), slurred speech, adrenalin rushes at the slightest provocation, seizures, sexual dysfunction, bloating and weight gain, endless ringing in the ears, burning or tingling in feet or legs, swelling in joints, heart flutter, and heart attacks are all being reported as physical reactions to Prozac.

One of the most obvious of glandular dysfunctions is the rebounding of the metabolic processes which have been revved up by Prozac. Far too many experience bloating and flatulence as this system shuts down its processes and the patient discovers his inability to digest. Male and female patients alike give the appearance of being pregnant as their bellies and abdomens become extended by the gas - a clear symptom of Cushing's syndrome. Then they begin to accumulate excess weight from the inability to digest and process the food. Many patients report these digestive problems after their Prozac use. Weight lifters as well as those seeking weight loss have been told that Prozac will speed up the metabolism. This revving up of the metabolic processes is produced by stimulant drugs. After being forced to perform beyond its capacity for an extended period of time the metabolism appears to just shut down or "crash" along with the other body systems.

An area causing great concern now is that of blood platelet disorders. Patients are reporting that after using Prozac their white blood counts as well as red blood counts are continuing to test low. Some of these disorders are "terminal." Suzanne Johnson of Atlanta, Georgia testified to the FDA in September of 1991, warning that something must be done about Prozac or the blood of many more victims would be on their hands because her blood already was on their hands. Suzanne died a year later in November, 1992 of a blood disease listed as a side-effect of Prozac where the patient can no longer produce their own blood. She was transfusion dependent for over a year and a half before she died. She, as many others, did not live long enough to fight her legal battle with Lilly. Richard Kapit, an FDA reviewer of Prozac, recommended product labeling for the drug to include warnings to physicians about "that certain signs and symptoms of depression may be exacerbated by this drug." And also should include warnings that "Patients exposed to this drug show higher rates of reduced hemoglobin..." and "a fluoxetine-induced elevation of LDH..." He felt further testing was necessary to determine the severity of these risks. Another antidepressant, Tegretol, causes an irreversible drop in the production of white blood cells.

Cancer is another concern. A study was released out of Canada showing that the antidepressants Elavil and Prozac are tumor promoters, "...amitriptyline and fluoxetine inhibit normal lymphocyte proliferation in vitro and promote tumor growth in three out of three...fluoxetine (20-40 mg/day) has been associated with 21 reported cases of reactivation of herpes...suggesting that even at the lowest range of prescribed doses, it can impair normal human immune function in vivo..." It also demonstrated that Prozac was "more potent than amitriptyline" in promoting tumors. When we understand the effects of these two drugs upon serotonin with Prozac being the more potent of the two and the subsequent increase produced by serotonin of body steroids, we can see why Prozac would have a more potent adverse effect upon the immune system. This study was published in the July 1st issue of *CANCER RESEARCH*. The study shows that the drugs accelerate the growth of tumors. Lorne Brandes, the oncologist from the Manitoba Institute of Cell Biology in Winnipeg, who led the team in this study feels that the tumor growth is being promoted by these drugs binding to the intracellular histamine receptor. If this is the case, it is beginning to raise questions about the antihistamines and cancer as well. This new information will have a great impact upon a physician's decision to put a cancer patient on antidepressants and could change the standard procedure of placing post-operative patients on antidepressants at a time when the immune system is more vulnerable. There have been additional reports of accelerated growths, such as endometriosis. One patient who underwent surgery to completely clean out her endometriosis surprised her doctor a year later when he opened her up to find her completely full of endometriosis again. She had been on Prozac for two years.

Alcohol has been associated with cancer because of its action upon the hormones. Perhaps as we come to understand even more about the action of antidepressants and other psychoactive drugs upon hormones it will help us to understand their association with cancer as well. Certainly all of the antidepressants are suspect because of the fact that they all raise serotonin and thereby increase hormonal output.

The obvious conclusion to draw from these reactions is that Prozac is causing a strong adverse reaction on the immune system, as so many of our new wonder drugs are appearing to do. When the cortisol levels are doubled with just one dose, this type of adverse reaction with the immune system should be expected. Using many of these drugs which cause stress responses from their toxic effects over several generations would naturally cause us to build up a tolerance level which would require larger doses to accomplish what lower doses have done in the past. All of these new drugs have such a highly increased potency in order to achieve the results we used to achieve with milder doses. It is having a strong adverse impact upon our immune systems. Beyond the risk it would pose for a healthy individual, Prozac's effect upon the immune system should be a clear message, a warning, to those taking Prozac for Chronic Fatigue Syndrome or AIDS or any other of our newer diseases, which involve disorders of the immune system. It should accelerate these diseases. At what rate it does that remains to be seen. (It is popular among some physicians to prescribe Prozac for these diseases because of its energizing [stimulant] effect.)

The diagnosis of chemically induced Lupus has become so common that a special support group for those individuals is now being formed, PAIN, headquartered in Hawaii. One woman who attended a lecture I gave this last summer kept saying, "After doctors being baffled for quite some time now, I have just been diagnosed as having Lupus. I have never been on Prozac, but all of the reactions you speak of are almost identical to my symptoms." She stated that the only difference in her life before the symptoms appeared was the use of a natural product, blue-green algae. When I asked where the algae was grown, if it might have been grown in heavily fluoridated water, she did not know, but said she would find out. My curiosity as to whether the fluorine molecule in Prozac might be breaking loose from the Prozac compound to produce many of these adverse reactions had been aroused nearly two years before this. Her voice was full of excitement when she called me early the next morning to inform me that she had looked through her information she had been gathering on this particular brand of algae and had found that it was indeed extremely high in fluoride concentrations. She immediately informed her physician of the discovery of this toxic chemical connection to her symptoms. Anyone wanting to follow up on the psychiatric effects of fluoride may want to refer to "What Looks Like a Neurosis May be a Fluorosis," (Forman, 1963).

Long term, latent or tardive effects are beginning to appear with Prozac. The type of "burn out" seen with stimulant type drugs is being reported regularly in conjunction with Prozac. At this point I have four people within four blocks of my home who have lost their jobs because of physical and mental disability after using Prozac at least two years. One has an inability to read or write and has moved her children back to live with her parents until she can recuperate. One is still in a drug-induced stupor, unable to cope with anything. Her children lost their mother four years ago when a doctor prescribed Prozac after a divorce. She was a vibrant, happy, good mother before this. Another cannot focus thinking clearly enough to write the reports necessary in his type of employment. The other, in an emergency medical position, was given Prozac to cope with the death of her sister from cancer. She became so physically ill from the adverse effects of Prozac that she nearly lost her own life. She became unable to handle her job any longer, but after two years of being on the drug and now two years off of Prozac and using many alternative treatments to restore her health, she is able to work again.

Tardive dyskinesia should be a concern with any of the psychoactive drugs. Although it took years for the profession to acknowledge this drug-induced disorder, the American Psychiatric Association figures predict half or more of elderly patients or long-term users of psychoactive drugs will develop tardive dyskinesia. This is an impairment of voluntary movement resulting in fragmentary or incomplete movements, involuntary and uncontrollable muscle twitches or contractions. The body muscles contract throwing the whole body into spasms. Legs and arms fly about and heads bob around and up and down as if they were puppets with someone violently jerking the attached strings. The facial muscles contract causing grotesque facial grimaces and contortions, involuntary protrusions of the tongue, etc. - all those gestures we have come to associate with mental illness, which we now know to be a side effect of the mind-altering drugs these patients have been treated with over the years. Dr. Breggin uses as a standard rule of thumb, there is a 5% increase in the possibility of the development of tardive dyskinesia with each year of psychoactive drug use. For the elderly and chronically ill the percentage is closer to 25% per year chance of developing this disabling adverse reaction. If this is an outward manifestation of what is happening within the brain itself...what types of involuntary actions and disruptions are also happening within the brain itself? Tardive dystonia is very closely associated with tardive dyskinesia. It is described as a condition wherein muscles tense up or contract involuntarily.

Involuntary muscle contractions of Prozac patients is often reported and could develop into either of these serious and apparently permanent disorders. Two lawsuits that have already been filed against Lilly for damages associated with Prozac involve this side effect. In association with Prozac these conditions are appearing to develop far more rapidly than with previous drugs. An Iowa woman took the drug for only eight days before she began to experience severe muscle spasms in her arms. Two and a half years later she still has TD. A Texas woman has sued because of suffering permanent neurological damage after taking two capsules of Prozac a day for a total of only two days.

Even Dr. Kramer acknowledges this very real possibility with Prozac, "Psychotherapeutic drugs can sometimes cause tardive neurological disorders, which may appear years after a drug is discontinued; and questions have already been raised whether Prozac can cause such syndromes...Concern over unforseen or tardive effects is realistic, because Prozac has been around too briefly for anyone to know its long-term effects." (*LISTENING TO PROZAC*, p. 312)

Parkinson's disease is another motor disability that can follow the use of psychoactive drugs. Unfortunately depression is generally associated with this disorder as well. Dr. Ernst Jansen Steur of Holland conducted a study published in January 1993 on the increase of motor disability in Parkinson's patients in conjunction with Prozac. The most frequently increased symptoms were: tremor at rest, fingertaps, hand movements, and body bradykinesia which is an abnormal slowness or sluggishness of physical responses. Because the increase in symptoms was transient and was reversible after the withdrawal from Prozac, it was concluded that it was Prozac induced rather than a natural progression of the disease process. In none of his patients was depression substantially alleviated by Prozac while "Parkinson disability definitely increased." Dr. Steur concludes that "The increase of Parkinson disability after fluoxetine exposure can easily be explained on the basis of a dopamine-antagonistic activity of fluoxetine." (Steur, 1993)

Tardive akathisia is another serious latent disorder, believed to be associated with tardive dyskinesia, which should be considered the most dangerous and tragic of any of the long-term effects. Panic attacks, anxiety attacks and adrenalin rushes are very common post drug effects reported in conjunction with the use of Prozac and the other SSRIs. It is my opinion that all of these latent or after effects are closely intertwined and produced through similar means. In order to understand the cause of these reactions we will need to cover at length many body processes so we will discuss akathisia and tardive akathisia in detail in the chapter REVERBERATIONS THROUGHOUT THE MEDICAL COMMUNITY.

CHAPTER 4

SEROTONIN DOUBLETALK
THE INCREDIBLE SEROTONIN BLUNDER

The chemical imbalance theory is centered in the story that certain behaviors and moods, including depression, are present because serotonin levels are low. To me the questions seemed more than obvious. Why was no one asking them? I am still not sure why the questions were not asked unless it was because the theory itself seemed too complicated for many to see the obvious questions. The most obvious and most critical questions are: If we are chemically forcing the level of serotonin to rise in the brain, when do we know to stop? What are the signs and symptoms of too much serotonin? If the brain requires such a fine balance, too much should pose as many problems as too little, right? And then if we are using a chemical to block serotonin in the brain and not allow it to leave, will the chemical blocking agent (Prozac, Zoloft, Paxil, Lovan, Luvox, etc.) itself interfere with the utilization of the neurotransmitter held in the brain in this way?

"Serotonin turnover" is an extremely critical matter to be understood in this theory of using various chemicals to raise serotonin levels as any disruption in the metabolism or turnover of serotonin within the brain can have very drastic repercussions. This term, "serotonin turnover," refers to the resynthesis or the remanufacturing and release of a neurotransmitter by the presynaptic neurons. Even though the brain may have a normal amount of serotonin, if the neurons fail to release the serotonin or manufacture replacement serotonin, the serotonin in the brain becomes essentially inactive, resulting in low serotonin turnover. Serotonin turnover is determined by the levels of a serotonin metabolite or by product known as 5HIAA (5-hydroxyindoleacetic acid). If 5HIAA levels are low, serotonin turnover is also low. The SSRIs were designed to inhibit the reuptake of 5HT serotonin because it was assumed that if you raise 5HT serotonin, an increase in serotonin turnover, metabolism, or 5HIAA serotonin would be the end result.

The concern over abnormally low serotonin stems from studies whcih have found that people with lower than normal serotonin turnover (or 5HIAA serotonin) tend to have histories of violent behavior (Brown, Goodwin, Ballenger, Goyer, & Major, 1979; Yarura-Tobias & Neziroglu, 1981). Valzelli found that rats with low serotonin turnover (5HIAA) would attack and kill while those with an increase in serotonin turnover became friendly and almost motherly toward others (Valzelli & Garattini, 1972). Those with the lowest serotonin turnover fought the most (Valzelli & Bernasconi, 1979).

Research indicates that serotonin turnover is depressed in those:

(1) who have committed suicide, especially those who have committed suicide by violent means (G. Brown et al. 1982; Edman et al. 1986; Mann et al. 1990);

(2) who have committed arson and other violent crimes (Virkkunen et al. 1987), in fact, one study predicted violent crime with an 84% accuracy by measuring serotonin turnover (Virkkunen, DeJong, Bartko, Goodwin, & Linnoila, 1989);

(3) who are most likely to commit suicide or violent acts (Traskman, Asberg, Bertilsson, & Sjostrand, 1981);

(4) who experience depression, insomnia or those who abuse alcohol (Depue & Spoont, 1986; Charney, Woods, Krystal, & Heninger, 1990);

(5) who act impulsively without any concern for punishment, as noted in sociopathic behavior (Depue & Spoont, 1986; Charney, Woods, Krystal, & Heninger, 1990);

(6) who make additional suicide attempts even after surviving a previous attempt (Roy, DeJong, & Linnoila, 1989).

(7) who engage in exhibitionism, drive recklessly or engage in pathological gambling

(8) who suffer bulimia or dependence upon various substances (Sources: *SEROTONIN RELATED PSYCHIATRIC SYNDROMES,* p. 39, *BIOLOGICAL PSYCHOLOGY,* p. 479-481)

It has been demonstrated throughout medical literature that the inhibition of 5HT serotonin results in a marked DECREASE of the critical 5HIAA serotonin or serotonin turnover (Buus et al., 1975; Nabeshima et al., 1983). Everyone of the above indications of depressed serotonin activity is exactly what many Prozac patients are reporting to the FDA and the various other groups collecting data on adverse reactions from Prozac patients. The reports are consistent in their content and rising in their numbers. Some of the symptoms of depressed serotonin turnover are even listed side effects in the Prozac package insert. All of these reactions should be considered further evidence that Prozac's action within the brain is causing a depression in 5HIAA (serotonin turnover) both rapidly in a particular group of patients, or for the larger majority, over a period of time as the drug accumulates and the brain becomes unable to fight the effects.

Because Prozac and the other SSRIs are being used in the treatment of obsessive-compulsive disorders, it should be noted at this point that a drug which quickly and directly stimulates the serotonin receptors will make obsessive-compulsive disorders (OCD) worse, not better (Zohar, Insel, Zohar-Kadouch, Hill, & Murphy, 1988). In light of this study what efficacy serotonergic drugs would have in the treatment of obsessive-compulsive behavior becomes more than highly questionable. It also makes the FDA's most recent approval of Prozac for use in OCD seem absolutely beyond comprehension. The reports coming in from ex-Prozac patients of the many developments of various overwhelming compulsions would support the findings of the above study. They also support the idea of paradoxical effect. Or as Dr. Breggin has said, the "drugs are too likely to achieve the opposite of what we intend" as the brain works to compensate for the imbalance which has been created by the drug itself.

The medical evidence does exist to prove that this raising of 5HT serotonin and lowering of the critical 5HIAA serotonin is also the action of the SSRIs upon serotonin. These drugs, the SSRIs, raise 5HT serotonin. They are 5HT reuptake inhibitors. Yet the SSRIs consistently *lower* the 5HIAA serotonin metabolite clearly indicating a lowering of serotonin turnover. Although it is generally believed among medical professionals that when 5HT serotonin goes up or down that the 5HIAA serotonin turnover follows along in the same direction, hence when one rises, the other rises or when one falls, the other falls, according to medical studies, this does not hold true for the psychedelic drugs, nor for the SSRI antidepressants. *The psychedelic drugs and the SSRIs all raise 5HT serotonin, yet lower 5HIAA serotonin or serotonin turnover.* Let me repeat this very critical point. Inhibition of 5HT serotonin results in the decrease of 5HIAA or serotonin turnover (Buus et al., 1975; Nabeshima et al., 1983). The tricyclic antidepressants and others are also known to actually lower the concentration of the critical 5HIAA serotonin levels. Imipramine and Chloroimipramine which were the strongest 5HT reuptake inhibitors as of 1975 both demonstrate a decrease in 5HIAA levels. Even though a drug may increase the 5HT serotonin, it is obvious that the chemicals are interfering with the metabolism which would produce the essential 5HIAA serotonin. In other words, they are apparently interfering with serotonin turnover and should produce the effects of low serotonin turnover we have just listed. *"Interestingly, all tricyclic antidepressants, even the putatively norepinephrine-selective desipramine, reduce concentrations of 5HIAA in the CSF [cerebrospinal fluid] following chronic administration...An early study reports a similar effect even after fenfluramine administration (Shoulson and Chase 1975). As expected, the second-generation*

5HT uptake inhibitors also consistently reduce 5HIAA levels." (SEROTONIN IN MAJOR PSYCHIATRIC DISORDERS, p. 240).

Some of the second-generation 5HT serotonin reuptake inhibitors which have been shown to reduce 5HIAA serotonin levels are: Fluoxetine (Prozac), Zimelidine, Clomipramine (Anafranil), Fenfluramine, Sertraline (Zoloft), Citalopram, Trazadone (Deseryl), Femoxetine, Paroxetine (Paxil), Indalpine, Fluvoxamine (Luvox), etc. Some of the tricyclic antidepressants are: Amitriptyline, Clomipramine, Imipramine, Desipramine, Nortriptyline, etc. The percentage at which a few of them reduce 5HIAA is: Imipramine 21-22%, Desipramine 32%, Amitriptyline 21-37%, Nortriptyline 10-25%, Clomipramine 44-47%, Zimelidine 20-39%, Citlopram 29%, and Fluvoxamine 24%. (Asberg et al. 1973; Bertilsson et al. 1974, 1980; Bjerkenstedt et al. 1985a; Bowden et al. 1985; Martin et al. 1987; Potter et al. 1985; Traskman et al. 1979.)

Additional evidence of the lowering of serotonin levels was brought out very clearly in the Yale study submitted in March 1991 to the Journal of the American Academy of Child and Adolescent Psychiatry which will discus in detail in CHAPTER 6. We find that drastic drops in serotonin levels were reported, in Case #1 the patient's serotonin tested at 11.1 ng/ml, down from 170 ng/ml, after one month's use of Prozac. In Case #2 the patient's serotonin level dropped from 140 ng/ml to 9.3 ng/ml within eight weeks of starting on Prozac.

All of these drugs by reducing 5HIAA serotonin levels should, therefore, produce any or all of the listed behaviors associated with low 5HIAA serotonin levels, ie: suicide, arson, violence, alcoholism, depression, insomnia, impulsive behavior, etc. These are many of the symptoms which patients are encouraged to take these drugs to alleviate. They actually lower the type of serotonin level patients are lead to believe they are raising, while they raise the level of 5Ht serotonin which we are about to discover is found in *serious* mental disorders. This has been the most incredible deception. Whatever the reason for patients, many physicians, the FDA, Congress, any of us, to have been kept in dark about the critical similarity of these antidepressant drugs to the psychedelic drugs and their potential to induce these behaviors is absolutely inexcusable. This issue is far too significant to ignore. This is solid scientific evidence that these drugs are actually *causing* what they are touted to cure. The general public have been encouraged by their physicians for several years now to use the SSRIs, which work on serotonin in the same way as the hallucinogenic drugs. And then to understand that the older so called *anti*depressants actually lower 5HIAA, thus setting the foundation for a multitude of psychiatric disorders, is almost beyond belief. Yet this scenario only follows the example of what has happened with each new psychiatric biochemical "breakthrough" we have seen for decades. Perhaps even worse than being kept in the dark about these drugs by the pharmaceutical companies is the subtly of the action of these drugs. Patients are caught of guard. For most patients, the effects seem milder at first and then build slowly over time as the drugs accumulate in the brain and the body. Although subtle, the impact this accumulation has upon the glandular system and behavior is devastating physically as well as mentally. The end result with all of these chemicals appears to be the same overall - serious organic brain disease and various chronic illnesses. How does this happen? Much to our surprise we find it happens first of all in *elevating* 5HT serotonin - exactly what the SSRIs are designed to do.

Higher 5HT serotonin levels can cause schizophrenia, organic brain disease, etc. and be hazardous to your physical health as well. Elevated serotonin (5HT) concentrations are as great a cause for concern as low 5HIAA serotonin turnover. *"A recurring finding has been elevated platelet concentrations in schizophrenic patients (for review, see Meltzer 1987). However, elevated platelet 5HT (serotonin) concentrations are not specific for schizophrenia; they are also found in mood disorders, organic brain disease (especially mental retardation), and childhood autism* (Partington et al. 1973)..." (*SEROTONIN IN MAJOR PSYCHIATRIC DISORDERS*, p. 214) Elevated serotonin levels are also found in old age and Alzheimer's disease. With the serotonergic agents, those which block the reuptake of serotonin, those which are agonists, those which enhance serotonin in any way, a condition is being chemically induced within the brain in which we *consistently* find such serious mental disorders as: "schizophrenia" (psychosis or insanity), "mood disorders" (exactly what the antidepressants are being prescribed to alleviate), "organic brain disease" (causing structural damage to the brain), "mental retardation" and "autism." It should be pointed out again that *LSD not only enhances the serotonin levels, but was originally marketed by Sandoz to chemically induce schizophrenia in "normal subjects. "* In fact the very first antidepressant, Iproniazid, "did indeed elevate levels of norepinephrine and serotonin (just as the new Effexor claims to do)...and might *reverse the antischizophrenic effects*" of other drugs (*DRUGS AND THE BRAIN,* p. 97). The process of reversing the antischizophrenic effect, should leave the patient open to the schizophrenic process - full blown psychosis. Instead of realizing that this excited state this first antidepressant produced was possibly the beginnings of schizophrenia, it was decided that this energizing action, more appropriately called a stimulant effect, produced by the drug might be useful in treating depression. The percentage of serotonin increase for a few of the serotonin enhancing drugs are: citalopram 450%, paroxetine (Paxil) 420%, fluoxetine (Prozac) 300%, fluvoxamine (Luvox) 270%, Clomipramine (Anafranil) 200%, imipramine 150%, and sertraline (Zoloft) was too variable to determine *(SEROTONIN-RELATED PSYCHIATRIC SYNDROMES*, p. 18). Results from another study demonstrated that sertraline (Zoloft) was five times more potent in serotonin reuptake as Prozac and Paxil to be more potent than either Prozac or Zoloft (Davane, 1992).

"In 1961 Schain and Freedman reported the presence of elevated levels of 5HT [serotonin] in the whole blood of 6 of 23 autistic children. Since then, a number of studies (Anderson et al. 1987; Hanley et al. 1977; Ritvo et al. 1970; Takahashi et al. 1976) have confirmed that mean concentrations of 5HT in blood are significantly higher in groups of age- and gender-matched normal control subjects...The finding of elevated whole-blood 5HT content is not specific to autistic disorder. Hyperserotonemia is present in medical disorders, most notably carcinoid syndrome (Crawford et al. 1967), and has been reported in other neuropsychiatric disorders, including schizophrenia (DeLisi et al. 1981). Approximately one-half of severely retarded children...without prominent autistic symptoms have elevated blood 5HT levels (Hanley et al. 1977; Tu and Partington 1972)." *(SEROTONIN IN MAJOR PSYCHIATRIC DISORDERS*, p. 50-51)

When a drug increases 5HT serotonin and decreases 5HIAA serotonin what is the end result? We have just covered an incredible amount of research in a few short pages so let's review what this research demonstrates. When 5HT serontonin levels are high what is consistantly found is:

> #1 schizophrenia (psychosis, mania, etc.)
> #2 mood disorders (depression, anxiety, etc.)
> #3 organic brain disease - especially mental retardation at a greater incident rate in children
> #4 autism (believed to be a form of childhood schizophrenia autism is a self-centered or self-focused mental state with no basis in reality)
> #5 Alzheimer's disease
> #6 old age

When 5HIAA serotonin levels are low we consistantly find:

> #1 suicide (especially violent suicide)
> #2 arson
> #3 violent crime
> #4 insomnia
> #5 depression

#6 alcohol abuse

#7 impulsive acts with no concern for punishment

#8 reckless driving

#9 exhibitionism

#10 dependence upon various substances

#11 bulemia

#12 multiple suicide attempts

#13 more contact with police

#14 more hostility

#15 arguments with spouses, friends and relatives

#16 obesessive compulsive behavior

#17 impaired employment due to arguments, etc.

Controlled double blind medical studies have demonstrated repeatedly that when a drug raises 5HT serotonin it lowers the essential 5HIAA serotonin. We even know at what percentages many of these drugs produce this action. Therefore, when the Specific Serotonin Reuptake Inhibitors, Prozac, Zoloft, Paxil, Lovan and Luvox, raise 5HT serotonin and lower 5HIAA serotonin we should expect the preceeding to be the result. We should expect the other antidepressants to do the same, perhaps over a longer period of use, since they are not as serotonin specific. The psychedelic drugs have this same action upon serotonin and this considered to be the means by which they produce the psychedelic experience.

The psychedelic drugs directly target serotonin and they chemically induce psychosis in normal human beings. These drugs are referred to as the instant insanity drugs. Hofmann, who developed LSD for Sandoz, described his first LSD experience, "a remarkable restlessness combined with a slight dizziness...characterized by an extremely stimulated imagination." He described his second dose of LSD (a high dose) as "demonic transformations of the outer world" which made him believe he was going insane or dying. LSD brings one to the brink of panic even while bringing on feelings of more intense beauty or deeper meaning. The panic can be devastating. "Terror and confusion have caused many people in these circumstances to jump from windows to their deaths. Others have suffered psychotic breakdowns from which they failed to emerge when the drug's effects wore off. Hundreds of cases of schizophrenic illness have been precipitated by a *single* psychedelic drug experience. The possibility that they may initiate a long-term mental illness is perhaps the most serious danger presented by psychedelic drugs." *(DRUGS AND THE BRAIN,* p. 182)

How does LSD produce insanity? Scientists have long suspected that LSD might act as a trigger mechanism to release or inhibit a *naturally occurring substance* in the brain as the means by which it produces its effects. We now know that serotonin is the target chemical in the brain for LSD. Dr. Solomon Snyder is considered one of the foremost authorities on bio-psychiatry and is a man whose name is often mentioned for the Nobel Prize. In fact, many major developments in American biological psychiatry are connected in some way to his work. Dr. Snyder's belief is that *the action of all hallucinogenic drugs upon thought processes, mood, consciousness, behavior, etc. is a direct result of their action upon serotonin. He points out that psychedelic drugs mimic the effects of serotonin and that changes in the activity of serotonin are directly related to the action of the psychedelic drugs. In other words, SEROTONIN IS THE KEY TO THE PSYCHEDELIC EXPERIENCE. (DRUGS AND THE BRAIN,* p. 19, 205)

Freedman in 1961 reported that LSD initially causes an *increase* in the level of serotonin (5HT). This serotonergic effect of LSD was found to include not only the rise of serotonin (5HT) levels, but was accompanied by a *fall* in the concentration of the primary metabolite of serotonin (5HIAA) as well, clearly indicating a decrease in serotonin turnover. In 1954 Wooley and Shaw reported the neurophysiological aspects of serotonin and its importance in normal mental function. *These researchers suggested that LSD's effect upon serotonin is the method by which LSD produces the mental changes it does produce within the brain.* Mescaline, Ditran and PCP (Angel Dust) all have this same action upon serotonin levels. They all increase serotonin (5HT) and decrease the primary serotonin metabolite (5HIAA) (Tongue and Keonard 1969).

Dr. D. W. Wooley was first to suggest that an abnormality of brain serotonin levels may be involved in the development of schizophrenia (Wooley & Shaw 1954, Wooley and Campbell 1962). The theory was based upon the similarity in structure between the neurotransmitter serotonin and the hallucinogenic ergot alkaloids - LSD, DMT, psilocybin, etc. (LSD mimics serotonin and there is a strikingly close chemical resemblance between LSD and serotonin.) The hypotheses took two directions in investigation. The first theory was that schizophrenics somehow produce larger amounts of these types of compounds through abnormal metabolism. The second theory was that the action these compounds have upon serotonin, by producing either an over-production or under-production of serotonin, may be what causes the production of schizophrenic symptoms. What did they learn about these schizophrenic affects of LSD upon serotonin? "The actions of LSD on brain 5HT (serotonin) have been most widely studied. In classic work by several investigators, it was shown that LSD suppressed the firing rate of serotonergic neurons in the raphe nucleus, causing *increases in brain 5HT concentrations and decreases in 5-*

113

hydroxyindoleacetic acid (5HIAA) concentrations (Aghajanian et al. 1968, 1970; Freedman 1961; Freedman and Giarman 1962)." (*SEROTONIN IN MAJOR PSYCHIATRIC DISORDERS*, p. 211-212)

Many drugs of abuse mimic serotonin in chemical structure. It has been shown that LSD causing an increase in serotonin, acts much the same as a SSRI. One young man who had used LSD in his past said that taking Prozac was for him like taking "half a hit" of LSD, except that it made him angry and aggressive. This "half a hit" of LSD has been described by other LSD users as more of a "body rush" rather than an immediate strong psychedelic effect.

In 1958 Hofman, the man who discovered LSD, announced that he had synthesized psilocybin and psilocin. These drugs are indole compounds with a striking similarity to serotonin. Cocaine blocks serotonin reuptake leading to an initial increase in serotonin levels. Alcohol increases levels of serotonin. The levels then subsequently drop just as they do with LSD. Steroids (cortisone, prednisone, etc.) directly affect serotonin and are known to create psychotic behavior. It appears that all drugs which cause this initial rise in serotonin levels, no matter by which means they do so, produce an accompanying fall in serotonin. Why, when we know all this about serotonin and the effects produced by the drugs of abuse upon serotonin would our latest new fad in psychoactive drugs be those which are designed to raise serotonin levels?

Hyperserotonemia (elevated serotonin levels) can produce very serious complications medically, as well as serious neurologic and psychiatric disorders. Carcinoid syndrome and the serotonin syndrome are two medical conditions in which elevated serotonin levels are present. Carcinoid syndrome is a set of symptoms caused by the secretion of serotonin by carcinoid tumors, prostaglandins, etc. Symptoms include attacks of severe cyanotic flushing of the skin lasting from minutes to days, diarrhea, bronchoconstrictive attacks, sudden drops in blood pressure, edema, and ascites, which is an abnormal accumulation of serous fluid in the abdominal cavity, also known as abdominal or peritoneal dropsy.

The serotonin syndrome is a hypersotonergic state which is a very dangerous and potentially fatal side effect of serotonergic enhancing drugs which can have multiple psychiatric and non-psychiatric symptoms. It is a condition which has been on the rise since the 1960's when we began using more and more drugs which directly affect serotonin. This is a toxic condition which requires heightened clinical awareness in order to prevent, recognize, and treat the condition promptly. Promptness is vital because, as we just mentioned, the serotonin syndrome can be fatal and death from this side effect can come very rapidly. This syndrome is a toxic hyperserotonergic state whose rate of incidence is unknown, but is on the rise. The suspected cause of that increase is the introduction of the new specific serotonergic enhancing agents in clinical practice - the SSRIs. This disorder brought on by excessive levels of serotonin is difficult to distinguish from the neuroleptic malignant syndrome because the symptoms are so similar. The neuroleptic malignant syndrome is a serious condition brought on by the use of the neuroleptic drugs: Thorazine (chlorpromazine), Mellaril (thioridazine), Haldol (haloperidol), Stelazine (trifluoperazine), Verprin (trifluopromazine), Prolixin or Permitil (fluphenazine), Orap (pimozide), Navane (thiothixene), Compazine (prochlorperazine), Repoise (butaperazine), Serentil (mesoridazine), Dartal (thiopropazate), Trilafon (perphenazine), Quide (piperacetazine), Tindal (acetophenazine), Taractan (chlorprothixene), Loxitane or Daxolin (loxapine), Moban or Lidone (molindone), and Clozaril (clozapine). Dr. Breggin points out that there are several antihistamines, antinausea drugs, antihypertensive drugs and some used in conjunction with anesthesia which are also neuroleptics and need to be used cautiously (refer to *TOXIC PSYCHIATRY*, p. 51). The symptoms of the serotonin syndrome are: euphoria, drowsiness, sustained rapid eye movement, overreaction of the reflexes, rapid muscle contraction and relaxation in the ankle causing abnormal movements of the foot, clumsiness, restlessness, feeling drunk and dizzy, muscle contraction and relaxation in the jaw, sweating, intoxication, muscle twitching, rigidity, high body temperature, mental status changes were frequent (including confusion and hypomania), shivering, diarrhea, loss of consciousness and death. (*The Serotonin Syndrome, AM J PSYCHIATRY,* June 1991)

The serotonin syndrome is generally caused by a combination of two or more drugs, one of which is often a specific sertonergic medication. The drugs which we know most frequently contribute to this condition are the combining of MAOIs with Prozac (this should also include the other SSRIs) or clomipramine (Anafranil), etc. The combination of lithium with these specific serotonergic agents has been implicated in enhancing the serotonin syndrome. The tricyclic antidepressants, lithium, MAOIs, SSRIs, ECT (electric shock treatment), tryptophan, and the serotonin agonists all enhance serotonin neurotransmission and can contribute to this syndrome. Anything which will raise the level of serotonin can bring on this hyperserotonergic condition. The optimal treatment for the serotonin syndrome is discontinuation of the offending medication or medications, offer supportive measures, and wait for the symptoms to resolve. If the offending medication is discontinued, the condition will often resolve on its own within a 24 hour period. If the medication is not discontinued the condition can progress rapidly to a more serious state and become fatal. It should be apparent that the greater the enhancement of serotonin levels, the greater the chances of producing the serotonin syndrome. Therefore it is recommended that Zoloft, Prozac, Paxil, etc. not be used concurrently with each other or any other serotonergic drugs and that these serious adverse reactions should be expected with these combinations (Callahan, 1993).

Just how serotonin specific are the SSRIs? Serotonin is the most prevalent neurotransmitter system in the brain, yet the theory behind raising serotonin levels is that this procedure is *only* going to affect specific areas of the brain causing changes in mood to alleviate depression and other mood disorders. The petition made to the FDA by Ralph Nader's consumer protection group, Public Citizen, voiced concern that Prozac may also inhibit the synthesis of the neurotransmitter dopamine in some areas of the brain. It has been demonstrated in research that 5HT serotonin will enhance dopamine levels (Yi et al. 1991; Blandina et al. 1989). If serotonin is being raised or lowered dopamine will be affected by the increased or decreased serotonin levels. This effect upon dopamine in turn affects adrenalin (epinephrine) production and so on down the line. Any change in the levels of one of the types of neurotransmitters will have a domino effect. All the other neurotransmitters rush to readjust their levels in order to compensate for the changes in the one. Any theory which suggests that only one neurotransmitter can be affected by a particular chemical becomes an extremely weak theory when this compensation process is considered.

Dopamine is not the only other neurotransmitter system believed to be affected by Prozac and the SSRIs. Several studies (Frances et al. 1987; Manier et al. 1987; Potter et al. 1985) began an accumulation of data which indicates that drugs affecting serotonergic systems will affect noradrenalin (norepinephrine) and visa versa..."there is an increasing body of data showing neuroanatomical and functional links between the noradrenergic and serotonergic systems in the CNS such that drugs affecting one are likely to affect the other." (*SEROTONIN IN MAJOR PSYCHIATRIC DISORDERS,* p 242)

In fact, the brain's attempt to compensate for the imbalance brought on by the drug can create the opposite effect that was initially expected to be produced by the drug, thus creating a paradoxical reaction. In his university text book, *BIOLOGICAL PSYCHOLOGY,* James Kalat ends his section on the SSRIs and the other antidepressants with, "You are excused if you feel confused at this point. *Prolonged use of antidepressant drugs produces effects in opposite directions:* It increases the amount of neurotransmitter released while decreasing receptor sensitivity to the neurotransmitter." (p. 563) As we get this domino type effect many other neurotransmitter systems are affected. Researchers are

116

questioning the phenomenon produced through the effects upon other neurotransmitters by serotonergic agents as evidence of either nonspecificity or compensatory changes stemming from the direct effect upon serotonin. "These findings bring us to a consideration of whether chronic effects on other neurotransmitters should be interpreted as evidence of nonspecificity or of secondary compensatory changes resulting from a primary serotonergic effect." *(SEROTONIN IN MAJOR PSYCHIATRIC DISORDERS,* p.239)

The delicate balance involved in brain chemistry is demonstrated by the fact that an excess of one vital chemical can cause shortages in the other neurotransmitters. This domino effect can be very dangerous when we consider that the repercussions can cause these paradoxical reactions. Since the nervous system has many redundant pathways and is so incredibly complex, we should not assume that one neurotransmitter will produce a given behavior. Yet, one particular type of synapse appears to be more important for certain functions. Therefore an excess or deficit of any particular type of synapse may create in the patient altered or even abnormal behavior. In discussing the newest antidepressant on the market, Effexor, with a pharmacist I asked if the drug shouldn't be considered a tricyclic, rather than an SSRI. He said that it all depended in how you look at it. I agreed and mentioned that I felt that the SSRIs were about as specific as a shotgun blast. After a very boisterous laugh his reply was a very emphatic, "You got it!"

Mixing SSRIs with other antidepressants can be very dangerous for several reasons, the most obvious would be toxicity and an increase in side effects. Mixing drugs can increase the dosage of drugs within the blood because of the impaired function of the liver. For example, Prozac can quickly raise the level of tricyclic antidepressants and MAOIs (Monoamine Oxidase Inhibitors) to toxic levels. It has been demonstrated to increase the levels of Valium and Xanex (Lemberger et al., 1988; Lasher et al., 1991) and many other drugs. Xanex and Prozac in combination has been reported by patients for quite some time now to be a dangerous combination. Now we know that Prozac has been shown to increase blood levels of Xanex by 30% and decrease its elimination of Xanex from the system by an additional 21%. Presently there is more information available on the mixing of the SSRIs with tricyclic antidepressants than there is information on other drugs. Dr. Michael Lowry, director of the Mood Disorder Clinic at Wasatch Canyons Hospital, Salt Lake City, Utah warns, "Prozac can increase tricyclic levels in the blood by three-fold or more. So a usually small dose of amitriptyline (100 mg.) could result in toxicity if added to Prozac."

As it turned out Dr. Lowry greatly underestimated the effect of Prozac upon tricyclics. According to a study done by Lilly (a study few doctors or pharmacists are aware of), we find that a single dose of 50mg of imipramine (Tofranil) and desipramine (Norpramin) in conjunction with Prozac demonstrates a *ten fold* increase in tricyclic blood concentrations (Bergstrom et al. 1992). This study was conducted by giving six subjects one 50mg of imipramine and six other subjects 50mg of desipramine. Blood levels of these drugs were taken at intervals over the next 144 hours. The next test was to give the men one single 60mg dose of Prozac and three hours later one 50mg dose of either tricyclic and test blood levels again. The last stage of the study was to give 60mg of Prozac daily for eight days and then three hours after the last dose of Prozac they once again were given one single 50mg dose of either tricyclic. They point out the fact that only single doses were administered and yet they found a ten fold increase in tricyclic concentrations..."it is possible that our findings underestimate the full impact of this interaction when both floxetine and imipramine or desipramine are given under steady-state multiple-dose conditions." In other words this may be much greater if you take these drugs the way patients generally take them on a daily basis. The symptoms to watch for in a toxic overdose to these drugs are: nausea and vomiting are predominant, agitation, restlessness, hypomania, and other CNS excitation. Nausea is the first sign of liver malfunction and should not be ignored. Yet many doctors will tell their patients to just take the drug at a different time of day to see if they can avoid the nausea that way, instead of heeding that warning given through his patient's reaction. (Another interesting sideline is that Lilly did not bother to include the warning of their own researchers in the Prozac product labeling. They state only that, "There have been greater than 2-fold increases..." in combination with tricyclics. Ten fold is greater than two fold - five times greater.)

These researchers also state that even though the study did not note an increase in side effects the reason for that was because only single doses were administered. They add, "...the possibility exists that if the subjects had received multiple doses of the tricyclic the concentrations of these agents may have reached levels that could have produced an undesirable degree of adverse reactions." Once again they are stating that if these drugs are taken in the way patients are being prescribed to take the drugs on a regular basis, greater possibility of adverse reactions could be expected. In fact as they conclude their report they repeat that although there have been reports of the emergence of increased side effects with the combination of Prozac and tricyclic antidepressants they did not note an increase, "undoubtedly because only single doses" of these drugs were given. Another study refers to this increase in side effects in conjunction with the combination of Prozac and the tricyclics, "...the marked pharmacologic interactions observed between fluoxetine and tricyclics can often lead to toxicity even when tricyclics are used in dosages within the normal range, suggesting that adverse central nervous system (CNS) reactions to this combination are quite possible." (Fava & Rossenbaum, 1991) Patients and physicians, as well, should be alert to the possibility of increased side effects with this combination. In fact, the Fava & Rossenbaum study demonstrated the highest number of suicidal ideation reactions in patients who had never experienced suicidality before in those patients who were taking this combination.

This increase in tricyclic concentrations is believed to happen because of Prozac's interference with the metabolic processes of the P-450 liver enzyme. Both Prozac and the tricyclics are metabolized by the P450 system. They go on to warn that, "These facts and evidence of a drug interaction lead to the postulate that fluoxetine may interfere in the metabolism of other drugs that are metabolized by common P450 isozymes." Translated that means Prozac may interfere or cause increases in other drugs metabolized by the P450 enzyme. Which drugs are metabolized by that system of liver enzymes? A very large majority of drugs are involved. The list is so long that we do not have the space to include them all, but it should be kept in mind that using Prozac in conjunction with any of these drugs could cause an increase in dosage beyond a safe level. Caution should always be used when combining drugs. Even more startling are the findings with Paxil. It demonstrates a *forty fold* increase in levels of the tricyclics and possibly any other drugs metabolized by the P450 enzyme (Davene, 1992).

In April of 1990 the American Journal of Psychiatry reported three cases of serious adverse reactions with the combination of Prozac and several tricyclic antidepressants and benzodiazepines. A 28 year old woman using Xanex and imipramine had Prozac added to it. After 10 weeks she suffered a grand mal seizure. All medications were stopped and she had not suffered a seizure within a year after. A 37 year old woman on doxepin, lithium and Xanex suffered a grand mal seizure two months after Prozac was added to the combination. A 69 year old man who had been taking desipramine for two months began on one Prozac a day and within 10 days developed delirium, marked short-term memory impairment, confusion, agitation, became mildly unable to speak or move and showed impairment in calculations. They emphasize that none of these patients had prior seizures or delirium.

These drugs which inhibit the P450 liver enzyme system also nullify the effects of the antiarrhythmic medications. Those with heart conditions who are using antiarrhythmics should be alerted to this danger as this effect can produce fatal results.

119

And because of the general caution taken with lithium because of its propensity to produce toxicity, adding it to Prozac would cause an ever greater concern for closer observation. These combinations would cause even greater possibility of producing the serious life threatening disorder, the serotonin syndrome. This may be a the reason so many ex-Prozac patients report that they can no longer tolerate other drugs the doctor has attempted to use after Prozac. They often continue to have the same reactions brought on in the past by Prozac. Most patients relate a fear of using any other drugs because of their reactions to Prozac and turn to alternative treatments. With the combination of the 100 fold accumulation of Prozac within the brain that Dr. Karson has found and this at least 10 fold magnification of other drugs, these reactions could continue indefinitely.

With the combination of fluoxetine [Prozac] and alcohol or other drugs, which all have a strong impact upon liver function, or excessive intake of processed sugars or the inability of the body to maintain balanced blood sugar levels the liver could go into overload and not be able to function normally. This would create much higher drug levels in the blood, thus producing the "nightmarish" results we are witnessing from this drug. It helps us to understand why patients and families report that the suicidal or homicidal impulses came on suddenly, without warning. Who knows how long the liver will maintain the ability to control the level of Prozac in the blood? Patients should be aware of this aspect of Prozac and realize that they are playing Russian Roulette with not only their own lives but considering the ramifications of these toxic reactions, the lives of their loved ones and those with whom they associate can be affected by their uncontrolled violent out of character behavior.

Physical weakness impairs both the metabolism and the excretion of drugs, thus enhancing the possibility of toxicity. So patients who would also be at higher risk are those prescribed Prozac for a physical ailment involving general debility, such as Chronic Fatigue Syndrome, Lupus, cancer, etc. (those with chronic diseases), or the elderly whose organs are no longer functioning at top capacity. In the December 23, 1990, issue of PARADE Dr. Jerry Avorn, an associate professor of social medicine at the Harvard Medical School said, "Drugs can have dangerous side effects for persons of any age" yet, "The efficiency of the kidney and liver can decline with age, hampering the ability to excrete drugs, which in turn can lead to a drug build-up in the body." Stress placed upon these organs from chronic disease can also hamper their ability to excrete drugs. He further explains that, "many organs of the body, from the heart to the bladder to the brain, can undergo change in their sensitivity to medication."

120

Additionally Dr. Avorn cautions us that even aspirin can pose serious problems if mixed with medications because it can intensify the effects of those medications. Dr. Bruce Janiak's information quoted in the following chapter ties in very closely with this as he discusses the high incidence of drug interaction and toxicity. Dr. Janiak wants patients to understand that *caffeine and nicotine are drugs which will interact with medications and increase one's chances of drug interaction, and over the counter medications will do the same.* He stresses that certain foods can also affect how drugs react. He says that *mixing only three chemicals and/or medications can give the patient a 50% chance of a drug interaction and mixing six raises the chance to "extremely likely!"* This drug interaction within the blood then produces the adverse reactions from those drugs. To see choices of reactions to the various drugs being combined just turn to "Warnings - Adverse Effects" listed in the package insert with each drug. Unfortunately the patient does not get to make the choice of reactions, circumstances do that for him and he gets a chance to experience any of them.

As we can see there are many variables that determine the efficacy and safety of a drug. Patients who are not made aware of the seriousness of combining various foods and chemicals stand the chance of suffering drug interactions or drug intoxication. In particular, patients who have been rendered completely unsuspecting of any possibility of the problems of such combinations, (when they are constantly reassured by their doctors that their medication has no side effects - which would be a "first" in medical science), end up being victims of drug interaction or drug intoxication. The patient should *carefully and closely, with a medical dictionary in hand*, read the warnings in the package insert or in a *PHYSICIAN'S DESK REFERENCE*. (The reader may check appendix A for a few of the side effects produced by Prozac and the other SSRIs and their medical description in laymen's terms.) *One must remember that with a combination of drugs a patient can suffer even the **rare** side effects of a drug at a **higher incidence rate**, so be sure to read all warnings if you are combining drugs. Also keep in mind that Prozac has been demonstrated to greatly multiply the effects of many other drugs, which also greatly increases the possibility of adverse reactions.*

How long a waiting period is safe to add other drugs after using any of the SSRIs? Fatalities have been reported in conjunction with the serotonin syndrome even in cases where some of these other serotonin enhancing drugs or methods were used after the discontinuation of Prozac or other SSRI. Extreme caution should be used with ECT (electric shock) or when prescribing any drug which enhances serotonin as a follow up medication to Prozac or any other SSRI. How long a period of time between medications is safe is not yet known, even though some doctors presume to be sure that a few weeks or months is sufficient. The actual truth is - there is little research that has been completed that would give us an answer yet. The Zoloft warnings to prescribing physicians from its manufacturer, Pfizer, indicate "There is limited controlled experience regarding the optimal timing of switching from other antidepressants to Zoloft. Care and prudent medical judgment should be exercised when switching, particularly from long-acting agents. The duration of an appropriate washout period which should intervene before switching from one selective serotonin reuptake inhibitor (SSRI) to another has not been established." The latest research in this area was just published in the summer of 1993. Dr. Craig N. Karson, who is a professor of psychiatry and pathology at the University of Arkansas and Chief of Psychiatry at John Mc Clellan Memorial Veterans Hospital has been researching the issue of Prozac accumulation for several years now. His research involves the use of a nuclear magnetic resonance spectroscopy (NMRS). This is a process whereby the magnetic sensitivity of the chemicals is measured. It requires a special type of lab and building special coils. Because Prozac has fluorine molecules and fluorine has a magnetic sensitivity, it can be detected with a magnetic resonance spectroscopy. Fluvoxamine (Luvox) has three fluorine molecules, Fluoxetine (Prozac) has three fluorine molecules, which means Lovan also has three, Paxil has one fluorine molecule, but Zoloft has none, so it cannot be tested this way to determine the extent to which it is accumulating in the brain. Dr. Karson's results are staggering, "The results are the brain Prozac levels are maybe even a hundred times higher than serum levels and that they accumulate much more gradually over time and probably don't reach their peak until about six to eight months, in contrast to about two weeks for serum levels. So they're there and they'll stick around in the brain for a long time. So a hundred times more in brain...I think what it means is that the stuff concentrates in the brain and sticks around for a pretty long time."

Me: "Well, that's what I have been finding with patients. They seem to report that if they start having side effects those side effects just continue for so long."

Dr. Karson: "And that's why."

Me: "So that would also explain why I continue to get reports of delayed withdrawal from patients?"

Dr. Karson: "Yes, yes, yes...Those are the type of issues we would like to sort out using this technique, is not only clinical response linked to this, but when you have basically some kind of a medication - a very serious medication side effect, which is relatively rare, such as neuroleptic malignant syndrome or perhaps, if it exists, this Prozac suicidal behavior or whatever, is that somehow linked to the brain levels?...if we can link this somehow to clinical response or terrible side effects, if you will, then it will be very useful. If we can get the therapeutic level - the level at which the drug usually works, then we could help physicians dose correctly. Blood levels are useless. Blood levels generically have turned out to be not so great."

Dr. Karson's research on the massive build up of Prozac in the brain would suggest the time period for flushing Prozac, in order to avoid post drug interaction, could be incredibly long. It should be clearly emphasized that it is not known just how long a waiting period is safe. Patients have reported consistently that other drugs cause a variety of adverse reactions for them long after their use of Prozac. When we combine Dr. Karson's information with the study which demonstrates a magnification of other drugs, we understand that Prozac will continue to magnify the effects of those drugs until it is entirely flushed from the brain and body. It is also unbelievable that six years after Prozac has been on the market that Dr. Karson's research demonstrates that we have not had the correct knowledge of what is a therapeutic (safe) level of Prozac.

CHAPTER 5

ADDICTION, DEPENDENCE & WITHDRAWAL

Former Prozac patients have repeatedly reported an addictive pattern or dependence in conjunction with Prozac. They also report cravings for the drug, both physically and psychologically, long after discontinuation of use. They will often state, "I can't live without it!" or "One day without it and I really know it!" They are reporting horrible withdrawal symptoms lasting for months and even years, generally depending upon the length of use. They also often describe developing overwhelming cravings for one or all of the following substances: alcohol, sugary sweets, caffeine in the form of caffeinated soft drinks or coffee, over-the-counter drugs, other pain killing and mind-altering psychiatric prescription drugs or even illegal drugs. Those who have stopped smoking often report that they have started smoking again.

Patients on Prozac consistently report developing an overwhelming compulsion to consume alcohol. These reports are coming even from those who have never previously used alcohol. Patients who have been reformed alcoholics with their addictions under control for many years report that they are returning to alcoholism while using Prozac. This compulsion for alcohol was also one of the observations made by Harvard's, Dr. Martin Teicher who submitted the first medical report that began warnings to practitioners and the public about suicide and violence. (*AMERICAN JOURNAL OF PSYCHIATRY*, 147:2, February 1990, Case #4) The package insert on Paxil lists this as a side effect. This alcohol compulsion is also reported with the benzodiazephines, ie. Valium, Halcion, Xanex, Librium, Dalmane, Ativan, Centrax, Paxipam, Restoril, Serax, Tranxene, etc. Psychiatrist Ruth Richter reports that she will not use the benzodiazepines for this reason. You will recall that we have already referred to studies which demonstrate that low levels of 5HIAA serotonin are linked to alcoholism and that the SSRIs and all of the tricyclic antidepressants have this effect.

Eli Lilly and other major drug manufactures who are rushing to get their cut of the profits from the latest fad in anti-depressants by releasing their own version of an SSRI, have apparently overlooked medical studies completed in the late 60's and early 70's...studies which link higher levels of the neurotransmitter serotonin to cravings for alcohol. As we have already stated, Prozac was the first in this new class of anti-depressants designed to chemically raise the level of brain serotonin. The evidence from the following double blind medical studies indicates that this serotonergic increase produces a *craving* for alcohol. In a study conducted by Liisa Ahtee and Kalervo

Eriksson (*Physiology and Behavior*, Vol. 8, pp. 123-126, 1972) rats which preferred alcohol had 15-20% higher concentrations of serotonin in the brain. One month into the study those showing an addiction to alcohol had 31% higher levels of serotonin concentrations.

Another study linking alcohol preference to serotonin levels was conducted by Myers and Veale and reported June 28, 1968 in Science, pp. 1469-1471. They reported that when serotonin levels were lowered, the preference for alcohol was reduced. Dr. James Milam in his revolutionary and remarkably informative best selling book on alcoholism, *UNDER THE INFLUENCE* (p. 38) discusses this serotonin-link to alcoholism. He additionally states that alcohol, like Prozac, raises the brain's serotonin concentrations, which levels subsequently drop during withdrawal from alcohol. It is known that alcohol acutely and chronically releases serotonin which subsequently lowers serotonin levels (Ballenger et al. 1979).

These serotonergic drugs, the SSRIs, were designed to *raise, not normalize*, the levels of this neurotransmitter. Drug manufacturers, including Lilly, did not go on to explain to consumers the possible effects as the level of serotonin rises abnormally high. They have focused only on informing us of the effects of low levels of serotonin. America already has an estimated 10 -15 million alcoholics. To increase that number with a reaction from prescription drugs which causes a compulsion to drink is a tragedy! What a sad state of affairs that a drug which is actually being promoted as a treatment for alcoholism has the potential to create alcohol craving behavior. What a self-defeating and terribly frustrating scenario for those who are working so hard to overcome alcoholism.

Mixing alcohol with Prozac or any SSRI can be very dangerous by magnifying the possibility of side effects. Beyond chemically inducing an overwhelming urge to drink in patients through chemically raising the serotonin level are additionally mixing alcohol with a powerful anti-depressant. Any physician is aware of the extreme dangers of this combination and its potential for producing psychotic behavior. This information raises serious overall questions about the efficacy of this new class of serotonergic drugs, especially in those patients with a family history of alcoholism or as Dr. Milam's book would emphasize, in those who have a family history of blood sugar disorders such as diabetes or hypoglycemia.

We all understand the dangers posed by a drug showing evidence of being addictive. What we need to understand is the additional danger posed to the patient and society by the implications that Prozac is inducing a compulsion to mix other substances which would bring on a synergistic or multiplying effect of the drug. An article which appeared in the August 8, 1990 issue of the Salt Lake *Deseret News* gives us an idea of the seriousness of mixing Prozac with alcohol. It says, *"The dangers of combining Prozac with other drugs have not been fully studied. Of particular concern to physicians are drugs that affect the central nervous system, such as narcotics or alcohol."*

In November of 1986 Noreen Ackerman wrote an extremely informative article for the *FRIENDLY EXCHANGE.* Because this article sets an excellent basic foundation for understanding the overwhelming seriousness of this particular aspect of Prozac, we will review this information very closely. The article is entitled, "A Mixture for Trouble" with the sub heading: "Mixing your medicines...can be hazardous to your health. If you mix medicine and alcohol, the result can be deadly."

It continues, "The National Safety Council reports that misuse of medicines ...accounts for 40 percent of the 2 million accidental poisonings that occur annually...Some combinations can cause the medicine to have far too great an effect; other combinations might prevent a medicine from working at all.

"'The public is beginning to realize the dangers of drug interaction,' says Margaret Gladden, a technical specialist for the National Safety Council. But there are still many people who disregard the warnings or just do not give drug interaction much thought.'

*"Alcohol is the worst culprit. When alcohol and drugs are combined, one can compound the effects of the other so the resulting impairment is **far worse** than if the two were taken separately...**even small amounts, mixed with some medicines, will deaden your senses or change your perceptions.*** [This changing of perceptions is exactly what patients report when mixing Prozac with alcohol or one of the benzodiazepines such as Xanex, Halcion, etc.] *Alcohol depresses the central nervous system, and if you use it along with other depressants, such as narcotics, tranquilizers, or barbiturates, the effect is multiplied...Caffeine and nicotine are drugs, too, and can cause an adverse drug reaction in your body...* [It is very rare to see an individual on Prozac without a large diet Coke or Pepsi in their hand every second of the day or drinking 10 to 15 cups of coffee to start their day - another indication of the obsession for caffeine, sweets, alcohol, nicotine or other drugs reported by ex-Prozac patients.]

Ingesting several chemicals can cause an unintentional intoxication. When Dr. Bruce Janiak was interviewed for this article he was head of the department of emergency medicine at The Toledo Hospital, past president of the American

College of Emergency Physicians and handled drug-interaction accidents every day. Dr. Janiak stresses, "The victims of these accidents most commonly mix a drug that has the same type depressant effect as alcohol...*the individuals appear to be intoxicated because they are*...in essence they are intoxicated because there are several drugs producing the same effect. Their reaction time slows and their judgment is impaired ...both signs of alcohol intoxication.' [This intoxication Dr. Janiak speaks of which the patient is experiencing unbeknown to him, is what our legal system refers to as "involuntary intoxication" which some states as yet do not allow as a defence.]...*the more drugs you mix, the greater your chances of having a drug interaction.* If you take *two drugs*, for example, there is a *small chance* of a drug interaction, Janiak explains. However, if you take *three kinds of drugs*, your chances approach *50 percent*, and if you take *six drugs*, it is *extremely likely* you will have some sort of drug interaction." (Emphasis added)

Dr. Fred Riehmerr who heads the Mood Disorder Clinic at the University of Utah and was involved in the clinical trials on Prozac adds that *any anti-depressant will cause problems in long term use and all should be used short term*. (It is well known that one of those problems is that the antidepressants can activate mania.) He has also voiced concern over Prozac being prescribed in high doses.

Common chemicals used on a daily basis can pose serious risks when combined with prescription drug use. How many people use caffeine, nicotine, excess sugar or alcohol on a regular basis or any other prescription medication, and do not even think of discontinuing the use of these when prescribed Prozac? How many are on high doses of Prozac? How many have taken the drug long-term? And how many had already suffered diseases which could have affected their liver or pancreatic function, which, as we discussed in the last chapter, can increase drug concentrations in the blood?

Using Dr. Janiak's formula we can estimate what a patients' chances are of experiencing an adverse reaction. As an example, a personal friend, with a highly stressful occupation as an investigative news reporter, took Prozac for one year then switched to Zoloft for the past one and a half years. This person smokes, drinks coffee, drinks alcohol, does not avoid sugar, and was on double the average 20 mg. dose of Prozac. As we count the number of variables which would affect my friend we find: alcohol, caffeine, nicotine, sugar, high Prozac intake, long term use of SSRIs, slight liver impairment, which would be indicated by years of alcohol use and then magnified over the past year by combining the alcohol with Prozac and Zoloft. So from the number of determining factors we see that the chances of an adverse reaction from a drug interaction are *very high* and my friend and anyone around this person would be in danger, if that reaction proved to be a violent outburst.

Another personal friend who has a very strict health code and does not use caffeine or nicotine or alcohol or other medications took Prozac for one year. She doesn't use much sugar because of her concern over some indications of having a slight case of hypoglycemia. She was on low doses of Prozac (20 mg. every other day) and mixed no other substances during her period of Prozac use. The only adverse reactions she experienced were headaches and withdrawal when trying to discontinue the drug "cold turkey", along with feelings of addictiveness.

What we understand from all this is: *If* the patient is not too old, nor too young, *if* the patient has not had a drug reaction to a psychiatric drug in the past, *if* the patient has not had extensive use of a mind-altering drug in the past (do not forget that anti-histamines, sleeping agents, painkillers, hormones, etc. are all common mind altering drugs), *if* the patient is not under a lot of stress, *if* the patient is in excellent physical health, *if* the patient is not using any other medications, *if* the patient does not regularly use the common chemical stimulants and depressants: caffeine, tobacco or alcohol, and *if* the drug is used in low doses and extremely short-term, the drug *may* produce the desired effect rather than a dangerous adverse paradoxical reaction. For most people there are too many *ifs*. When one combines this information on drug interactions with the continued reports of Prozac causing an obsession for other chemicals which would cause a mixing of various mind altering substances, it becomes a very alarming and dangerous situation. This combining of substances would, in turn produce drug interactions, thereby insuring the adverse reactions from Prozac.

It is extremely rare for me to find a reformed alcoholic, who after using Prozac, has been able to stay away from alcohol because, as they describe it, either the overwhelming drive to drink they experience becomes too overpowering. One exception was a young mother in her late twenties who was able to prevent returning to her alcohol addiction during eight months of Prozac use by attending AA meetings every day. She reported that she was not sure how much longer she would have been able to resist the strong compulsion she was feeling to drink again and had not realized until discontinuing Prozac that the compulsion was related to her use of the drug. Another was a psychologist and the wife of a well known author and entrepreneur. Their marriage did not survive her Prozac reactions. When he told me his wife was an ex-alcoholic and I asked about her ability to avoid returning to alcohol, he explained that she also was attending AA daily - three times a day!

Is Prozac removing inhibitions and thereby causing a compulsion for alcohol or is this a physical reaction through altering blood sugar? Drug and alcohol abuse officials are theorizing that this Prozac-Addiction or Dependence connection is brought on by Prozac's mood altering effect. They feel it may be removing the inhibitions that individuals have placed upon themselves to stop their addictions to alcohol and other substances. (In light of how many state that "nothing mattered" to them and the consequences of their actions made no impression upon them - no feelings of guilt, this theory is plausible.) Once the inhibitions are removed in this way, the patient feels no desire to exercise control over his addiction. Individuals who have a history of abusing various substances will, according to the theory, revert to that addiction or begin abusing Prozac by increasing their dose.

Dr. Vogel explains in his book *THE NATURE DOCTOR,* "Alcohol and drugs can influence the brain to the extent that several centers are slowed down while others accelerate. Hence the person may lose his inhibitions and temporarily act and feel differently to how he would under normal circumstances." If we are using a substance that removes feelings and inhibitions, how do we have any control over our lives? What is our contact with reality if it is not our feelings? If we are not completely aware of what is happening around us and how we are being affected by it, how do we know how to react or respond to life? Isn't that awareness what determines our level of intelligence? Isn't awareness the key factor in generating change in our lives? Without that awareness, how can any growth take place within us, and because of this inability to grow, how would any counseling or therapy be effective? How does one make rational choices about anything he is doing? How does one exercise his agency to act of his own free will and choice if his own internal "check and balance" system is removed? This distancing us from reality is the reason society considers alcohol to be a very dangerous mind-altering substance. Prozac patients who have come off the drug report that they are now able to see that reality and imagination had become so scrambled in their minds that they could not detect what was real and what was a dream. (See the description of the side-effect "depersonalization" in Appendix A for an understanding of this adverse reaction.)

Beyond this mood altering effect of Prozac which would, in turn, remove inhibitions, there seems to be a physiological cause for the alcoholic obsession or craving for other addictive substances. As mentioned previously, we have many reports of people who rarely drank or never drank before Prozac, consuming excessive amounts of alcohol after starting the use of the drug. One example is the case of a young newly wed who was given Prozac for a hormonal imbalance which appeared soon after her marriage. This hormonal imbalance produced effects similar to PMS. Before this she would have two or three social drinks a year, yet after Prozac she began bringing alcohol home by the case.

With Prozac being so obviously hard on the pancreas, even to the extent of pushing a healthy pancreas into a diabetic or hypoglycemic state, causing the pancreas to malfunction, thereby upsetting the blood sugar balance in the body. This blood sugar imbalance would in turn cause the "craving" for alcohol patients are reporting as the body reaches out for a "quick fix" to raise the blood sugar level. Then begins a vicious self-perpetuating cycle as the alcohol pushes the blood sugar level even lower after a brief high. This would be a very logical explanation of these reports coming in from so many patients of feeling *"overwhelming compulsions"* to drink while using Prozac. (For a greater understanding of this reaction refer to the discussion on hypoglycemic reactions in the chapter CHEMICAL DEPRESSION.)

Is the concentration of alcohol magnified in combination with Prozac or other SSRIs? To compound all of the above information on alcohol compulsions, we are beginning to receive very reports from Prozac patients who, after only a couple of mild alcoholic drinks, are discovering their blood alcohol count is extremely high. For quite some time we have received reports that patients were noticing that just a little alcohol would give them a high that previously would have required far more alcohol than the amount they had just consumed in combination with Prozac. Now these reports are beginning to provide documentation about how Prozac is affecting blood alcohol levels.

One young woman in her early twenties was stopped and charged with a DUI after having one glass of champagne. Her blood alcohol was not consistent with the amount of alcohol she consumed. Her test results showed her blood alcohol level far above the legal limit. She was on a very low dose of Prozac, only one 20 mg. capsule every three days. To get an idea of how she was reacting to a combination of Prozac and alcohol as a test she was given three drinks of vodka in grapefruit juice - one inch of vodka with the remainder of the glass containing grapefruit juice. Two hours later she was given one glass of wine. The local hospital emergency room then ran a blood alcohol test. The doctor administering the test was clearly shocked when her blood alcohol level registered 2.2. He wanted to know how she was still on her feet and functioning and "appearing" alert with that much alcohol in her blood. When they explained that she was on Prozac he was even more bewildered. She could walk. She could get into a car and drive, obviously not safely or she would not have been pulled over by the police, but she could drive. And she could carry on a comparatively intelligent conversation without any noticeable slurred speech. With an alcohol level high enough to knock her flat on her back, she was functioning! At what capacity was she functioning? What areas of the brain were being affected? How was it affecting her judgement? How was it affecting her reflexes? We have no answers to any of these questions. No one knows yet because no one has tested those areas.

The facial expressions of the emergency room doctor in this case clearly demonstrated that he wondered if the patient was from another planet. The patient's blood alcohol level was so totally inconsistent with the amount of alcohol consumed and had jumped so rapidly he was baffled. This same type of situation can happen with a diabetic who drinks, which would make us look again at what effect Prozac is having on the pancreas and how it is affecting blood sugar balance.

This case would also raise questions about abnormal liver function. Is Prozac inhibiting liver function to the extent that alcohol metabolism is being inhibited? January 1, 1992, a study was submitted to *THE JOURNAL OF THE AMERICAN MEDICAL ASSOCIATION* showing that the popular drugs Tagamet and Zantac inhibit the production of an enzyme in the liver which metabolizes alcohol. The liver would normally function by breaking down the alcohol so that only a portion would be allowed to enter the blood stream. With the liver function being inhibited, the alcohol is dumped directly into the blood stream. What would have been considered a "safe" amount for the patient before would prove *dangerously high* when taken in combination with either of these medications. According to the report the patient could unexpectedly find himself suddenly losing consciousness. It showed that Zantac increased blood alcohol concentrations by 34% and Tagamet caused increases of a staggering 92%. Even after a small amount of alcohol the individuals using these drugs are finding that they pass out or become staggering drunk. The authors of this study, Dr. Carlo Dipadova of the Bronx Veterans Affairs Medical Center in New York and Dr. Charles Liever at the Mount Sinai School of Medicine in New York warned, "The blood alcohol levels achieved have been clearly shown to impair tasks that require a high degree of attention and motor coordination."

Prozac is known to be a highly accumulative drug and especially long-acting which affects metabolism. It will not wash out for quite some time, and the side effects may continue to persist during the entire washing out period, even though the patient has stopped taking the drug. This can force the liver, kidneys, pancreas, etc. to work far beyond what should be required of them. Could it be that this excess stress upon the liver is causing it also to inhibit the production of the same alcohol metabolizing enzyme? As we consider the high number of people using Prozac and driving or working jobs that require motor coordination and judgement, this could pose very serious problems in a multitude of areas which would affect us all. Dr. Corsten who was also involved in the study above reported that he believes that most drugs raise the level of alcohol and affect the patient's alcohol metabolism in this way. In his opinion it is most likely that Prozac would do the same. A study published on this issue has proved Dr. Corsten's opinion to be correct. The study done by Lilly reports an almost unbelievable increase of 1000% with Prozac (Bergstrom, 1990). Another study demonstrates that the problem of interactions with Paxil would be much greater. It indicates a 4000% increase with Paxil for any chemical metabolized by the P450 liver enzyme, which includes ethanol or alcohol and a very large majority of other chemical substances (Davane, 1992). This should signify that one alcoholic drink would have the impact of ten with Prozac and 40 with Paxil.

We must add to this information of alcohol metabolism another area of concern which presents a real danger. This is that Prozac appears to be raising the tolerance level to alcohol for Prozac patients, making it possible to consume large amounts. In feeling this *"drive to drink"* some patients are consuming *amazing* amounts of alcohol very rapidly. (Refer to cases reported in chapter entitled THE LEGAL REPERCUSSIONS.) Is this made possible because Prozac has such a strong stimulant effect of doubling the adrenalin flow added to the cortisol increase from the alcohol that the drinker is kept functioning enough to continue drinking when he should have already passed out? Does this have such a powerful stimulant effect that the patient with high blood alcohol levels is given the energy to stay on their feet when they should be out cold? When one passes out it is a safety gage for the drinker and anyone around him. Who wants a drunk up and moving?

The brain wave patterns in this book also indicate that this is what is happening. The brain is effectively "nonfunctioning" on a conscious level, but the patient is functioning physically. So, exactly who is handling the controls? Diabetics report a similar experience when they drink. A diabetic can drink alcohol and have multiplied effects in one instance and the next time they drink feel no effect from the alcohol consumption. There seems to be no ability to predict how the alcohol will affect them. As we begin to gather additional information concerning the adverse effects produced by Prozac upon the pancreas, perhaps we will begin to understand the reason for this very similar reaction in Prozac patients. If Prozac causes an overwhelming compulsion to consume alcohol, then raises one's alcohol tolerance level and then, on top of all that, is boosting the blood alcohol count, it is producing a "super drunk" and keeping him on his feet after he should have passed out. Why would extreme violence, terrible and bizarre accidents, etc., as a result of this, be surprising to anyone?

Prozac is highly protein bound (94.5%), binding to albumin and other body proteins (Zoloft and Paxil are both approximately 98% protein binding. This binding process may be part of the reason that evidence is mounting to indicate that Prozac accumulates in the body. This binding process puts additional stress on the liver in metabolizing the drug. The liver must go through the process of breaking down the larger more complex chemical structures, which are formed by Prozac binding to the body proteins (in the past referred to as cross-linked proteins), before it can eliminate them. This process of overworking the liver would also magnify the effect of the alcohol and most likely magnify the amount of alcohol in the blood. All of which would greatly increase any damaging effects of either the alcohol and/or the Prozac. This means that those suffering a tendency toward alcoholism or any chemical addiction would suffer the most disastrous repercussions of Prozac (including the suicidal ideation and violence) faster than most.

Listening to reformed alcoholics who have had years of sobriety destroyed almost overnight and those who have never touched alcohol before Prozac, yet began drinking compulsively because of a medication prescribed by doctors unfamiliar with this alcohol connection is not a simple task. Knowing that Prozac is being promoted by some as a way for alcoholics to overcome their alcohol dependence becomes, not only frightening, but *absurd*, especially in light of the fact that so many who have never used alcohol before felt "driven to drink" on Prozac! And in light of the results of the studies which show higher levels of serotonin causing compulsive alcohol consumption.

We also need to ask how Prozac is affecting those who suffer from various other addictions or compulsions. In our society so plagued by a multitude of addictions, we need for much more research to be done in all the many areas of addictive patterns. The majority of these compulsions are related to the far too common antidepressant side effect of mania. What about the *compulsive spending* reports? Most patients who suffer adverse reactions find themselves financially destitute when they finally discontinue their use of Prozac. They generally discover that they have given away everything or used poor judgement financially and lost it all. Or they find that they have sold all they have worked for throughout their lives and then spent the money. They have also used credit to the limit in order to purchase items they cannot even remember buying. (Beware, once they have used their own cards to the limit, they often borrow cards from others and use them to the limit.) One wife reported that her retired husband who was taking Prozac for Chronic Fatigue Syndrome, sold all they had, used their

133

retirement savings and bought a large boat. Then a few days after the purchase, as he walked past the boat he asked her where it came from. He didn't even recall the purchase. They also report that the items purchased were nothing they needed or really even wanted. They state that they have no idea why they have bought the things they have.

Then there are the reports of sexual compulsions - young people firmly committed to reserve sex for marriage find themselves expecting a child after starting on Prozac, previously faithful wives and husbands committing adultery, heterosexuals having homosexual sex, etc. There are many other reports of people with a background of high morals and values and strong marriages suffering the same reaction. The PDR lists "increased libido" as a side effect. One theory suggests that when there is an increase in the dopamine level in the brain to the point where it exceeds the amount of 5HIAA serotonin, there is a higher chance of sexual activity and responsiveness. 5HT serotonin has been demonstrated to increase the release of dopamine (Yi et al. 1991; Blandina et al. 1989).

The risks involved with a drug induced increase in libido are great and certainly not advantageous as some might think. Cocaine, which is known to initially increase serotonin, also increases libido, but in long term use it "can make it difficult for men to maintain erection or to ejaculate, and for women to reach orgasm. It is also addictive and in some cases can cause heart failure and death." We also know that serum androgenic hormones (steroids) motivate sexual behavior in adolescent boys. But there is always a catch when drugs produce these effects "Overall, psychoactive drugs make sexual promises they are unable to keep. Though some may lower inhibitions, or increase desire, there is usually a trade-off in performance. In some cases, there is even permanent damage to sexuality, fertility, and reproduction...*the risk and dangers involved...far outweigh any temporary pleasurable effects...*" (*THE ENCYCLOPEDIA OF PSYCHOACTIVE DRUGS, DRUGS AND SEXUAL BEHAVIOR*, p.57)

A local psychiatrist informed me that one of his female colleagues had discovered that Deseryl, a fairly potent enhancer of serotonin levels, increased sexual desire in her female patients. He quickly added that it was important that the information not get out to the wrong people. My first thought was, perhaps it already is in the wrong hands as I had just heard University of Utah psychologist Donald Strassberg, who specializes in sex therapy, state in an interview with KTKK radio the summer of 1992 that recent figures show that 40% of therapists believe that having sex with their patients is "therapeutic." Of course the question remains, "For *whom* is it therapeutic?" This increase in sexual desire seems to hold true with this newer serotonin enhancer, Prozac, as well. This could stem from its ability to produce mania or its suppression of REM sleep. Remember that excessive spending and promiscuous behavior are both symptoms of mania or a manic reaction. The repercussions of this side effect are cause for great concern when considering the massive problem our society is facing with AIDS. A drug that can reportedly produce as a side-effect in some patients an obsession to have *any type of sex with anyone* is all we needed. Remember that Prozac causes a disruption in the level of serotonin which is believed to be the neurotransmitter which regulates the driving sexual forces in an individual. We do know that low levels of serotonin can cause impulsive behavior with no ability to think clearly before acting or any concern for consequences.

A young woman I assisted two years ago had a tragic experience because of this increased libido reaction which changed the rest of her life. This was a young woman with high moral standards who had always worked very hard to set a perfect example for her six younger brothers and sisters to follow. When she was having a rough time in her life (that is what life as a teenager is generally all about for many of us) her mother, on Prozac herself, encouraged her daughter's use of the drug. It took nothing to find a doctor to prescribe it for her. It seldom does. The manic reaction began rapidly for her and three months later she was pregnant. She had two babies out of wedlock before she learned on her own that she was experiencing a manic reaction to Prozac. She immediately stopped using the drug. It has been a long and painful road back, but she has made it. Prozac certainly did help her overcome her shyness and become very out going. I sat with her as she explained to her brother what had happened to her. They cried together for a while. He understood her experience though. He understood because their mother had persuaded him to take the drug as well. Luckily for him, he became aware of the adverse effects of the drug right away and got off before the effects became too great for him to handle. But he used the drug long enough to understand how it could cause such a reaction. Let me add that this is a very, very religious family.

I wish I could say that this was an isolated incident. It is not. I heard a radio show last year on a station for adolescents. There were calls from young people who reported that they and their entire family were on Prozac. Two young women called in during the short one half hour open for calls to ask if their use of Prozac could have had anything to do with them becoming "out going" enough to find themselves pregnant at such an early age. The pain in their voices was clear. The confusion they felt about their own actions was very apparent. Unfortunately no one on the show knew enough about this drug to answer their question. How terrible to have your life so drastically changed forever at such a tender age. I have read many reports like this of unwanted pregnancies reported to the FDA by physicians as adverse reaction reports on Prozac.

Increased libido or decreased libido? Although some patients report increased libido, a side effect listed in the Prozac package insert, a recent study (*JOURNAL OF CLINICAL PSYCHIATRY*, April, 1993) shows the opposite. It reports that 34% of patients said that their sexual desire or response had diminished after taking Prozac. Overall, 43% of women taking antidepressants report less sexual desire. The quote above also talks of a "trade-off" in sexual performance even the drug may increase sexual desire. The general trend in patient reports is showing a higher rate of decreased interest shown by men. Male patients have also reported extremely painful erection. In light of these reports of sexual drive dysfunction in men it becomes very puzzling that in the Fall of 1992 articles were printed both in the *ENQUIRER* and *PLAYBOY* touting Prozac as a treatment for premature ejaculation. Remember that cocaine can make it difficult to ejaculate as well. Of course if Prozac robs one of any desire for sex or makes it too painful to consider, ejaculation, premature or otherwise, should not be a problem at all. That would take care of the problem of premature ejaculation, but what kind of "cure" or "treatment" is that?

What is odd is that Prozac reportedly affects the patient in one extreme or the other. The reaction can either be an increase in sexual activity or just the opposite of not even wanting to be touched (This not wanting to be touched is a classically autistic symptom, a condition in which higher levels of serotonin are a marker.) So we find another indication of a paradoxical or opposite effect brought on as a drug reaction. To demonstrate this aspect I will include quotes from a couple of interviews with patient family members: "When my husband was taking 40 mg. a day he would become very cold sometimes - extremely distant and untouching. I began to think he was having an affair and I ended up in a hospital myself." (This situation where the mate falls apart watching their loved one go through this is something I have heard repeatedly from couples.)

Another elderly man reported, "I have a daughter-in-law that I think is still using Prozac. In the process she divorced her husband, my son. Now two young boys are without their father. I don't know of her becoming violent, but I do know she is real cold. We are hearing about a lot of divorces on Prozac - by the thousands right here in this valley. If you could trace it you would find out that Prozac had a lot to do with it. My wife took it for a while and she is the most kind and loving person I have ever known, but she became very mean while on Prozac."

136

Can Prozac chemically induce obsessive-compulsive behavior? If the reader will check Appendix B he will find medical reports of Prozac chemically inducing a variety of "obsessive - compulsive" type disorders in patients. People with this disease are generally very acutely aware that their behavior is not "normal" or "right," but they feel powerless to do anything to control it. According to Dr. Peter Roy-Byrne, director of the Anxiety Disorders Program at the University of Washington, patients with obsessive - compulsive behavior feel guilty and ashamed of their behavior and deny or hide the behaviors. So do not expect a patient on Prozac who might be going into obsessive - compulsive behaviors to be very open or honest about any obsessive-compulsive symptoms they are experiencing. It is certainly understandable why one would react this way to something so foreign to them. This disease, obsessive - compulsive disorder (OCD), was rare in the past, but has seen an explosion in growth during the last decade. Doctors postulate that stress could be the contributing factor since stress can bring on compulsive symptoms. Those with OCD have also been found to have abnormally low levels of 5HIAA serotonin. "We do know that the low levels of this substance [serotonin] affect one's sense of certainty...they suffer from terrible doubt and uncertainty", continues Dr. Roy-Bryne. This uncertainty and doubt are the cause of the patient's repetitious actions.

From this information we find several reasons for the obsessive - compulsive disorders in Prozac patients. The first reason for these chemically induced compulsions is that we have medical studies showing that Prozac can cause great *decreases* in 5HIAA serotonin levels. The second reason would be demonstrated to us by the drug induced sleep deficit (which we discuss in detail in the chapter on sleep) robbing the patient of a peaceful or restful state. Another is increase in cortisol which chemically determines stress. All of this combined would cause feelings of stress or anxiety to precipitate obsessive-compulsive behavior.

None of the SSRIs were tested for drug abuse potential, dependence, tolerance or withdrawal. We know that other serotonin enhancing drugs produce dependence, for example, imipramine and fenfluramine (Oswald, 1971), clomipramine (Anafranil), etc. are all milder serotonin enhancing drugs and are known to produce dependence. As we continue our look at Prozac's addiction or dependence connection in light of the problems in our society with addictions, I was appalled to discover that the FDA would approve a drug that has the following statement listed in the PDR, yet they have done so over and over, time and time again. This is the statement from the Prozac package insert, but each of the package inserts on the SSRIs contain almost identical statements on drug abuse and dependence.

"Drug Abuse and Dependence:

"Physical and Psychologic Dependence - Prozac has not been systematically studied, in animals or humans, for its potential for abuse, tolerance, or physical dependence. While the pre-marketing clinical experience with Prozac did not reveal any tendency for withdrawal syndrome or any drug seeking behavior, these observations were not systematic, and it is not possible to predict on the basis of this limited experience [Keep in mind that the studies submitted to the FDA were only 5 and 6 week trials.] the extent to which a CNS-active drug will be misused, diverted, and/or abused once marketed. Consequently, physicians should carefully evaluate patients for history of drug abuse and follow such patients closely, observing them for signs of misuse or abuse of Prozac (eg, development of tolerance, incrementation of dose, drug-seeking behavior)."

Evidence of drug abuse, dependence and withdrawal coming from patient reports. After feeling as though we have been used as the guinea pigs in this particular area of insufficient testing, as has been the case with so many so called "wonder drugs" in the past, we the public can report to Eli Lilly many evidences of drug abuse and dependence:

1) There is withdrawal, not in every patient, but in many patients. Patient after patient is reporting withdrawal and in many cases it is *horrendous withdrawal - lasting in some degree for as long a period of time as the patient used Prozac or even longer* - with: even more intense suicidal ideation and rages, single words racing through the mind, crying non-stop (this could be referred to as "rebound emotions" - after a period of suppression the emotions come flooding out such as crying for no apparent reason, laughing for no apparent reason and becoming angry for no apparent reason), an upheaval of emotion - "like a roller coaster", hives, headaches, seizures, the shakes, mania and hypomania, rashes, itching, joint pain, nausea, vomiting, general flu-like symptoms, sweating and chills, dizziness, symptoms of panic attack, insomnia and/or total exhaustion or feeling as if they have Chronic Fatigue Syndrome, intense irritability, bloating, involuntarily cursing and swearing (This odd occurrence even surprises most patients and their families.), rambling, slurred speech, etc. Rest and sleep become most critical in overcoming the withdrawal.

One patient described her withdrawal experience after her doctor had her drop immediately off Prozac because he felt she had suffered a toxic reaction from a combination of Prozac and Lithium. "I gained twelve pounds of water in a day and a half. My ankles looked like they had tea cups hanging on them. Now my knees and my feet and my hands are still numb. I am so tired. My poor husband is so shocked at me because I've started swearing "shit" and "hell" around here. Suicidal tendencies? I'll tell you! You have to put up with the dizziness. I just throw up and throw up and there is this terrible numbness and pain shooting through my joints. I guess Prozac and Lithium aren't the greatest combination."

It is most important to realize that these withdrawal symptoms, although they mimic signs of insanity, are a toxic drug state. The symptoms should leave as the drug is flushed out of the system. The patient returns to "normal" after the withdrawal period. The withdrawal also includes the brain's period of adjustment to normalize its production of serotonin after it was interrupted by Prozac. It additionally includes "rebound depression" (the intensification of depression which often follows the use of anti-depressants) and "REM rebound" causing the patient to sleep excessively to compensate for sleep loss which we will discuss in the chapter on sleep. Of critical importance in withdrawal is helping the adrenal system to normalize after drug use. Physical, mental and emotional stress should be avoided. A quiet and peaceful surrounding is critical. Nerves are very much "on the edge" during this period. Love, support and understanding from family and friends is essential.

The withdrawal is often long-term and is quite often delayed for several weeks or months (especially in long-term use) after discontinuing Prozac, causing much confusion for both the doctor and the patient. The benzodiazepines (Valium, Xanex, Halcion, etc.) also possess this unique feature of delayed and long-term withdrawal. These drugs are also very highly protein bound which still raises curiosity in my mind about this being the central reason for the long period of time it takes to flush them out of the system, and therefore, the long-term withdrawal period. "The fact that these drugs' clinical effects appear and disappear quickly, however, does not mean that the drugs are eradicated from the body rapidly. As a person uses them over a prolonged period of time, there is a build-up of unmetabolized or partly metabolized drug in the tissues and central nervous system...to delay the onset of withdrawal symptoms...Such people, unless warned, may be devastated by the onset of withdrawal symptoms when they *do* begin, usually suddenly...What are the withdrawal symptoms? The most notable is the exact opposite of the nervous system depressant effect of the drug - a sense of nervousness, jitteriness, anxiety, and sleeplessness, as if the nervous system is suddenly running in high gear. And this in fact, is precisely what is happening...Some people exhibit all sorts of peculiar or disordered thinking, developing false ideas, thinking in circles, and coming up with a long series of wrong answers...one of the most common and difficult of all benzodiazepine withdrawal symptoms: a free-floating sense of anxiety and fearfulness of something terrible about to happen...they don't know what they are afraid of, but they are afraid...A second common element of benzodiazepine withdrawal is depression - the same symptom that we see in withdrawal from virtually every addictive drug...One final aspect of benzodiazepine withdrawal is the matter of duration: it tends to hang on." (*THE HIDDEN ADDICTION*, p. 179, 180)

Many of these same withdrawal symptoms are experienced in Prozac patients. One of my neighbors went to the hospital one night in withdrawal because of overwhelming feelings that she was dying. This type of intense fear is common. Depression is very common. Prozac withdrawal is also very long term in some patients. One woman who was on several psychoactive drugs along with high doses of Prozac for a back injury over a three year period is still in withdrawal three years later. How long the withdrawal takes tends to depend first of all upon the strength of your on constitution, then the number and type of other drugs used in conjunction with Prozac and the length of use. After abrupt discontinuation of Prozac after several years of use I have witnesses the onset of withdrawal being delayed for five to six months. Tapering slowly off the drug is much safer and can minimize withdrawal symptoms. A patient who discontinues the drug "cold turkey" is more likely to find withdrawal so difficult as to compel the patient to restart the drug and encounter a more delayed withdrawal later on after more extensive use. A study was done on this "cold turkey" withdrawal approach to Prozac by Don Black. His report published in the July 1993 issue of *CURRENTS IN AFFECTIVE ILLNESS* showed that patients who rode out the withdrawal symptoms felt better in a few weeks. Many patients are reporting flashbacks, just as we have seen with LSD which also raises serotonin levels. Generally this occurs during illness or stressful situations.

Withdrawal can prove to have serious physical effects as well, as the body rushes to do its job of flushing this foreign toxic substance out of the system and the brain goes into a rebound where it over reacts to restore all the normal brain functions and compensate for any losses brought on by interference with normal function. Reports of kidney failure or kidney and bladder pain, liver and gall bladder pain, heart problems, etc. are quite common reports. Many who experienced the intense gall bladder pain have had these organs removed surgically, only to discover later that for others the pain subsided a month or two after discontinuation of Prozac.

How should a patient withdraw from these drugs? Doctors at the University of Utah who are tapering patients on to the drug or slowly tapering them off of the drug are recommending that the patient empty the Prozac capsule into a glass of cranberry juice, drink a portion of it and refrigerate the rest for the next day. In

140

this way you can closely regulate and slowly taper off the amount of the drug being consumed. Those having the most success are those who are tapering off very slowly, i.e., from 20 mg. daily to 15 mg. daily for several weeks to a month or longer depending upon the effects they feel and severity of withdrawal symptoms, then to 10 mg., etc. Slow and easy is the best policy. The general rule of thumb is the longer you have used the drug, the longer you should take to come off. In this way the brain and the body systems, especially the adrenal system, which can trigger serious reactions, are less likely to go into shock from such an abrupt change. Possible serious life-threatening results such as seizures or embarrassing and dangerous results like mania can more easily be avoided in this way.

I have seen very little success in the use of drug therapy for the withdrawal symptoms after Prozac. The patients tend to continue to suffer from these Prozac reactions as other drugs are introduced into their systems. There are many reasons why this could be happening. Part of it could be that the other drugs prevent Prozac from flushing out. Another could be the extensive amount of time Prozac takes to flush out of the body causing drug interactions as other drugs are added to one's system. Recent information would show this to be the case. According to Dr. Karson's study using functional MRI scans with Prozac accumulating in the brain at a rate 100 times greater than the blood and taking so long to wash out, any drug prescribed to the patient for quite a long period of time would be mixing with Prozac still in the body and possibly having its effects multiplied. This is incredibly significant in understanding why withdrawal is delayed, why such a long withdrawal, and why such strong reactions to other drugs are experienced after Prozac use. It should also change decisions in a number of court cases. In these cases the blood was tested for "therapeutic levels" of Prozac when it should have been considered that there was 100 times that amount affecting the person's brain to alter behavior.

Where do you turn for help in withdrawal? Withdrawal from a drug can have many serious and dangerous aspects and it is unfortunate that Prozac patients can rarely find a professional to turn to who understands this or wants to deal with it. All too often they have to withdraw themselves from these drugs. Dr. Jonathon Wright, M.D. and Dr. Brad Weeks, psychiatrist, work together in Kent, Washington and report that since Prozac's release they have had many many patients addicted to Prozac come to them for assistance in withdrawal. They attribute their success to the implimentation of alternative treatments in assisting their patients.

Dr. Peter Breggin emphasizes the importance of support from family, friends and physician. "As in withdrawing from the neuroleptics, patients trying to stop taking antidepressants may need emotional support and patience. The patient and the doctor, and members of the patient's inner circle of friends and family, may have to put up with troublesome symptoms and behavior during the withdrawal period. There is an ominous aspect to these withdrawal symptoms, most of which are produced by rebound hyperactivity of the suppressed cholinergic nerves...when they rebound, they cause mental disturbances, such as anxiety, depression, or mania." (*TOXIC PSYCHIATRY*, p. 154-5)

There are those researchers who believe that there is damage incurred by the brain from these reactions to Prozac which could prove to be permanent damage. Yet, after observing the results, both in cutting the length and the severity of this withdrawal and the readjustment period, by a patient's use of the alternative methods mentioned in the "SOLUTIONS" section, it is my opinion that even though there can be damage, this damage is not necessarily permanent and can be repaired over time if the period of drug use is not too long.

Withdrawal from the SSRIs produces rebound depression which is all too often diagnosed as returning disease symptoms leading to a reintroduction to the drugs, which produced the withdrawal. What is so terrible about this withdrawal syndrome or the delayed withdrawal not being brought to the attention of the patient or his doctor is that the withdrawal itself brings on such an upheaval of emotions that the patient, as well as the doctor, interprets this emotional response as a necessity to go back on Prozac! Of course the use of the chemical substance that created the withdrawal reaction will certainly stop the withdrawal. Alcohol will stop D.T.'s. So often the reason why many patients state that "Prozac saved my life and I cannot live without it," is that every time they have tried to go without it and have gone into this withdrawal, readministration of the drug has stopped the withdrawal and they feel they have been "saved."

An additional dose of a toxin will stop a toxic reaction. Unfortunately this is only a temporary cessation of the toxic drug reaction. The down side of stopping an adverse reaction this way is that the drug will continue to be toxic to the patient even though it will *temporarily* alleviate the withdrawal symptoms. As the amount of the drug increases within his system, the patient reacting to the higher drug concentrations will have an even stronger reaction the next time he experiences an adverse reaction to the drug. He can also experience an even more severe withdrawal the next time he tries to quit.

Dr. Breggin addresses this issue in his book also, "The questions must be asked, Are we producing permanent symptoms of mental dysfunction, including anxiety, depression, or mania, by giving patients antidepressants? How often do we induce a vicious circle in which patients attempt to come off the medications and then experience withdrawal symptoms that are mistaken for a recurrence of depression or other mental dysfunction - leading to further treatment with the offending medication?" (*TOXIC PSYCHIATRY*, p. 156)

Accumulation may be another indication of the higher possibility of dependence. A Neuropsychopharmacologist, Dr. Bruce Wooley who teaches psychiatrists how to use psychoactive drugs, explains that we have no idea just how long it takes for Prozac to flush out of the system. It is his opinion that it is most likely very long term.

Dr. Karson's research, which we discussed in the last chapter is the strongest support of Dr. Wooley's statement. His results demonstrate that the brain Prozac levels are a hundred times higher than serum levels after using the drug for about six months. He says Prozac "concentrates in the brain and sticks around for a long time." He said that his research would confirm that this accumulation aspect of Prozac would also explain why there are so many reports of delayed withdrawal with Prozac. Patients who have been on the drug for long periods or have been on high doses or have been mixing it with other drugs or have impaired liver function or general poor health, such as a debilitating disease, have a stronger possibility of accumulation. These individuals will often experience delayed withdrawal. It can be several weeks or months before they begin to notice withdrawal symptoms begin to appear. The benzodiazephines are also are known to have a delayed withdrawal action. This can prove to be very confusing for the patient and physician alike as the delayed withdrawal obscures the connection of between Prozac and the withdrawal symptoms. Demanding to know the origin of these symptoms and why they are in such physical and mental pain, the patients go through extensive medical and psychological tests. Many have ended up having surgery to remove various organs suffering trauma from the flushing of the drug from the body. Kidney, bladder, liver and gallbladder problems indicated as a burning pain are reported. The large majority of patients have no knowledge of withdrawal and the symptoms associated with withdrawal. And they certainly have no knowledge of delayed withdrawal. Many physicians are unaware of delayed drug withdrawal. As this delayed withdrawal begins long after discontinuation of the drug and as the "rebound depression" sets in (this medical term refers to the even more intense depression than the initial depression the drug was prescribed for which comes after discontinuation of an anti-depressant), the patients are set up for a "my depression is returning and I must really need Prozac" scenario. What a terrible shame that they do not realize this is all drug-induced and will pass with time. One young man in his mid thirties has been very uncharacteristically aware and alert about his experience. He was prescribed Prozac for something other than depression and had never experienced a bout with depression before his two and one half years of Prozac use. When I asked how he was doing five months after he dropped off Prozac "cold turkey", he replied, "Very well! The unexplained depressions that would hit me for absolutely no reason are now coming only every two weeks instead of every week as they were previously and I am now able to sleep through the entire night again." He explained that he felt confident that things would continue to improve as he got plenty of rest and waited it out. That type of understanding is unfortunately *very rare*. He told me he was appalled to learn how many patients were being mislead to believe that the rebound depression and the withdrawal symptoms were symptoms of a mental disease for which they would need to begin using Prozac or another psychiatric drug to "cure".

Dr. Walter Afield states that it is "amazing and appalling" that doctors are so ignorant of these various aspects of drug use. When we consider the tremendous amounts of drugs utilized in their profession, it should be considered a disgrace that they do not understand or recognize drug reactions or drug interactions or drug withdrawal! Because of this ignorance the vicious cycle begins all over again as the patient is reintroduced to the drug and it becomes even *more disastrous, dangerous and damaging the second, third, etc. time around.*

Additional evidence of addiction and dependence:

2) The patients when faced with possible discontinuation of the drug are defending the drug ["It has saved my life" and "I can't live without it."], even to the point of threatening to kill anyone who takes it from them. Or patients faced with discontinuation by their doctors will change doctors in order to continue their use of the drug.

3) Patients, family, friends and doctors are reporting that the patients are going to two and three doctors to insure they have an ample supply of the drug or "stockpiling," and patients are increasing their own doses and even badgering their doctors to increase the dosage. And many are admitting to falsifying prescriptions in order to continue use of the drug or increase their dose. One patient was stealing from her offering plate at church as it passed in order to fund her Prozac use.

4) Many patients who are using or have discontinued the use of Prozac admit that they were addicted, but confused by the fact that a drug their family physician had given them would be addictive. They claim they did not know what they

should do about it. They wanted help but did not know where to turn because Prozac is not addictive according to most doctors. *As we have just seen from Eli Lilly's own literature (p. 56) there is no evidence for non-addictiveness, but doctors continue to re-affirm this "fact" to their patients - patients who inside are crying out for help and finding it **nowhere**.* Dr. Kramer, speaking of the other anti-depressants, states, "But they have not inspired the sort of enthusiasm and loyalty patients have shown for Prozac." Drug enforcement officials generally would read this "loyalty" as a clear sign of "addiction" or "dependence."

5) A very good source for discovering addictiveness is from the teenage population. And according to reports from teenagers, Prozac is a drug being sold among them as a street drug. They report that it is common knowledge among them just how much Prozac one can take for a "high" without overdosing. Unfortunately, as with other drugs, they do not always get only the "high" they are looking for and often end up in the emergency room of the local hospital with tubes connecting them to a stomach pump.

What do we find when we compare Prozac withdrawal to withdrawal from illegal substances? To gather more information about the typical characteristics and the severity of withdrawal from street drugs in comparison to what I had been having reported to me about withdrawal from Prozac I called Ed Wilson with The Volunteers of America drug detoxification program in Salt Lake City. This was about a year after I began to assist those in trouble on Prozac. After discussing the withdrawal from various street drugs, which almost sounded like a picnic compared to the reports coming in on Prozac withdrawal, he told me that they regularly drop those with addiction to illegal substances right off the drugs, "cold turkey", but he explained that this "cold turkey" approach cannot be taken with the prescription drugs. He stated that this procedure is much too dangerous. *"We will not even deal with the prescription drugs because these people withdrawing from these drugs become far too violent and aggressive for us to handle. They must be monitored closely 24 hours a day and often need to be restrained. We don't have the facilities or capability."*

I was shocked! I struggled in an attempt to catch my breath without gasping out loud as the whole picture came together in my mind. The thought ran through my head, "What a 'con job' we have been given on the issue of illegal drugs vs. prescription drugs!" "Why", I asked him, "wasn't I aware of this before? Why don't others seem to be aware that this is the case? Why is the general public so completely unaware of this situation? Is this whole drug war just a diversion to keep us from realizing how dangerous prescription drugs can be, while giant pharmaceutical companies make their profits off such extremely addictive *legal* drugs, those drugs that you will not even consider in assisting with the detoxification process? Are they just using us and our tax money to win us over to their side of the battle and fight off their competition when their drugs are as deadly or, from what you are telling me, even worse? How can we have this 'Just Say No To Drugs' campaign nationwide and be so completely oblivious to the danger of prescription drugs? Where are these people suppose to turn for help now that they are addicted? Who will help them withdraw if it is as dangerous as you say? The large majority of us know nothing of addictive drugs and how to deal with withdrawal. Why aren't all of you in drug rehabilitation and drug enforcement doing something about this situation if these prescription drugs can be so addictive and dangerous? Why are you not more vocal in alerting the public?" (As you can see, I ask a lot of questions.)

He replied, "You don't understand, it wouldn't do any good for us to try. The pharmaceutical lobbyists are far too powerful. You can't fight them. They have too much influence with the FDA." I asked him if he thought that doctors may be keeping their patients on Prozac because they too are so frightened of dealing with the withdrawal and too busy to take the amount of time involved in the withdrawal process. He replied that he was sure that was the case. He strongly reaffirmed his position on prescription drugs again by stressing that they would not be the least bit interested in dealing with patients coming off Prozac and said goodby.

Yet the misinformation continues to be perpetrated that the drugs in the street are so different from anything we get from a doctor. From a little book on drugs for children we read, "Dope is not for sale in any store. You can't get it from a doctor. Dope is bought from someone called a 'dealer' or a 'pusher' because using, buying, or selling dope is against the law. That doesn't stop some people from using dope. They say *they do it to change the way they feel. Often, that means they are trying to run away from their problems. But when the dope wears off, the problems are still there - and they are often worse than before.*" These are the same reasons people use the psychiatric drugs and they too find that their problems are still there when they come off the drugs, plus they are often addicted to the drugs - drugs with such terribly violent withdrawal that the largest drug withdrawal center in Salt Lake City will not admit them to their program.

Valium was one of the worst prescription drugs for producing severe withdrawal. I was so disturbed by my conversation with Ed Wilson that I immediately called Jiff Wise with Salt Lake County Drug and Alcohol Abuse. My question for Jiff was, "Why Jiff, with all the information I have shared with you over the last couple of years about what is being reported to me by patients on Prozac, have you not told me how far out of line Prozac withdrawal is compared to withdrawal from illegal drugs?" His answer was that he too was so surprised by the reports of withdrawal from Prozac that he still was not quite sure how to respond. He informed me that so far Valium had proven to be the worst for withdrawal they have ever seen and it lasts for about two months. Once again reaffirming that another psychiatric prescription drug has worse withdrawal than the street drugs - drugs we have been led to believe are such a terrible menace to society, while these dangerously addictive prescription drugs come in our back doors through our family physician with ever stronger more addictive effects! (Drs. Phelps and Nourse in their book, *THE HIDDEN ADDICTION,* mention a patient they treated for Valium withdrawal five years after being on Valium only three or four months.)

For those wanting to know more about Valium withdrawal there is an excellent book written by Barbara Gordon about her own experience entitled, *I'M DANCING AS FAST AS I CAN.* A movie by the same title was also made and should be available at your local video store. Here are a few excerpts from her book: "I didn't know why Valium worked when it did, or why it didn't [Barbara was not alone. Researchers proved many years after Valium had been on the market that it did not do what it was assumed to do within the brain. And no one was aware of the terrible withdrawal associated with Valium until years after it hit the market. And now we have discovered that Xanex, which was developed to take the place of Valium because of its very terrible addictive potential, is far more addictive than Valium - one third of the users have been unable to withdraw from it.] Nor did I know that withdrawal from Valium can cause more serious complications than withdrawing from heroin...I was taking thirty milligrams a day and I went off it cold. I didn't know I wasn't supposed to do it that way. I only knew I had to change things, I knew I wanted to stop...I could say no to the pills...In a few days I'd be fine, rested, refreshed, ready to face a new day,...Instead I blew my head open...By early afternoon I began to feel a creeping sense of anxiety. But it was different from my usual bouts of terror. It felt like little jolts of electricity, as if charged pins and needles were shooting through my body. My breathing became rapid and I began to perspire...Restaurants were too noisy, streets too wide, stores to crowded, buildings too tall, elevators too fast. But home, home had to be safe. It couldn't happen here...My scalp started to burn as if I had hot coals under my hair. Then I began to experience funny little twitches, spasms, a jerk of a leg, a flying arm, tiny tremors that soon turned into convulsions. I held on to the bed, trying to relax. It was impossible. I told myself it was just a twenty-four hour withdrawal, that it was nothing. I could take it..." Then she was committed to a mental institution. (What a way to handle drug withdrawal!) "I clutched at the letters and cards I did receive. I read them over and over again...They reminded me of a Barbara I wasn't anymore, reminded me of love and happiness and doing. But I also used them as an affirmation of my being. 'I must be Barbara,' I said to myself (This depersonalization is so difficult for the patient to handle. How often I hear people say, "I'd give anything to be the me before I took Prozac!")...But I still couldn't speak to anyone of the phone, couldn't write back. To respond would mean that I understood what had happened to my life, and I still didn't have a clue to how to put it back together...Besides, how could I care about their lives? I was too sick to care about anything. But the guilt I felt about not caring was enormous." Finally Barbara found a good doctor who put her experience in the proper perspective for her to begin to rebuild her life. "You're going to feel lousy for a while, maybe a long time, but I think you can beat this...*But let me emphasize, you are not psychotic. You had a psychotic reaction to drug withdrawal.* You have a lot of unresolved conflicts, but you could have lived the rest of your life and not ended up in a mental hospital." Barbara Gordon's experience with Valium was very similar to what I hear daily from Prozac patients, except that they report their withdrawal symptoms as lasting far longer.

Does Prozac have a stimulant effect? Fred Gardner noted the symptoms of a stimulant effect in an article for the *ANDERSON VALLEY ADVERTISER*. "Dennis says that whenever he asks somebody if they're on Prozac, it turns out that they are. The obvious symptoms, he says, include 'chatteriness, a phoney self-assurance, almost a braggart-type behavior where they're not willing to stop and listen because they're going a lot faster than we are...Mark S. says: 'It felt as if I had done speed. You take it for a few days and then it kicks in after you've achieved an appropriate blood level. [This is most likely the effect produced when the serotonin level has increased enough to raise the body's steroids.] It was the fourth day that I started feeling it and felt this sensation of acceleration. By the seventh day I was getting ready to explode. I thought they were going to have to scrape me off the roof. I was so wound up. The effect was similar to speed with none of the euphoria that makes speed pleasing. It was just this feeling of impending destruction...'"

This issue of a stimulant profile for Prozac was addressed extensively by the FDA reviewer of Prozac for product safety, Richard Kapit. In an official report dated March, 1986 he stated that, *"fluoxetine's [Prozac] profile of adverse effects more closely resembles that of a stimulant drug..."* He pointed out that this stimulant action of "fluoxetine may negatively affect patients with depression." Mr. Kapit has proved himself correct as the evidence is rapidly proving his observation of the stimulant aspect of Prozac to be correct. His report to the FDA was made before Prozac was approved. Why were physicians and patients not warned about this stimulant effect with subsequent withdrawal? Why was the drug not made a "controlled" substance at that time? A lesson in politics and finance is the most likely place to find the answer to that question. These issues are addressed in the chapter LILLY AND POLITICS.

Dr. Peter Breggin emphatically states that Prozac is a stimulant which produces dependence and addiction and "crashing" (withdrawal) and that the FDA had knowledge of that fact before approving the drug. He points out that the two main criteria in testing for stimulant effects are an energizing effect and an appetite suppression effect and Prozac has both. We quote from the *RIGHTS TENET*: Winter/ Spring 1992, Pg. 4:

THE PROZAC STIMULANT EFFECT

"The Prozac-induced toxicity reported by the survivor groups closely resembles the brain disorders caused by amphetamines and related stimulants such as PCP and cocaine. In the 'Diagnostic and Statistical Manual of Mental Disorders, Third Edition, Revised (DSM III-R)', the 'organic mental syndromes' caused by these stimulants include intoxication 9305.70), delirium (292.81) and delusional disorder (292.11). For example, amphetamine stimulant intoxication is described as follows: "The maladaptive behavioral changes include fighting, grandiosity, hypervigilance, psychomotor agitation, impaired judgment, and impaired social or occupational functioning' (p. 134)."

"...Amphetamine intoxicated patients often develop manic symptoms (p. 135). They also frequently crash into depression with compulsive suicidal behavior (p. 136). These reactions are again characteristic of the Prozac patients. Both amphetamine-like drugs and Prozac produce dependence and addiction."

"As I describe in 'Toxic Psychiatry', the detailed unpublished FDA evaluation of Prozac twice remarks that the drug possesses a 'stimulant profile', meaning that it produces amphetamine-like effects. This would have alerted doctors to the possibility that Prozac carried with it the danger of producing hostility, violence, suicide, agitation, depression, a withdrawal syndrome, addiction and other problems typically associated with stimulants. But the FDA backed down and did not require inclusion of this potentially important warning in the official labeling of the drug."

"Eventually psychiatry and medicine will have to recognize that Prozac

organic mental syndromes (brain disorders) and that the mental effects are similar to those induced by amphetamine-like stimulants. Further delay in recognition of the Prozac stimulant effect will result in considerable harm to patients, their families and any victims of their violent or out-of-control behavior."

Dr. Breggin also just recently had a case report published in the *INTERNATIONAL JOURNAL OF RISK AND SAFETY IN MEDICINE*, (1992)325-328 entitled, "A case of fluoxetine-induced stimulant side effects with suicidal ideation associated with a possible withdrawal reaction ('crashing')". As the title indicates the report discusses the stimulant profile of Prozac and the typical stimulant reactions associated with its use in this particular case. It also discusses the evidence of withdrawal.

Dr. Peter Kramer explains, "It is not unusual for a person beginning to take an antidepressant to experience an amphetamine like effect on the third or fourth day - the feeling of having drunk too much coffee. Often this sensation disappears spontaneously. Sometimes it is necessary to lower the medication dose or to add a second, sedating medication at bedtime or to select a different antidepressant." (*LISTENING TO PROZAC*, p. xi) If the antidepressants are so stimulating as to require the addition of a sedating medication to overcome the strong stimulant effects, is it any wonder that many commit suicides on these medications? It should always be kept in mind that adding a second medication to treat a drug reaction can be dangerous because of possible drug interactions.

The doubling of adrenalin with only one single 30 mg. dose of Prozac demonstrates a strong stimulant effect. We should keep in mind the repercussions of a stimulant effect: "Stimulants like caffeine, amphetamines and cocaine can cause severe damage to the nervous system, liver, kidneys, immune system, adrenal glands, heart and circulatory system. Extreme stimulation of the nervous system, adrenal glands and metabolism creates severe deficiencies of the neurotransmitters, calcium, magnesium, fatty acids, and B vitamins. Heavy users often develop serious mental disorders, including acute paranoia." (*ADDICTIONS, A NUTRITIONAL APPROACH TO RECOVERY*, P. 29) It should seem extremely irrational to be using drugs with a strong stimulant effect to treat mental disorders when in the long run they create mental disorders.

Drugs which produce a stimulant effect although they appear to enhance ability and help depression in short term use, they impair learning and cause increased depression in the long term. Dr. Vernon H. Mark and Jeffery P. Mark, M.Sc. in their book *REVERSING MEMORY LOSS*, p. 78, bring to our attention some very interesting data on stimulants: "Repeated use of stimulants only enhances their negative effects. The elevation of mood proceeds too far, to hyperexcitability, which in turn leads to distraction, not concentration, and consequent difficulty in acquiring new information." They go on to discuss cocaine and bring up some aspects of this drug which are very similar to Prozac. "Cocaine is often used for this purpose, [to reverse depression] especially if the depression is of the bipolar variety called manic-depressive illness. *All too often the euphoria produced by a dose of cocaine is followed by a depression that is much worse than the original one.* [Sugar has the same effect with a hypoglycemic related depression.] The anxiety and hyperactivity associated with cocaine effects, however, may not disappear even when the rebound depression is full-blown. Of course *the effects on every aspect of memory, concentration, and new learning are devastating.* As with amphetamines, cocaine can also lead to *states of increased suspiciousness and even paranoid delusions.*

"Some cocaine users go on to become *aggressive and even dangerous in initiating unprovoked attack behavior.* Their *memories are selectively and sometimes randomly inhibited during these episodes, and they may not remember their actions afterward.*"

It has been reported that Prozac is not considered an acceptable medical treatment by several drug and alcohol treatment centers because of its cocaine-like effects. One young man who had previously used cocaine as well as Prozac in the past and was now actively involved in drug rehabilitation told me, there is no difference in the way you are affected by Prozac or cocaine. The only difference is that Prozac is more powerful than cocaine and more subtle. "Prozac sneaks up on you and you don't know what's happening to you until it's too late." Another young woman who had previous problems with illegal drugs was introduced to Prozac when her father, a licensed social worker, shared his prescription with her. She returned the pills explaining to her father that she could not take the drug because it gave her the same sensation as being on a combination of speed and cocaine.

151

CHAPTER 6

REVERBERATIONS WITHIN THE MEDICAL COMMUNITY

What has been the reaction of the medical community to all this Prozac clamor? As *NEWSWEEK* so accurately stated in their April 1, 1991, article on Prozac, "Antidepressants are not cough drops. Dr. Joseph Lipinski of Harvard Medical School and McLean Hospital likens them to loaded pistols. *They all pose hazards.*" Dr. Frederick K. Goodwin, while director of the Alcohol, Drug Abuse and Mental Health Administration, a psychiatrist, said, in the August 16, 1990, issue of *THE NEW YORK TIMES,* "*But this is a powerful drug, and any powerful drug will have powerful side effects. The backlash effect of all this adverse publicity probably will lead to a correction that won't hurt.*" In the January/February 1991 issue of *IN HEALTH* Dr. Jere Goyan, who is the head of the school of pharmacy for the University of California at San Francisco and a former FDA commissioner stated, "Some people misconstrue the word 'safe' in 'safe and effective' as meaning no potential harm, but when you're talking about drugs, safety is always relative."

Dr. John Tilden has said, "Not one [physician] can say with any certainty that the drug he prescribes will have the action he hopes to experience. *Not one can tell, after the first 24 hours of medication whether the symptoms presenting themselves are those of disease proper or are due to the drug.*" Apparently this is exactly what we are witnessing with Prozac - a chemically induced insanity. It seems we have created a new disease, "Prozaculosis", with its own specific symptomatic profile - all of which are emotional side-effects of this drug. Logic should lead us to believe that if we are dealing with a drug that directly affects the neurotransmitter, serotonin, which in turn determines activity in the mood center of the brain, that the side effects would naturally be *primarily emotional* rather than physical with this drug. Yet few families or close friends of patients are even encouraged to watch for emotional reactions in a patient on Prozac.

Dr. Martin Teicher began bringing to the attention of mental health practitioners these severe emotional reactions to Prozac in a 1990 published report to the AMERICAN JOURNAL OF PSYCHIATRY. These patients Teicher observed, "developed intense, violent, suicidal preoccupation". Although several had contemplated suicide before starting on Prozac, none had experienced this intensely powerful compulsion to self-destruct. Some became obsessed with specifically violent methods: blowing their brains out, driving into bridge abutments, turning on gas ovens to blow up their

152

apartments. In October 1990 Teicher stated in an article in *AMERICAN HEALTH*, "As a scientist, it's easy to remain skeptical and say it hasn't been proved, one should rechallenge these patients with Prozac and see if it happens again. But that would be largely unethical...Those who develop the extreme reaction seem very strange when they're on this medication - their thoughts are so intrusive, and completely out of character. Some of these patients I've known five or six years and I've never known them to be this way before. Take them off the drug and they say 'How could I have thought that way? Boy, I was really feeling strange on that medication.' As a clinician, *I do feel it's some strange adverse response to the medication, and not just a coincidence.*"

Teicher said this *suicidal obsession* *"was unlike anything they had ever experienced either before or since.* It really seemed to be something out of the expected pattern...While they were on the medication it became an *irresistible impulse*." Perhaps this observation of an irresistible impulse would explain why the large majority of those patients who commit suicide on Prozac do not tend to show signs of depression, instead they appear happy and jovial just before taking their own lives. It comes on suddenly, without warning. *Just at the time when patients are planning for the future and psychiatrists would not believe they would consider taking their own life is exactly when someone on Prozac does.* A pharmaceutical rep was in a hotel in Belgium eating dinner and visiting with friends, laughing and joking, when he excused himself, went to the seventh floor, put a gun to his head and pulled the trigger. A mother was fixing dinner when she stopped to hang herself. Although it often follows a warm flush throughout the body oran outburst of anger (another clear sign of an adrenalin rush), most families report that there was just no warning. In fact Teicher pointed out that "No patient was actively suicidal at the time fluoxetine [Prozac] treatment began. Rather *all were hopeful and optimistic...*"

A quote from the above reports' conclusion indicates the researchers' amazement at what they found, "A great deal has been written on the possible role of serotonin in violence, suicide, and obsessive behavior, and fluoxetine [Prozac] is known to be a potent and selective serotonergic uptake inhibitor. Given this background, *we were especially surprised to witness the emergence of intense, obsessive, and violent suicidal thoughts in these patients. Their suicidal thoughts appear to have been obsessive as they were recurrent, persistent, and intrusive. They emerged without reason but were the patient's own thoughts. It was also remarkable how violent these thoughts were.*"

These are researchers from one of the finest medical facilities in the country. These are doctors who regularly are involved in these types of studies who are expressing shock and amazement at the results of their own study. But it is shocking and amazing to see the intensity of the violence as these reports come in from patients and their friends and families, no matter how many times you hear them. Each story is unbelievably violent and ever more shocking. The suicides almost always involve a gunshot wound, generally to the head. Other reports list patients stabbing and slashing themselves to death, jumping off high buildings, throwing themselves in front of trains, trucks or cars, or lying down on train tracks or freeways, hanging, burning themselves alive, zipping themselves up in a plastic bag and spraying it full of Raid, etc. All generally tend to be violent and/or bizarre.

Teicher and his colleagues went on to recommend that, "the practitioner be attentive to the possible emergence of suicidal ideation, even in those patients without a previous history of suicidal thoughts or actions. Patients who have previously been treated with other antidepressants or who develop intense fatigue, hypersomnia, or restlessness while taking fluoxetine [Prozac] may be at risk."

What is akathisia and what connection does it have to violence and suicide? The reason the restlessness Dr. Teicher refers to above poses a risk is because it is indicative of a more intense form of restlessness known as akathisia (Opler, 1991). This is a drug-induced insanity brought on by a number of various psychoactive drugs including Prozac and the other SSRIs. Akathisia is a Greek term signifying "can't sit down". It is an urgent need of movement" or "a vague disturbing inner restlessness" that brings on severe anxiety. The patients report experiencing an inner "jitteriness" or muscle quivering, mental and physical restlessness - constantly racing thoughts coupled with an inability to sit or rest, feeling "driven" non-stop. They often express that they can "feel no peace." It is often associated with strong feelings of terror, hostility, anger or rage which produce extremely violent behavior. Inner jitteriness or muscle quivering, mental and physical restlessness, constant movement, aggression, rage, hostility, anger, self-destructive outbursts, anxiety, somatic complaints, constant movement, terror, hatred, violence, feelings of impending loss of mental control, increased psychotic symptoms, hallucinations, etc., are all signs of akathisia. The increasing feelings of hostility are often very puzzling to the patient. These feelings of hostility can progress to violent physical attacks. Patients begin to believe they are going insane and attempt to find reason for their chemically induced hostility. They often assign blame to others for these feelings leading to false accusations toward others, generally those closest to the patient.

Akathisia is somewhat difficult to detect and is often overlooked in diagnosis.

Dr. Jerome L. Schulte states in the *AMERICAN JOURNAL OF FORENSIC PSYCHIATRY*, 1985, Vol. 6, p. 3-7, *"Homicide and Suicide Associated With Akathisia and Haloperidol [Haldol],"* that akathisia is "the least understood and appreciated side-effect" of psychoactive drugs. *Akathisia can be extremely dangerous and it is very critical that this side effect not go unrecognized. It is often intermittent, switching on and off again (a transient psychosis), and although a common side effect, it is all too often overlooked, endangering the lives of the patient and those around him or her* (Crowner et al.). Without education about this serious side-effect patients do not recognize that akathisia is being produced by the medication they are taking and do not seek treatment. Instead they rationalize this drug-induced anger and aggression by assigning blame to someone near them and focus the rage toward them. If their ability to be alert or astute has not been fully chemically cut off when akathisia is experienced, they recognize these feelings as strange and puzzling and they begin to believe they are going insane. The previous study points out that many doctors also very often confuse akathisia with other psychiatric complaints and do not recognize the symptoms as being drug-induced. The doctors, therefore, do not take the proper steps to remedy the situation by discontinuing the drug which is causing the akathisia.

Unfortunately the large majority of physicians cause a intensification of an akathisia reaction by prescribing additional drugs to treat the symptoms of akathisia. This treating a drug with a drug is far too common a practice, especially when akathisia is experienced in withdrawal. When the patient is prescribed additional drugs to "cure" what is actually a drug reaction he becomes a patient caught up in an endless cycle of psychiatric drugs being prescribed for one drug-induced reaction after another. Or he ends up in prison for an action taken which he has no logical explanation for and often has little recall of the incident. This is more especially the case when additional drugs are given for akathisia during withdrawal when doctors are not suspecting a continuum of drug reactions. Yet we now know that the reactions can continue long-term and the effects of additional drugs are often magnified.

This violence producing side-effect of akathisia has not been given the attention it deserves. It is extremely dangerous. There are reports in medical literature of terribly violent crimes being attributed to akathisia. For instance, a psychiatrist from the Washington School of Medicine, Dr. Walter Keckich, related a case about a male patient who became uncontrollably agitated. The report, made in 1978, was titled, "Violence as a Manifestation of Akathisia." He experienced "violent urges to assault anyone near him" and attempted to kill his dog - all was attributed to the drug reaction of akathisia.

The *JOURNAL OF CLINICAL PSYCHOPHARMACOLOGY* included a case report by psychiatrist M. Katherine Shear, et al., 1983, of two suicides that were thought to be brought on by akathisia-like symptoms from a neuroleptic drug.

THE AMERICAN JOURNAL OF FORENSIC PSYCHIATRY, 1985, Vol. 6, No. 2, pgs. 3-7, described five cases of violence which were attributed to akathisia. In one of the cases a man who had been taken to an emergency room suffering paranoia and disorganized behavior was given an injection of the psychiatric tranquilizer, Haldol. He ran out of the emergency room, totally disrobed and then within the next 45 minutes he assaulted and attempted to rape a woman on the street. He was stopped by the woman's husband, then broke down the door of an 81 year old woman, he attacked her while she was sleeping and beat and stabbed her to death. He was sprayed with maze as he exited through the front door, turned and ran out the back door, started stabbing another woman in front of her child, left her and began stabbing another before he was stopped. This last victim suffered the loss of an eye and a colostomy as a result of her wounds.

It took eight officers to subdue the patient. He described feeling as though he were watching himself in a movie, with no sense of caring about anyone nor any feeling of physical sensation. The study calls this an evidence of the side-effect of akathisia. It goes on to mention a second patient who repeatedly stabbed a grocer and a third patient suffering akathisia who beat his mother to death with a hammer. The study concludes that *akathisia is "the least understood and appreciated side-effect" of psychoactive drugs, warning clinicians to be careful about ruling out its presence.*

The same year psychiatrist Robert E. Drake reported on two more akathisia related suicide attempts. Both patients felt that because their mental conditions had so rapidly deteriorated, their lives were "no longer worth living." Yet the deterioration of their mental condition was akathisia.

A 1986 report published in the *JOURNAL OF CLINICAL PSYCHOPHARMACOLOGY* linked akathisia to suicidal and homicidal thoughts in a double-blind clinical trial.

Then in 1990 the *PSYCHOPHARMACOLOGY BULLETIN* published a two-year study on akathisia and its association with violence. They found a higher incidence rate of akathisia among those who commit violent acts.

Another example attributed to akathisia is the case of David Peterson in Connecticut who walked out of a mental institution, bought a hunting knife and

156

started stabbing the first person he saw, a nine year old girl. He stabbed her 34 times, killing her. He stated that he had done this for revenge against his psychiatrist who would not change his medication which was causing him pain.

What percentage of patients experience akathisia as a result of Prozac or the other SSRIs? Teicher had *four out of six patients* in his 1990 report develop akathisia. *THE JOURNAL OF CLINICAL PSYCHIATRY* reported in the September 1989 issue a study by Lipinski, Mallya, Zimmerman and Pope in which they discussed five cases of akathisia associated with Prozac. The report states that it is appearing that Prozac is converting a nonagitated depression to agitated depression and that agitated depression and severe akathisia are indistinguishable. They indicated that their observance of the incidence of akathisia induced by Prozac is a rate of 10 - 25% of the patients - up to one fourth of the patients. Although Lilly admits that akathisia is a side-effect of Prozac, they claim the incidence rate is only 1%, not even close to what studies are showing after Prozac gained its FDA approval for marketing. Lipinski who headed this study is one of the top researchers in the country and his figures would classify akathisia as a"common" side effect of both Prozac and the other SSRIs. The rage and violent feelings are often refereed to by the patients as: "indescribable," "an anger unlike I have ever felt before," "after only two weeks on Paxil I cannot believe I did not kill myself or someone else."

The akathisia incidence rate associated with the SSRIs could prove to be much, much higher over time if our history with other psychoactive drugs is any indicator. It has been shown now that up to one half of those taking the neuroleptic drugs which have been on the market for many years experience akathisia. It is a common side effect of these drugs. In the study we just mentioned Dr. Lipinski reported an akathisia rate of 71% in the patients at Boston's McLean Hospital who are suffering from this side-effect, which, if not recognized and treated immediately in the beginning stages, can result in disastrous and tragic results. A leading researcher in tranquilizer addiction, Dr. Carl Essig of the Addiction Research Center of the National Institute of Mental Health, has said that many tranquilizers must be considered "drugs of addiction" and told the American Association for the Advancement of Science in 1963 they *"can lead to violent behavior."* Van Putten et al. cite studies which demonstrate that akathisia leads to suicidal ideation and/or homicidal thought. They refer to this as a "behavioral toxicity" produced by the mind altering drugs.

Dr. Barbara Geller, psychiatrist, from the University of South Carolina reported that she had to abruptly terminate a Prozac study in adolescent patients because of the emergence of intense violent suicidal and/or homicidal ideation which appeared de novo (appearing for the first time, not a pre-existing condition) in a staggering five out of eight patients. Many experts feel that these intense suicidal and homicidal feelings are caused by the side-effect of akathisia. This study would certainly indicate an extremely high incidence of akathisia. We must keep in mind though that these drugs generally have a somewhat stronger impact upon adolescents.

Dr. William C. Wirshing, psychiatrist, in a report entitled, *"Floxetine [Prozac] and Suicidality, A Consequence of Akathisia"* addressed the issue of Prozac producing this dangerous psychiatric side effect and concluded that akathisia was the cause for contemplation of suicide in these patients. He and his colleagues state, "We have observed the development of agitation...pacing, and internal sense of desperation, and suicidal ideation."

Another report entitled, "Reexposure to Fluoxetine After Serious Suicide Attempts by Three Patients: The Role of Akathisia", was made to the *JOURNAL OF CLINICAL PSYCHIATRY* 52:12 in December, 1991 from McLean Hospital at Harvard. It appears to be one of the most conclusive case studies yet in indicating that Prozac actually is chemically inducing these self destructive behaviors. Three patients who had previously made a serious suicide attempt while on Prozac and did not die were re-introduced to the drug. Once again each of those patients became *intensely suicidal*. (This is the type of test Dr. Teicher mentioned above stating that it would be the best evidence to conclude that these behaviors are actually "drug induced" behaviors.) These patients noticed the feelings produced by the side-effect "akathisia" associated with the suicidal impulse they were experiencing and recalled that these same feelings were manifested just before their first suicide attempt as well. *Patients experiencing akathisia in precipitation of a suicide attempt relate that they had no desire to die but would have done anything to escape these totally intolerable drug-induced feelings.* The study concludes that the reason for suicide in Prozac patients is this side-effect of akathisia repeatedly reported by the patients and known to be produced by the drug.

Masand, Gupta and Dewan, 1991, Department of Psychiatry State University of New York Health Science Center, Syracuse, New York, reported two patients who became intensely suicidal on Prozac. Although depressed, neither had and history of suicidal ideation or attempt. One, a 58 year old man with a 13 year history of depression, attempted suicide by hanging *only three days* after starting on only one capsule (20 mg.) of Prozac daily. Four days after medication was discontinued his suicidal thoughts disappeared. The other patient, a 28 year old woman suffered intense akathisia while receiving Prozac and Xanex (alprazolam) for depression and bulimia. She began fantasizing about jumping out the hospital window one week after her Prozac dosage was raised from one pill (20 mg.) to three pills (60 mg.). Ten days after discontinuing both medications her suicidal thoughts also disappeared.

In Vol 49, July, 1992 issue of *ARCHIVES OF GENERAL PSYCHIATRY,* akathisia associated with Prozac is further discussed in another study. It states: *"akathisia has been associated with psychotic exacerbation and deterioration, medication non-compliance, and homicidal and suicidal behaviors. "* The letter to the editor which introduces the report reads: "We thank Drs. Mann and Kapur for their thoughtful and cogent treatment of the antidepressant-suicidality question. Their central neurochemical hypothesis was that *fluoxetine [Prozac] (or any selective serotonergic reuptake blocker) might cause the presynaptic serotonergic neuron to temporarily decrease its firing rates. Such temporary serotonergic hypofunction would, in effect, leave the patient more susceptible to depression and subsequent suicidal ideation.* The return of the depressive symptoms after experimental depletion of the serotonin precursor could be cited in support of the conjecture. However, the reemergence of original depressive symptoms or 'relapse' contrasts sharply with the presentation *of our patients who became suicidal during treatment with fluoxetine...None had a history of significant suicidal behavior; all described their distress as an intense and novel somatic emotional state; all reported an urge to pace that paralleled the intensity of the distress; all experienced suicidal thoughts at the peak of their restless agitation; and all experienced a remission of their agitation, restlessness, pacing urge, and suicidality after the fluoxetine was discontinued..."*

In November 1992 Hamilton et al. reported "adrenergic as well as dopaminergic and serotonergic mechanisms have been suggested as possible mechanisms for akathisia." These researchers conclude that the suicidal ideation reported by Prozac patients is not true suicidal ideation produced by depression, but is actually the side effect of akathisia produced by the drug. As we have already demonstrated that Prozac impacts each one of these mechanisms, it should be easy to see why it would most certainly produce akathisia. These researchers go on to note that Prozac in combination with the neuroleptic drugs (Haldol, Thorazine, Mellaril, etc.) will produce an increase in akathisia, Parkinson's, etc.

Prozac patients report these akathisia type reactions. The large majority of patients who begin to have paradoxical or adverse reactions to Prozac or one of the other SSRIs report this feeling of intense anger, aggression or rage and often associate those feelings with suicide attempts. A small handful of the many many examples (many have filed lawsuits) which demonstrate akathisia type reactions associated with Prozac use follow:

In Dane County, Wisconsin, in January of 1989, Catherine Rouse killed a friend and then committed suicide while on Prozac.

In that same month in Arizona James Bulfin shot and killed one and wounded two who were attempting to rescue him from a suicide attempt.

In April 1989 Abbie Hoffman of anti-Vietnam War fame committed suicide on Prozac.

Rebecca McStoots shot her doctor while on Prozac in March of 1990.

While attempting suicide after only ten days on Prozac Jiff Fortin shot himself in the head and arm in August 1990.

April of 1991 Tucker Moneymaker, of Halifax, Virginia, came home to find that his wife had shot and killed both of their sons and then turned the gun on herself, inflicting two gunshot wounds to her stomach. She had been on Prozac only three weeks.

That same month in San Diego County, California Hank Adams, a former sheriff's deputy also on Prozac murdered his wife and committed suicide in front of one of their five children.

November 1991 in Kittery, Maine Freda Howard murdered her husband with an ax, set her house on fire and then killed herself by a self inflicted gunshot. Blood tests revealed she was on Prozac at the time of the murder/suicide.

Seventeen-year-old Tracy Ann Ingstrom went through a dramatic change in personality after two months of Prozac use. Completely out of character she began verbally and even physically attacking friends and driving wildly. On January 24, 1991 she had one of these heated arguments with her boyfriend, drove home, kicked down a locked bedroom door and tore her parents bedroom apart until she found a gun and used it to kill herself by a gunshot to the mouth. Her father Rick, an investigator for the California Bar Association, says her "act was quick and violent and one that she would never, ever have thought of committing prior to taking the Prozac."

Barbara Wilson's experience gives us a lot of insight into the inner thoughts and feelings of someone experiencing this type of reaction. She had been prescribed Prozac for a hormone related depression following a hysterectomy. While yet in the hospital she felt compulsively suicidal and attempted to jump from the window, burn herself and hang herself. She describes these akathisia-like feelings, "I began pacing and racing. I felt strong as a locomotive. I felt like I could crash through the walls or fly. I started to try to kill myself...taking every opportunity to use blood pressure cuffs, cords, and electrical cords to strangle myself, and towels from the bathroom and shower curtains around my face and just bizarre things."

April 28, 1992 Kenneth Seguin slashed the wrists of his two children (5 and 7 years of age) after drugging them and taking them to a pond. After dumping their bodies in the water he drove home and hacked his wife to death with an axe while she slept.

The beautiful setting of San Luis Obispo and Morrow Bay, California became a holocaust in November of 1992 when Lynwood Drake, III shot and killed six before taking his own life.

March, 1993 in Kaanapali, Maui, Hawaii after only 10 days on Prozac as a treatment for Xanex induced depression William Forsyth stabbed to death his wife after 37 years of marriage. He then stabbed himself to death. After the third day he had begged to be hospitalized because he didn't want to do something strange and he didn't feel like himself. The hospital released him after five days. The following day he and his wife were dead. His actions were shocking to all who knew him. His son who spent the evening before the incident was completely bewildered. As so many other sons have declared of their fathers in almost identical instances, "My dad loved life and his family, he was a wonderful man of great character and integrity." All who knew the couple believed it must have been a double homicide and recommended a search for the murderer.

In Chelsea, Michigan in December of 1993, Stephen Leith walked into a school meeting and began shooting. He killed the school superintendent and wounded two others. He was found later calmly doing paperwork at his desk.

Over a nine month period in Dallas County, Texas their were 27 cases reported to the medical examiner with fluoxetine present. The proportion of suicide seemed to be "extremely high" (Bost, 1992). These researchers point out that the means of suicide were of particular note. The large majority of two thirds choose the violent means of a firearm. They state, "These data show that suicide occurs

161

in a significant proportion of people who die while taking antidepressant drugs. However, *it is apparent that the proportion taking fluoxetine and committing suicide is higher by an amount to be of concern to medical examiners and also to health care providers...The present report provides evidence that suicide has occurred more frequently in patients taking fluoxetine than in those taking tricyclic antidepressants...the possibility that fluoxetine has induced the idea of suicide must be considered. Furthermore, it is apparent that physicians prescribing fluoxetine must be cognizant of the possible association, must be cautious in prescribing the drug.* "

The evidence of this akathisia-like reaction will become very apparent in conjunction with Prozac use as we progress further into this chapter and discuss in detail a March 1991 study out of Yale. Let's listen to what patients are reporting in their own words to describe these feelings:

A caller on a radio show described it very well: "For the first month, two months, it worked real good. Instead of having a lot of thought, you know, like a barrage all the time, getting on my nerves, interfering with my work and what not, it smoothed it out. I didn't get excited. But then progressively instead of having the anxiety I would have had without any kind if medication, this stuff in time started to create a feeling of anger that was different than any other type of anger I've ever felt. It was really subtle and as time went on I got to where I could feel it coming on. It started to become kind of frightening. I would envision myself doing things I didn't want to do. It seemed to be real good, better than the rest. I didn't have any kind of sleeping problem, like being too sleepy, but the thing that was strange was this intense feeling of anger. I kept taking it. I thought it was just me or something, but it was totally unlike any other feeling I've ever had. I've been angry before, everybody has, but this type of anger was red hot! It was a type of feeling like something was taking over my mind. It made me feel feelings that I would never feel otherwise, feelings of doing unreasonable things. Like it would be reasonable if somebody got mad at me and I in turn would get irritated with them. But with this *I found myself just getting mad for absolutely no reason at all*. At first it had just kind of smoothed out my thinking so I wasn't interrupted during my work, but then in time it was like a monkey on my back! One thing I've noticed since I've been on this medicine that I haven't had for many years is the rages. But I have eaten lot more cookies and stuff like that since I've been on that. The urge for sweetness is definitely there. Stiffness in the muscles like charley horses and stuff."

"I was happy one minute, horribly depressed the next minute and very angry the ¬xt, with no apparent reason for any of these feelings."

162

"My husband had a hot temper before, but he never scared me. On Prozac the temper was indescribable! He really frightened me! I was afraid that if I said something, he would explode. I'd seen him get mad at me before, but never like that!"

"I'm constantly moving around and trying to find something to do. I haven't cut myself before. I have thought about it. I have a razor blade that I keep in my room just in case I decide to use it. I am really defiant too. People will tell me not to do something and I will go right out and do it anyway."

"They have me taking Prozac twice a day now since I saw my psychiatrist a couple of days ago. It seems like it will pick me up really fast for a while and then about the middle of the day it drops me down even faster. Then when I get mad it does not seem to stop and I get really mad really fast!"

"I was getting madder by the day. I hit the wall and I probably wouldn't have cared if I'd hit my wife. And we have been happily married for twenty years. That's the sad thing, you just don't give a hoot about what you are doing."

"My wife told me that while she was on Prozac she could have killed me once or twice. Yet she is the most gentle, kind and sympathetic person I've ever known in my life! Contrary to what Lily would have to say about it, it was not a pre-existing condition. Everybody has ups and downs and depression and so forth, but this is different. This is a thousand times worse than the original problem they took the Prozac for to begin with."

"I found that the Prozac was making me more angry. I just started going around looking for fights and stuff and I am not a violent person. I was on Prozac for about four or five months total. I felt good for about the first six weeks. I guess then all of a sudden things started getting crazy, really crazy. I mean nuts! I was acting like I wanted to kill people. I mean not just normal reactions, I wanted to go out there and break their necks. I was getting to the point where I thought I might. But it didn't make any sense. You see I am agoraphobic and when you are agoraphobic you are afraid of everybody. You don't want to hurt anyone cause you are afraid of everyone."

A nurse in Southern California put it this way, "I wanted to hide. I felt so drained. I didn't want to be around anyone. I especially did not want to be around someone who might require something of me because that might just be enough to push me over the edge and set me off." (an excellent example of the inability to control adrenalin levels or the activation of the "fight or flight" response)

163

"I always had a mask on that was smiling, but what was going on inside of me was indescribably horrifying!"

"The anger I felt was so intense!"

"I thought the entire world was out of line and I was the only one who was okay. I really thought I was Superman!"

"After two months on Prozac I had a terrible nightmare that involved me dismembering someone! Never have I experienced anything like that before! That was enough for me! I told my doctor I wasn't about to put up with that kind of side effect and I was getting off the stuff. His solution was that he wanted me to double my dose of Prozac!!! Can you believe it? I am so glad I got off it when I did!"

"I would wake up each morning thinking, 'Oh God, I'm still alive! I have to live another day of this hell of wanting to die!' I thought of running into trees at a high rate of speed."

"I traveled across the country to visit my family then spent all three days I had planned to visit barricaded in the basement. I told the whole family that if any one of them came near me I knew I would kill them. I couldn't stand having those feelings!"

"During the month I spent on Prozac I could think of nothing but various ways of killing those closest to me - my family, my mom, my dad and my brothers and sisters. (A very sweet and sensitive 14 year old girl who took herself off Prozac because of these thoughts it was causing her.)

"I found that I was blaming the person I loved the most, my husband, for this terrible upheaval of emotions. I took everything out on him. How could I have ever treated him the way I did?!"

"When my wife reached the point where she was sitting in our front window trying to decide which passerby to shoot, she finally realized that she had to get off prozac. Being frightened by the drug-induced rage she was feeling, she dropped off the drug 'cold turkey' and two weeks into withdrawal she committed suicide."

"On Prozac, my whole personality did a complete change. I started becoming intentionally self-destructive although I didn't know why and I didn't care. As my behavior got stranger and more destructive, the doctor didn't see that the behavior changes were due to the drug, and he increased the dosage from one to two and then to an occasional third a day."

"I became obsessed with hurting myself and developed an obsession with guns and knives."

"I felt I had to kill myself but I could not leave my family alone. I planned how I would accomplish the deaths of my husband and children in detail. How could I ever have had such thoughts?!"

"I was furious all the time!"

"Throughout my life I have always been known as 'Mr. Mellow,' but the rage I felt on Prozac helped me to understand how someone could murder another."

"Not many weeks after starting on prozac, I was visiting with a neighbor and I thought, 'I wonder what it would be like to pick up that yardstick and hit her up the side of the head'. My thoughts were just so odd!!!"

"Everything felt like a personal attack!"

"I felt there was something bad inside of me and cutting myself with razor blades would let it out. So instead of me doing the cutting myself I became heavily involved in plastic surgery so someone else would cut me up."

"I became obsessed with dying. I thought dying was the only way out, and I never contemplated suicide before that time."

"After taking only one pill I sat with my arms wrapped around me the rest of the day to stop myself from doing anything to my children! Needless to say, I never ever took a second pill!"

"Wicked! That's exactly how you feel on Prozac, wicked, just plain wicked!"

"It worked okay at first. I seemed to have more energy and felt okay but after about six weeks it turned on me. I was mad but I didn't know why! It was like a monkey on my back! I felt a rage unlike anything I have ever felt before or since."

"I threw all caution to the wind. I started doing many life threatening things, i.e., driving at high speeds, participating in life-threatening sports, exposing myself to aids, etc. I thought I was invincible!"

"Nothing mattered to me, especially my life or anyone else's. I didn't care about anyone or anything!"

"Someone snoring was reason enough to commit murder when I was on Prozac!"

"I felt possessed!"

"I have been off Prozac for three years and still have thoughts of stabbing and slashing when I see a sharp object! Never in my life have I had such disturbing thoughts! Just today I was dicing potatoes while my little boy was playing with blocks on the floor nearby. The picture of stabbing him in the back over and over again kept flashing through my mind. The feelings were so intense I had to throw down the knife and leave the room. This was the third such incidence today and its been three long years!! How long can this go on?!!!"

"I would lay in bed and think of things I could do to hurt myself. I hurled myself down stairs, poured boiling water on myself and beat myself in the face, cut myself, and last week I even ran over my own arm with my car!"

"After being on Prozac for one week I had an argument with another motorist and attempted to run over him with my car!"

"I got to the point that I was mad, but I didn't know who I was mad at, and I took a ballpoint pen and tried to stab my wife. I was not aware that there was anything wrong with me, only those living in my house could see it."

"How anyone on Prozac can hold a marriage together is a puzzle to me! I became so rude, distant, arrogant, aggressive, so easily offended by what I interpreted as personal attacks, etc., that I lost or cut off my husband, family and most of my friends."

"I became enraged and despondent. I was hostile and aggressive toward my family and friends. I was obsessed with killing myself. The muscle spasms and suicidal despair continue. As each day goes by, I seem to be relieved of some symptoms and bothered by others. My primary concern is the hostility, because that's not my nature and I don't like having it in my life."

Later on in this chapter we will discuss in detail a Yale study published in

March, 1991 psychiatrists at Yale Medical School's Child Study Center where researchers observed the incidence of intense self-destructive thoughts in adolescents on Prozac who were given the drug because of obsessive - compulsive disorders. Dr. Robert King and Dr. Mark Riddle led the research and believe that the disruption of serotonin production by Prozac *"may directly affect the brain's ability to regulate aggression"*. When we consider the fact that when used on a regular basis it more than doubles the flow of adrenalin, the fight or flight hormone, that concept is certainly easy to believe. What on earth are we setting ourselves up for if one of the most popular drugs on the market is affecting the patient's ability to regulate aggression? How many more jails, prisons, morgues, etc, will we need to cope with this type of situation?

Various mind altering drugs can distort orientation toward the immediate present and cause disregard for long range consequences of his/her behavior thereby making it difficult for him/her to premeditate criminal acts. Yet these drugs can also produce a tendency to react strongly to sensory stimuli in the immediate environment, and develop an inclination to refer everything to oneself that often develops into paranoia, all this combined with the need to move or do something due to intense psychomotor stimulation can all produce an aggression-prone individual leading to the serious akathisia type reactions.

Akathisia needs to be addressed in far more depth than it has previously in conjunction with the violence associated with Prozac or any other psychiatric "medication". This type of drug reaction is one that the public has generally associated only with illegal drugs, not with prescription drugs.

Deseryl, the tricyclic antidepressants, the neuroleptics, monoamine oxidase inhibitors (MAO's) and the new group of serotonin uptake inhibitors (Prozac, Zoloft, Paxil, Lovan, Luvox, etc.) are all known to produce this potentially violent form of inner restlessness known as akathisia. All of these drugs powerfully enhance serotonergic and/or noradrenergic transmission. Some researchers believe that akathisia is caused by an enhancement of the adrenergic receptors in the brain activating the fight or flight response, or as in the case of the drugs which affect serotonin, the 5HT serotonin enhances dopamine release (Yi et al. 1991; Blandina et al. 1989). When serotonergic transmission is enhanced, that in turn is believed to inhibit the dopaminergic neurons. Akathisia would then be produced when the dopaminergic neurotransmission is impaired. As we learned in discussing the effects of higher levels of serotonin upon the glandular system, higher serotonin levels consistently increase the blood levels of ACTH and the adrenalin, cortisol. We also know that serotonin stimulates the hypothalamus/adrenal/cortical axis which, in turn, causes adrenal releases, ie.

167

"an enhancement of the adrenergic system" (Fuller 1981; Stark et al. 1985; Lesieur et al. 1985). It also bears repeating that *one single dose of 30 mg. of Prozac clearly doubles cortisol (adrenalin) levels (Petraglia et al. 1984).* If one single dose causes this drastic rise in adrenalin, the fight or flight reaction, what kind of increase can be expected when Prozac is used in more than one single dose as patients take it on a daily basis? Prozac has also been demonstrated to increase the release of CRF (Gibbes and Vale 1983), indicating an accompanying increase in ACTH and cortisol levels. This excess adrenalin or adrenalin rush would explain the "warm flush" (similar to the hot flashes brought on by menopause as the hormones become imbalanced) which patients so often report feeling just before committing murder or other violent acts or a suicide attempt while on Prozac.

As I said before, from the beginning it appeared obvious to me that Prozac was causing elevated levels of adrenalin (epinephrine) to activate the "fight or flight" response which, in turn, produced the feelings of uncontrollable rage patients were reporting. The information we have reviewed thus far should make it quite clear that if the corticosteroids are stimulated that the adrongenic steroids are as well. For instance, it has long been known that higher levels of testosterone will induce violent behavior (Maccoby & Jacklin, 1974; Moyer, 1974). A study done by Kreuz and Rose, 1972, discovered a significant correlation between the testosterone levels and violence among prisoners. The five with the highest steroid levels had a combined total of two murders, one attempted murder, one assault, and four armed robberies which they had committed. A more recent and even wider study of over 4000 military men found that those with higher steroid levels more frequently committed assault, abused alcohol and other drugs, were absent without leave and in general ended up in more trouble (Dabbs & Morris, 1990).

These many reports from patients about "feeling like a teenager again" should be a clear sign that hormones are being affected, ie., "I thought and acted just like a teenager again. At forty-five I grew my hair long and put psychedelic designs all over my car! I even grew a duck tail and bleached it blonde! I was very defiant toward everyone and about everything. No one could get anywhere with me. You couldn't tell me anything because 'I knew it all'!" Much has been written and many medical studies completed which link these feelings and behaviors we generally associate with adolescence to hormone levels. The parent of any teenager can relate to the behavioral problems produced by hormonal imbalances brought on during puberty - the cause for much stress and distress in many a family and many a teenager. Hormones alter temperament. From the time that researchers first looked at steroids as an answer for mental disorders they have felt that the "stress hormone" cortisol would be discovered to be the biochemical link between stress and depression. Dr. Peter Kramer discusses the importance of stress hormone levels (adrenalin, cortisol, etc.) in depression, suicide and violence "...not only depression but also temperament rests on and is sustained by levels of neurotransmitters and stress hormones...Indeed, we should be surprised if a medicine that resets the norepinephrine and serotonin systems does *not* directly alter temperament." *(LISTENING TO PROZAC*, p. 175) As we have already mentioned,, there is an increasing body of evidence to suggest that any drug which affects serotonin will affect the noradrenergic (norepinephrine) system (Frances et al. 1987; Manier et al. 1987; Potter et al. 1985).

Further evidence that increased adrenal stimulation is the key to understanding this side effect of akathisia is the fact that Inderal (propanalol), a high blood pressure medication which blocks the adrenalin flow, is the most widely recommended treatment in conjunction with dropping or lowering the dose of the medication which is chemically stimulating the rise. Lipinski, et al., suggest that if treatment other than discontinuation of the medication inducing akathisia is necessary, anti-akathisia treatment with various benzodiazephines, a standard treatment for akathisia, or propranolol (Inderal), may prove beneficial. Yet, in the interval between their research and the present, Prozac patients have consistently reported many serious adverse reactions to the benzodiazepines. This occurs both when Prozac is prescribed in conjunction with the benzodiazephines and even when benzodiazephines are prescribed long after a period of Prozac use. Although the other SSRIs because of their similar enhancement of serotonin should logically cause similar reactions, whether this will prove to be the case with other Specific Serotonin Uptake Blockers remains to be seen. These interactions would suggest that the first recommended treatment by Lipinski, et al., propranolol, may prove to be less problematic and more effective than the benzodiazepines. In a second and later study, "Reexposure to Fluoxetine After Serious Suicide Attempts by Three Patients: The Role of Akathisia", *JOURNAL OF CLINICAL PSYCHIATRY*, 1991, propranolol is the only recommended drug treatment. There are additional studies now to complicate that treatment and support the findings of significant reactions in combining Prozac with the benzodiazepines. Inderal is metabolized by the P450 enzyme and therefore its metabolism will be affected by Prozac.

We have already mentioned the side effect of hypoglycemia and we will discuss it in more detail as we go on, but for now it is important to understand the role of low blood sugar in producing akathisia reactions. The diverse symptoms of hypoglycemia generally stem from two sources. The first involves the reaction brought on through adrenalin. As the blood sugar is depleted to a certain level, the adrenals release adrenalin in an attempt to correct this potentially life threatening situation. The rush of adrenalin generates a flood of glucose which is necessary to produce the energy essential for the "fight or flight" response. This brings on symptoms of a pounding heart, feelings of anxiety or fear or anger, tremors, sweats, nervousness, nausea, intense hunger to replenish the blood sugar level, etc. The other symptoms: confusion, headaches, nervousness, insomnia, etc., come from the brain being deprived of glucose.

The question of neurotoxicity is an important one in connection with the SSRIs. Prozac's selective and powerful action on serotonin causes concern for Dr. Martin Teicher. His concern is brought on by our past experience with other drugs which have such an impact upon serotonin. This experience has demonstrated that these drugs cause permanent brain damage. He states that we have recently learned that over the course of time, other drugs which affect serotonin can have irreversible consequences. (The use of Prozac is demonstrating serious problems in the many patients I have interviewed when used over an extended period and Zoloft has been out just long enough now that many of the reports from these patients are sounding far too familiar. Paxil is so powerful that even for the short amount of time it has been out, the adverse reaction reports are incredible.) The drug Ecstasy [MDMA] is appearing to cause permanent damage to serotonin nerve terminals. Fenfluramine, which increases the release of serotonin to cause an increase in serotonin levels is a drug given to autistic kids and also used for appetite suppression, may have a similar effect. Both drugs appear to be fairly potent neurotoxins in animal studies.

Keep in mind the studies that demonstrate the danger of elevating serotonin levels as these drugs do. *"A recurring finding has been elevated platelet concentrations in schizophrenic patients (for review, see Meltzer 1987). However, elevated platelet 5HT (serotonin) concentrations are not specific for schizophrenia; they are also found in mood disorders, organic brain disease (especially mental retardation), and childhood autism* (Partington et al. 1973)..." (*SEROTONIN IN MAJOR PSYCHIATRIC DISORDERS*, p. 214) With serotonergic agents a situation is being chemically induced within the brain in which we *consistently* find such serious mental disorders as: schizophrenia (psychos or insanity), mood disorders, organic brain disease which is saying that the drugs are "neurotoxic" or causing structural damage to the brain), which produces mental retardation. It should be pointed out again that *LSD not only enhances the serotonin levels, but was originally marketed by Sandoz to chemically induce schizophrenia in "normal subjects."*

The U.S. Office of Technology Assessment warned that pesticides, insecticides, herbicides, disinfectants and petrochemical solvents found in synthetic building materials and other consumer products are also neurotoxins. This means that over time *they have the capacity to cause subtle damage to the brain without people being aware of it until it is too late. (NEUROTOXICITY REPORT*, April 1990) Are we creating this same subtle damage to the brain with the SSRIs without patients being aware of it?

Dr. Peter Breggin addresses this possibility of brain damage as well, "We have seen how a similar rebound hyperactivity of a different neurotransmitter produces permanent mental and neurological disorders after long-term exposure to the neuroleptics. The questions must be asked: Are we producing permanent symptoms of mental dysfunction, including anxiety, depression, or mania. by giving patients antidepressants? How often do we induce a vicious circle in which patients attempt to come off the medications and then experience withdrawal symptoms that are mistaken for a recurrence of depression or other mental dysfunction leading to further treatment with the offending medication?...If the lessons of neurophysiology hold true, the brain frequently does not fully revert to normal functioning after prolonged exposure to toxic medications...Patients diagnosed with 'affective disorders' (depression, manic-depression, and schizo affective disorder) are showing up with *atrophy on the brain scan, suggesting that antidepressants may play a role in causing brain damage." (TOXIC PSYCHIATRY*, p. 156)

Dr. Jack Gorman, Director of Psychological Studies at Columbia University College of Physicians and Surgeons, says *Teicher's concern about the possibility of neurotoxicity is reasonable and that we do not know what might happen if patients are kept on Prozac forever.* And the head of the University of Utah's Mood Disorder Clinic, Dr. Fred Reihmer states that if a patient is kept on consistently high doses of *any* anti-depressant for long periods he has seen problems with most of them and *this is not a safe thing to do.* Yet it is becoming more and more popular among physicians to keep patients on antidepressants long term in spite of the dangers involved. In light of these statements it is appalling that many doctors are telling their patients that they may have to stay on Prozac the rest of their lives. It appears clear to me that many doctors do not want to deal with their patients' withdrawal or have no understanding or recognition of this withdrawal state and therefore keep their patients on mind-altering drugs indefinitely, giving one drug after another for the effects brought on by the previous drug.

Dr. Teicher's report no longer stands alone to warn us of Prozac's adverse effects. In the February 7, 1991, issue of the *NEW ENGLAND JOURNAL OF MEDICINE* doctors reported two more cases of suicidal behavior in patients who had no previous history of suicidal thoughts. *The development of suicidal thoughts appeared rapidly in these cases. It happened in less than a week after starting on Prozac.* Even though they only used the drug for a week, it is interesting, yet shocking, to note that the suicidal preoccupation persisted for three or four days after the *discontinuation* of Prozac. In Dr. Teicher's study the patients used Prozac for only two to seven weeks, yet the intense suicidal mentality continued for two to three months. In light of these reports it is frightening to note that many doctors are denying any relation between Prozac and these suicidal feelings. They are telling their patients to ignore these drug-induced thoughts and feelings while assuring them that the Prozac they are taking just has not yet begun to start working for them and that if they will just continue to use the drug everything will be okay.

This lingering suicidal preoccupation after discontinuation of Prozac usage would indicate the necessity of monitoring the patient closely for some time after coming off the drug and encouraging them to abstain from the use of alcohol and other drugs for some time after discontinuing Prozac. As Prozac accumulates and is difficult to flush out, the patient would still be mixing these substances with Prozac for an extended period after discontinuation. We need to know if this lingering suicidal preoccupation is brought on by the effects of drug residues, sluggish metabolism of the drug because of liver impairment, or a permanent change in the serotonergic systems, the cholinergic nervous system, or the adrenal system and overall endocrine glandular system or a combination of them all. The possibility of kindling is an another theory that must be considered with this lingering preoccupation reported with Prozac. We have discussed the tardive effects of various psychoactive chemicals. Parkinson's, Tardive Dyskinesia and Tardive Dystonia are a few. Tardive Akathisia and Tardive Dementia are two more. I believe all of the knowledge we now have on the glandular system, stress and how stress causes various serious psychiatric effects because of its effect upon the adrenal system is sufficient for us to see what is the cause of these tardive effects of these drugs.

First lets review the facts about these tardive disorders. Parkinson's, Tardive dyskinesia, dystonia and akathisia are all disorders which are manifest by an inability to control muscle movement. Tardive dyskinesia is thought to be the result of inadequate release of acetylcholine. Acetylcholine helps to regulate adrenalin flow. We know that akathisia can be controlled through blocking adrenalin flow. Muscle movement is fueled through adrenalin flow and an inability to control movement, a symptom of all of these disorders, would then logically be a manifestation of an inability to control adrenalin. The ability to control our own steroid output is via the liver and/or acetylcholine. It is through noradrenaline and acetylcholine, two fundamentally antagonistic nerve hormones produced at nerve-endings, that the brain and the nerves exert their multitude of diverse actions. If either the liver which neutralizes excess adrenalins, or the balance of these two hormones, noradrenalin (the brain's adrenalin transported via the nerves) or acetylcholine, suffer permanent or long term impairment by the use of these drugs, or any other foreign chemical agent, or any other long term stressors, the patient no longer has an ability to control the flow of adrenalins in the body. This lowers resistance so that it takes less and less of a stressing stimulus to trigger a reaction and then the reaction is generally an over reaction. This processes is referred to as "kindling" or a magnification of one's responces or reactions to various stimuli.

Because of what I have seen in the lives of so many who have had reactions to these serotonergic agents, I feel confident that those researchers looking for the hormonal and chemical causes of kindling are on the right track. Kindling of hormonal responses is the most obvious cause for latent or tardive effects of these drugs - a kindling of the hormone system throughout the brain and body. Although this can cause apparent permanent damage to the glandular system and nervous system responsible for controlling the body's stress controls and adaptive powers, I feel that the body and brain can and will recover if given a rest from all the chemical and various other stimulants - not a simple task in our society today, but perhaps a patient's only hope for a normal life void of these latent reactions.

A study in the January, 1989 issue of the *AMERICAN JOURNAL OF PSYCHIATRY*, Dr. Alan Louie, a psychiatrist at the Langley Porter Psychiatric Clinic at the University of California Medical Center in San Francisco, reported that former cocaine users are experiencing the kindling of panic attacks even years after their drug use. We have already discussed the similarities between Prozac and cocaine. And it is important to note that many Prozac patients are also describing the same latent panic attacks as these ex-cocaine users. Dr. Louie's study includes one patient, a 33 year old male, who after using cocaine only on weekends over a four year period began to have such intense panic attacks that he thought he was going crazy. Another patient, a 25 year old female, who had used cocaine and amphetamines at least once a week during a three years period began having panic attacks *two years after discontinuing use* of the drugs. She described her attack as having light headedness, weak knees, racing heart, sweating and shaking, intense fear, even visual hallucinations, etc.

An article in *THE SEATTLE TIMES*, October 10, 1990 entitled, "Latent panic attacks reported among former cocaine users", quotes Richard Hessenflow, president of Beat It, a substance-abuse program, "Cocaine sets off a lot of fireworks in the brain, and something has to give...I don't think we've seen yet all of the medical problems associated with cocaine use." He has seen users with paranoia and those who years later felt such inner turmoil that they felt a need to seek counseling. We do not have any idea how far reaching the possibilities are of latent reactions to Prozac use (and the other SSRIs) years after drug treatment. The general public is currently acting as the guinea pigs to give us the answer. The information in the chapter about sleep disorders will help explain these latent reactions brought on by drugs.

We are a pill popping, "quick fix" seeking society. Dr. Walter Afield stated as a guest on the Geraldo show, that we would see more and more of these adverse effects cropping up. He says, "These drugs have to be carefully monitored and supervised by physicians who know what to do with them...It's amazing and appalling, across the nation, that they don't know how to prescribe, they don't know how to use the medication, they don't know how to supervise it; many of them, a large number." Asked if it isn't being marketed very aggressively Dr. Afield replied, "Very aggressively. When you've got these kinds of numbers and you've got the drug companies pushing it, you've got the detail men coming in and talking to the doctors and the doctors say, 'Gee, this is wonderful. I'm going to give it.' They'll give the medication, willy nilly, because *doctors have a need to give pills, and the public has a need to ask for pills in this society.*" He was then asked if he meant that if a doctor gives nothing the patient would feel gypped. He replied, "That's correct. You'll go to another doctor real quick. Basically, psychiatry is a noble profession. Medicine is a noble profession, but when it comes to looking for a drug or a rapid cure, *there are no wonder drugs. There is no magic pill. We ought to stay away from them, and let the buyer beware.*"

Dr. Glen Hanson in his Fall semester 1992 University of Utah course entitled "Common Medicine" stated, "Every drug will cause problems for somebody. There is no drug that is safe for everybody. If someone tells you that they are lying, either to sell their product or out of ignorance. There is no such thing."

Penicillin is the drug we all tend to look to as "the wonder drug" of all time. We have all heard what great strides have been made in medicine because of this drug. Yet, we now realize that to many people this drug spells death. There are many deadly allergic reactions to penicillin. Not even penicillin is considered a "wonder drug" for everyone. Yet, Prozac is expected to be just that. And what is extremely puzzling is that practitioners tend to be as guilty as their misguided patients. Years of medical training should have instilled far more reasoning abilities than what we have witnessed with the prescribing of Prozac.

Even more appalling is the fact that many doctors have been advising their patients to tell no one of their Prozac use. They are actually being told to lie if necessary to keep others from knowing they are on the drug. The excuse doctors are giving is that they do not want their patient to be upset by any adverse information about the drug. They tell their patients and their families not to listen to anything negative about Prozac. Isn't it harmful enough not to inform the patient about the risks surrounding a medication he is using? Do they have to make sure the patient does not get any additional information from any other source? What is going on? Why, why, why would a responsible health professional admonish his patient to not even investigate the available material on a new and controversial drug so that the patient could make a rational decision about using the product? Why would the doctor not want the patient's family, friends or acquaintances to be aware of this patient's Prozac use? These are all people who could suffer the most serious consequences of the drug indirectly and because of their close contact with the patient they are also the ones who could alert the patient of any problems they see in his condition.

Not with Valium, not with Thalidomide, not with PCP, or any other drug that has proven to be addictive or dangerous or even less than perfect have we seen a situation like this exist in the medical community. Why do doctors continue to hand Prozac out so quickly for any type of ailment and defend its safety? Why do they become so upset when nurses continue to take patients aside and warn them of the side effects of this drug when they notice the patients are having reactions to Prozac? Are they incapable of reading all the medical reports published on the drug because of lack of time or do they ever even consider reading research? Why does it take so long for research to be published? Why does it take so long for new research information to filter down to physicians? Do they rely solely upon the pharmaceutical reps to educate them about these new drugs? And how do pharmaceutical companies continue to get away with keeping new research, which may prove damaging to their sales, from the FDA and the public? Why is it so difficult to find a responsible, caring, knowledgeable physician anymore? It actually brings new meaning to the term "butt head" when we learn that proctologists are prescribing Prozac - what an insult to a patient's intelligence. It would also serve as evidence that some doctors don't have a clue as to which end is up.

Do doctors themselves have stock in Eli Lilly? We should keep in mind that many doctors are paid by Eli Lilly and other drug companies to do drug studies for them or they are affiliated with a university or hospital which do these studies. The "don't bite the hand that feeds you" philosophy plays a major role in their defending the safety of Prozac. Are the incentives being offered to them by Lilly to prescribe this drug so great that they feel it is worth "selling out" their own patients? What is it? Have they become totally irrational themselves from their own personal use of Prozac? We are aware that doctors in general have on of the highest rates of prescription drug abuse. Just how serious is the abuse of these mind-altering drugs among the individuals we are trusting with our lives? Psychiatric nurse, Joyce Strom-Paikin, puts her license and credentials on the line to fight the "conspiracy of silence" that exits in the medical profession with the use of drugs by doctors and nurses in her book, *MEDICAL TREASON.* She feels this is a practice which "threatens to corrupt the profession and cost lives of many patients."In defence of physicians it should be stated again that they receive very little training in medical school on the use of drugs. Our entire system is in desperate need of revamping.

A YALE CASE STUDY -EXAMPLE: The following case study, was published in the *JOURNAL OF THE AMERICAN ACADEMY OF CHILD AND ADOLESCENT PSYCHIATRY,* Volume 30, Number 2, March 1991. Because of the insight gained into the impact Prozac had upon these young patients we will discuss it at length along with the conclusions made by the doctors in charge. It is entitled *"Emergence of Self-Destructive phenomena in Children and Adolescents during Treatment".*

The study involved six patients, ages 10 to 17 years, out of 42 total who experienced self-injurious ideation or behavior de novo [for the first time] or had those feelings intensified during treatment with Prozac for obsessive-compulsive disorder. [Note that this figure is *one out of seven* or approximately 15% of these young patients who experienced the most serious side effects.]

They state that despite the widespread use of Prozac in children, there is little available data on the behavioral side effects of Prozac in this age group. Before going into the cases in detail, they mention that, although an additional child completed the double-blind placebo-controlled trial with no self-destructive compulsions during the initial phase of the study, obsessional thoughts of self injury appeared *after* she was restarted on Prozac.

Case 1 was "F", a 12-year-old male. During his first month of use he showed marked improvement in his mood. He claimed to have no suicidal thoughts. He became more willing to attend school and less easily upset. Yet, there was only

176

slight improvement in his obsessive compulsive disorder symptoms for which Prozac was being administered. He continued to report feeling 'high' since starting on Prozac and experienced increasing difficulty in falling asleep.

After thirty-eight days "F" had a violent nightmare. He dreamed about killing his classmates and in the end he, himself was shot in this nightmare. He stated that he had difficulty awakening from this nightmare, and that the dream continued to feel "very real." He went on to explain that he had experienced several days of increasingly vivid "bad dreams" before this particular nightmare which included "images of killing himself and of his parents dying." [In the following chapter we will discuss why and how these violent, vivid, very "real" dreams are such a significant, yet common adverse reaction and the connection between serotonin levels and nightmares.] Later that day he appeared agitated and anxious, refused to go to school. He reported increased intense suicidal ideation and felt unsafe at home as well. The study was then interrupted, revealing that he had been on 20 mg of Prozac. The medication was discontinued and *"examination of his laboratory studies revealed that his whole blood serotonin levels had fallen dramatically from 170 ng/ml just before receiving medication to 11.1 ng/ml after 1 month of fluoxetine treatment."* "F" was hospitalized for 3 days but he became more depressed and obsessional. Then on the 9th day after discontinuing the use of Prozac, he was again briefly hospitalized for further evaluation.

Because of the boy's "persistent obsessive thoughts of hurting himself (cutting himself with a knife)", he was admitted to a children's psychiatric inpatient unit 17 days after Prozac was discontinued. He continued to complain about hospitalization, suffered suicidal ideation and threatened to run away or hurt himself. Because of this he was transferred to a locked unit. Gradually the suicidal ideation subsided.

Case 2: "C, a 10-year-old girl...*did not appear depressed and had no reported history of self-injurious ideation or behavior."*

The child was diagnosed as having an obsessive compulsive disorder which seemed to show improvement during the first half of the trial. Her parents reported that she seemed less anxious or constricted in her activities, but more restless and active. They voiced concern that she was also frequently standing on her head. After six weeks her OCD symptoms had worsened to the point that the study was interrupted and the medication code was broken. It revealed that she too was receiving 20 mg. of Prozac daily. *"Her whole blood serotonin levels had fallen from a baseline of 140 ng/ml to 9.3 ng/ml after 8 weeks of treatment with fluoxetine..."*

Even after discovering how drastically her blood serotonin level had dropped during her initial Prozac treatment, she once again was started back on 20 mg of Prozac daily. Four weeks later her OCD symptoms appeared somewhat improved. But she stated that she was having very strong "increasing thoughts of wanting to bump into or fall off things in order to hurt herself or to pinch herself to experience pain..."

Case 3: "S", a 14-year-old female was given Prozac for "an exacerbation of longstanding obsessive-compulsive symptoms and perfectionistic tendencies that had begun to interfere with her school work and attendance. Always a model student and musician, S. had begun compulsively rereading homework, with the constant feeling she had not mastered it...was generally well behaved, even inhibited..." Throughout my life I have known many high achievers who could have easily qualified for this particular diagnosis. They were the class leaders, those who set an example for those who were not as motivated to apply themselves with such diligence. What about the stories of Lincoln studying late into the night by candlelight? Are such leadership qualities now considered "abnormal" and justification for "treatment?" Have we become so obsessed with forcing one another to conform to the norm and with labeling one another that it is now considered a "disorder" to have a strong desire to do our best?

Her compulsive feelings of self destruction appeared quickly. She began receiving 20 mg of Prozac per day, but she continued studying and rereading her assignments "compulsively" and was not able to return to school. After three weeks of being on the medication, she brought a knife to her room and scratched her wrists. "She revealed ruminative suicidal thoughts of 3 to 4 day's duration concerning violent ways of killing herself by cutting, shooting, or hurling herself downstairs." She stated that because of physical cowardice she would not kill herself in any of these violent ways, but she could not promise to refrain if she could find a less painful method.

At this point she was hospitalized in a children's inpatient psychiatric unit and was given a 50% increase in dosage of Prozac adding another 20 mg tablet every other day. "The following day, she spoke of wanting to hurt herself and die, drew a picture of a dead person on the ground, and picked and bit at her skin." After that she was given one-to-one supervision which continued throughout her hospital stay. During the next 10 days, she seemed "increasingly withdrawn, labile, and depressed. She spoke agitatedly of hurting herself and had to be restrained when she slammed her chair on her toes, excoriated her arms, and threw herself on the floor." The Prozac was discontinued, but over the next two weeks "she continued to be preoccupied with death. She banged her head and hands on the quiet room wall, picked at her arms to produce deep excoriations, and attempted to scald her hands, to choke herself, and to make herself vomit. Restraints, mitts, and behavioral techniques did little to relieve this relentless self-destructive preoccupation or her intermittent agitation. Periods of food and fluid refusal began, at times requiring IV rehydration." [The reader should recall that Lilly states in their informational literature that comes with Prozac that the drug remains in the system for at least 3 weeks after discontinuation of use. Now we know that there is substantial evidence to support that Prozac is *highly accumulative* and remains in the system for *far more extensive periods.*]

Two months after her admission, which would have been six and a half weeks after discontinuation of her four and a half week treatment with Prozac, she was intermittently anorexic, withdrawn and apathetic. The powerful self-destructive preoccupations continued with the patient repeating her attempts to injure herself; "she frequently insisted, 'I'm just waiting for the opportunity to kill myself,' and chanted, 'kill, kill, kill; die, die, die; pain, pain, pain' over and over." [Is it any wonder that ex-Prozac users refer to the drug as "Prozac - Hell and Back"?] She was then given imipramine for ten days which was discontinued because of dehydration. Now we know from recent studies that Imipramine, along with most other drugs are multiplied by at least 10 times by Prozac.

The patient was placed once again on 20 mg of Prozac daily at the beginning of the third hospital month. "She continued to chant and to attempt to hurt herself. Her behavior became increasingly bizarre, e.g., covering the floor with numbered paper squares. She choked and stamped on her teddy bear and cried out, 'Bear wants to die with me, don't you?'" Because of her violent reaction, a week after Prozac was restarted she was also started on trifluoperazine and benztropine. The dosage had to be adjusted because of dystonia, anticholinergic effects, and possible confusion. "She began to punch herself in the face and bang her head severely enough to inflict bruises and to require x-rays; she also began to strike out at the staff." She experienced only short-lived periods of being able to become more involved in the unit's activities and control her self-injurious impulses.

After a stay of 3 1/2 months, because of these unremitting symptoms, she was transferred to a longer-term adolescent psychiatric unit. Five days before her transfer the trifluoperazine and Prozac were discontinued. She was then treated with perphenazine, 20 mg/day. Her diagnoses at transfer were "OCD, overanxious disorder, and major depression; the staff was in disagreement about

179

the appropriateness of borderline personality disorder." [Please note that this was a child who in the beginning just studied too much and didn't want to go to school and was diagnosed only with OCD. The symptoms of a major depressive disorder and overanxious disorder or possible borderline personality disorder did not manifest until after treatment with Prozac. Depression is one of the most common adverse reactions to Prozac reported to the FDA.]

At the new hospital, she continued to take perphenazine. "During her first month after transfer, she continued to have prominent suicidal ideation and self-injurious behavior that frequently required restraints or seclusion." She was then placed on desipramine because of symptoms of a major depressive disorder. During the next several weeks this appeared to produce additional deterioration until she required restraints on a daily basis. She directed physical and verbal assaults toward others and injured some of the staff. She experienced frequent periods of agitation and compulsive driving self-destructive behavior. After an unproductive trial of lithium augmentation, the desipramine was discontinued, and to lithium was added chlorpromazine and lorazepam. Within the next few weeks, she gradually became calmer. Her aggression toward herself and others decreased. She no longer needed the restraints or seclusion. Her OCD symptoms did not appear to be as prominent.

After nine months the patient continued to remain at the second hospital and was being treated with chlorpromazine and lorazepam. She seemed calmer and to have more ability to participate in the daily hospital life. She was also better able to verbalize her feelings.

These researchers concluded, "...Alterations in serotonergic metabolism have been implicated in a variety of violent phenomena, including, in animals, certain types of aggressive behavior (Oliver et al., 1990) and, in humans, completed suicide, suicide attempts, impulsive violent acts, and obsessions of violence (Coccaro, 1989; Brown et al., 1990; Leckman et al., 1990; Roy and Linnoila, 1990)."

"Preclinical studies have shown that fluoxetine has complex effects on serotonin regulation that may vary over time. In rats, although presynaptic serotonin reuptake is promptly blocked by specific reuptake blockers, such as fluoxetine, there is an initial marked *decrease* in the firing activity of serotonergic neurons (Blier et al., 1987, 1988, 1990)...*fluoxetine may alter the balance between the serotonergic system and related neurotransmitter systems (Baldessarini and Marsh, 1990)."*

180

"Unfortunately, the time course and diversity of the fluoxetine's action in humans is less well studied...fluoxetine has diverse neuro-pharmacological effects that may vary over time and across individuals...It is not clear which of fluoxetine's many effects on serotonergic functioning might produce suicidal or preservative self-destructive symptoms or whether these possible side effects are shared by other serotonin reuptake blockers, such as clomipramine or fluvoxamine."

They concluded that Case 1's violent nightmares and the initial compulsive self-injurious preoccupations in Cases 2, 3, and 4 appear to be *"more than coincidentally related to fluoxetine* administration."

"Like all psychotropic agents, the behavioral and neuropharmacological effects of fluoxetine are complex and variable. Careful clinical scrutiny of patients both before and during treatment is essential both to understand better the drug's manifold effects and to detect adverse reactions. As fluoxetine and other medications are used in increasing numbers of younger patients with a wide range of psychopathology, vigilance is needed to detect potentially deleterious behavioral side effects."

This report, a controlled double - blind placebo - controlled scientific study, stands as a statement ringing out loudly and clearly to warn us of the adverse effects Prozac can have on patients. We have seen how a bright, well behaved, creative child and a model student, although perhaps overly concerned about her performance in life, can encounter a perpetual nightmare within her mind and find herself indefinitely committed to a psychiatric hospital after using Prozac.

The next time a psychiatrist or any physician makes the statement that they know of no psychiatrist or even any medical documentation which would substantiate Prozac's potential to induce violence or psychosis *PLEASE* refer them to this study, along with all the references which have been quoted throughout this chapter, then refer them to all references listed in Appendix B, and the REFERENCES section at the end of this book. Then refer them to each of the 28,623 adverse reaction reports filed with the FDA on individual cases. It should keep them busy for quite some time.

CHAPTER 7

SLEEP DISORDERS, SEROTONIN AND THE SSRIs

"Sounder and more restful sleep influences the mind and nerves, restoring emotional balance to people of a normally happy disposition and thus relieving constant depression and moods."

...Dr. H. C. A. Vogel

There is far too much specialization in medicine today. We must begin to understand that all parts of the body are connected and what affects the big toe can have a profound effect upon the head or any other part of the body. When we continue to deny these connections by separating research, knowledge and treatment of the body, we produce the same result as if those connections between the head and the body were literally severed - death. You cannot treat one area and not take care of other symptoms within the body as if they are not related. All fields of medicine have got to get together and compare notes. They have got to all come out of their separate corners and get together to discover what is actually happening in the various disease processes. Perhaps they need to sing the little song with their children we all sang in our youth about how the "knee bone's connected to the thigh bone," etc. They seem to be too busy trying to convince us that their particular field, whatever it happens to be from internal medicine to psychiatry, is the most important field of study and the crux of all disease. Doctors must look at every area of health to determine every area of a disease, why it is producing symptoms and which ones, and their effects upon their patient. These strong mind-altering chemicals are not the easy way out in treating patients. Glandular disorders, especially those affecting blood sugar, thyroid or hormones, can play a very big role in depression and other mental symptoms, but the origin is *glandular, not psychological*. As we will learn in this chapter, sleep disorders have an extremely profound detrimental affect upon both mental and physical health. Although sleep is such a crucial area of health, we will find that it has been almost virtually ignored until the last two or three decades. It is general knowledge that if an individual is kept awake long enough, several days or weeks depending upon the individual, they become psychotic. Stress which keys us up will keep us awake and accumulate a sleep debt for us. Research is now accumulating at a very rapid rate and the insight it is giving us, especially in the field of mental health, is both enlightening and exciting!

"The mystery of sleep lures us on, even tugs at us. Some of the mystery has been illuminated, but much remains. The facts we can discuss are fascinating in themselves; but more than that, they are crucial to each reader's health and longevity. Our society needs to assign a higher priority to discovering more about this uncharted path of our existence, these other states of being...Sleep is more important and worthy of study than wakefulness...[People] don't know about the insidious and unremitting nature of sleep debt." (William Dement, *THE SLEEPWATCHERS*)

Unsatisfactory sleep has been found to be a major cause of accidents on the job and many other types of accidents - a situation which is comparable to the effects of illegal drugs and alcohol. Sleep deprivation has been a key factor in many a tragedy in our society...the Exxon Valdez, the Challenger, Chernobl. Many questions might arise about other situations throughout history. D. Norman Edelman, dean of the Robert Wood Johnson School of Medicine said, "America is a sleep-deprived society, and [that] is interfering with its societal mission." Our understanding of this fact needs to be illuminated and heightened. Dr. Dement feels the day will come when it will be considered just as criminally negligent and reprehensible to drive or go to work while sleepy as it is now to be doing those things while drunk. He states, "The degree of impaired alertness - daytime sleepiness - that exists among individuals and in society as a whole should concern all. That such an epidemic could have been so steadfastly ignored for so long is especially amazing...The problem is so pervasive that it is not clearly perceived. Moreover, the known facts about how, and to what degree, sleep loss impedes waking performance are not presented at any educational level - not in middle-school health education classes; not in high-school or college biology or psychology classes; not even for the most part, in medical school. We have pinpointed chronic sleep deprivation and inadequate sleep as one of America's greatest health issues, causing problems in the workplace, in the classroom, and at home - yet this knowledge is unavailable to the public. As a result, *the way Americans conduct their lives and organize their work and rest schedules remains irrational and destructive.*"

Depriving ourselves of sleep accumulates a sleep deficit similar to a bank account. When the account becomes overdrawn we face the likelihood of falling asleep at a crucial moment which could cause a disastrous situation. Those suffering sleep deprivation seem to lose the ability to determine their level of alertness. Forty percent of the subjects in a random study tested "pathologically sleepy", while only ten percent of the ones who thought they were alert and feeling fine were optimally alert. Most of us remain unaware of the unremitting nature of sleep debt. We are aware that we are drowsy the day after we stay up late the night before. But few of us are aware that the deficit builds and must be compensated for in some way.

Most, if not all, psychiatric disorders characteristically include some type of sleep disturbance as a biological marker. Depressed patients enter REM sleep more rapidly than what is considered normal. This is referred to as "decreased REM latency". Other disorders which are characterized by short REM latency are: anorexia, obsessive-compulsive disorder, borderline personality disorder, schizophrenia, mania, and subaffective dysthymics have decreased REM latency. Panic disorder is characterized by a disturbance in sleep continuity and a decrease in sleep time. Anxiety disorder, posttraumatic stress disorder, schizophrenia and dementia all manifest both a disturbance in sleep continuity and decreased Delta wave sleep. Obsessive-compulsive disorder also manifests decreased sleep time and decreased delta wave sleep. With mania we find not only decreased REM latency, but increased REM density along with disturbance in sleep continuity. Overall the picture is very clear that there are many problems associated with sleep in conjunction with psychiatric disorders. The more we learn about the importance of REM sleep and sleep in general and the varying levels of consciousness a sleep deficit can produce, it should become apparent that sleep deprivation is the most logical cause, rather than a symptom, of these various mental disorders.

We accumulate a sleep debt in many ways. Alcohol induces severe levels of sleepiness and sleep debt, as do the majority of the mind-altering drugs, which links alcohol and drug related accidents to sleep deprivation as well. Prescription medications, especially those having a stimulant effect produce disturbed sleep (Oswald I. 1969, Knowles et al. 1968). Even medications taken to improve sleep, the sedatives, can cause withdrawal or manifest tolerance in the patient upon cessation of the medication. Withdrawal and tolerance cause the disruption in sleep patterns. Stimulants produce both withdrawal which induces fatigue during the day and they disrupt night-time sleep resulting in daytime sleepiness. Antihistamines do the same and in fact may cause excessive sleepiness. The effect medications have upon sleep patterns is not always apparent. Many types of drugs disrupt sleep. Anticonvulsants, pain medications and chemotherapeutic agents all can produce sleep disturbance in withdrawal and can alter sleep patterns for some time after their use.

It is important to remember that medications can cause sleep disturbance both during the period of use or upon discontinuation. Logically these drugs would continue to have such an effect until they are flushed out of the body. Respiratory disturbances have been a major factor leading to a rapid growth in sleep disorders. This rapid rise in sleep disorders caused by respiratory disturbances may soon be linked to our widespread use of tobacco over the last three or four generations. The use of tobacco will disrupt sleep and may cause respiratory disturbances to be brought on in the offspring of those using tobacco, thus inducing a disruption in the sleep patterns of those children. The toxic conditions in our environment play a significant role in sleep debt. As we pollute our world, we pollute ourselves. Toxic conditions in the body brought on by heavy metals or organic compounds disrupt our sleep patterns causing sleep disorders (Valciukas JA, et al. 1978, Kilburn KH, et al. 1985). [Dr. Luc DeSheffer, author of *PEAK IMMUNITY*, believes that Chronic Fatigue Syndrome is brought on by these toxic conditions. Considering the sleep debt these toxic conditions bring on his theory is a very valid one. As we have already mentioned, those coming off Prozac are often diagnosed as having Chronic Fatigue Syndrome.] Our diet naturally also affects our sleep. There are food allergy insomnias, for instance, cow's milk allergy which appears so often in children now (Kahn A, et al. 1985).

A sleep attack may occur without warning. Dr. Dement cautions us that if we are aware that we are drowsy it may already be too late. He then goes on to say in *THE SLEEPWATCHERS,* "Wake up, America - the alarm has sounded!...A sudden wave of drowsiness should be treated almost as seriously as chest pain. It is an urgent warning that *must not be ignored* - particularly in a potentially hazardous situation, when impaired performance, an error of inattention, even the briefest dozing off could lead to accident and catastrophe. The appropriate response is to get some sleep: Take a nap. Various parts of the world honor the afternoon siesta; America, too, should become a napping society..."

Sleep debt is very subtle and deceptive. Even if your sleep debt is very high, you may feel that you are not sleepy in the least, because your awareness of the sleep debt is offset by some type of stimulation. When stimulation is high a sleep deprived person may momentarily feel alert. The deception brought on by stimulation lies in the fact that the sleep debt has not been reduced at all and the brain remains on the verge of sleep, ready to check out at any time. A sleep attack can occur without warning. As we have just mentioned, sustained use or withdrawal from CNS (Central Nervous System) stimulants or depressants or other drugs, chronic alcoholism, or various toxic conditions can cause the onset of a sleep disorder. As our sleep becomes disrupted we are not always aware of the accumulating sleep debt. We live a life surrounded by stimulants. Every direction we turn there are bright lights, television shows and movies geared to stirs emotions, pump adrenalin and stimulate thought (not that this is all bad, but have we exceeded our limits?), stimulant drugs, video games, coffee, cigarettes, caffeinated drinks, diets filled to the brim with stimulants, fun centers, carnivals, the circus, endless meetings - business, school, church, its rush here and rush there, our entire lifestyle is overstimulating. With all the stimulants how can we be the least bit capable of detecting our individual sleep debt? How many of us are fully alert and capable to handle the responsibilities we are attempting to handle in life? Just how dangerous a position are we in? Why are sleep researchers sounding an alarm about our bankrupt sleep accounts? Let's see what this fast paced life style is doing to us as individuals and as a society as it raises our sleep debt.

REM is our dream state of sleep. REM is the stage of sleep with the highest level of brain activity containing vivid hallucinatory imagery known to us as "dreams". It generally entails about 20 -25% of our total sleep time. REM has proven to be *specifically essential* to good mental health. Full blown psychosis can be produced by depriving a person of REM sleep over a period of time. The average newborn would require eight hours daily of REM sleep. A fetus would require even more. Even brief periods of REM sleep deprivation in young animals can cause deleterious brain changes. It is interesting to note that animal studies show that chemically induced deprivation of REM in infancy can cause depression. Those deprived of REM over a period of time can become psychotic. In fact, sleep disturbance is a factor in many psychiatric disorders. Kupfer, et al. 1972 is a study involving manic-depression and hypersomnia. Depression is often associated with sleeping too much. With all the latest information on sleep disorders we need to start looking at the possibility that the sleep debt is what is causing the depression instead of the other way around. There is much evidence which has appeared in sleep research just in the last decade to strongly indicate that most psychiatric disorders are manifestations of sleep disorders brought on by an accumulated sleep debt. Hopefully this new information will bring understanding and solutions to many of these problems which have caused so much pain and suffering throughout history.

If our REM sleep debt is high enough we can actually go into a dream state while awake. When we are deprived of REM over a period of time we experience what is called REM-sleep rebound. This is our brain's attempt to make up the loss by lengthening and increasing both the frequency and density of this stage of sleep. Research has shown that the less time an individual spends sleeping, the less REM sleep will be experienced. Our bodies and our brains are so aware of our necessity for REM sleep that if we are not allowed to experience REM rebound to make up for this loss, our brain will compensate by forcing us into REM while we are awake.

A balance in serotonin is essential for normal REM sleep patterns. Serotonin not only helps to induce our REM sleep stage, but is crucial in maintaining REM throughout the night. Imbalances in serotonin levels will affect our sleep patterns. Some researchers have indicated that after chemical depletion of serotonin there

186

are decreases in the duration of sleep which would cut the amount of sleep period one would have in which to experience REM sleep (Laguzzi & Adrien, 1980; Pujol et al. 1971). It is also now considered that serotonin activity is essential throughout the sleeping and waking cycles for the utilization and the synthesis of other yet unknown sleep-promoting agents. (Sallanonm et al. 1983; Jouvet 1984) The link between serotonin and REM sleep, the dream stage of sleep, is critical in understanding the most extreme dangers of not only Prozac, but all the other drugs which interfere with sleep - the psychiatric drugs, hypnotics, sedatives, anesthesias, painkillers, some of the anti-histamines, etc. *Drugs which increase serotonin extracellular concentrations in the brain or inhibit another neurotransmitter, norepinephrine, will decrease REM sleep.* PCP is a strong inhibitor of REM sleep through its affect upon serotonin and the blockage of the reuptake of norepinephrine (Martin et al. 1979, Ary & Komiskey 1980). The SSRIs are all strong REM inhibitors as well because of their action upon serotonin. Some serotonin inhibitors have been found to increase both wakefulness during sleep and alertness during the day. *"It can be seen that as far as serotonin is concerned much remains to be clarified. Better understanding of the role of serotonin in sleep will be possible only when the physiological function of the various receptor subtypes now identified is determined." (HANDBOOK OF SLEEP DISORDERS*, p. 71).

This evidence of serotonin's critical role in sleep should specifically raise concern about any of the serotonergic drugs, those which are designed to directly and strongly affect serotonin levels, such as Prozac, Deseryl, Zoloft, Paxil, Luvox, Lovan, Anafranil, citalopram - all the drugs we have previously listed, and many other new drugs currently being tested and awaiting the FDA stamp of approval. Although not generally recognized or admitted to patients by physicians, clomipramine (Anafranil) is considered a powerful inhibitor of REM and is a potent serotonin uptake blocker (Linnoila et al. 1980). Jerking movements in the limbs and other side effects have been observed indicating sleep disruption. (Bental E. et al. 1979, Guilleminault C. et al. 1976, Cadihac J. et al. 1976) It is also a sedative. Tolerance also develops with clomipramine (Anafanil) which can produce withdrawal and the disruption in sleep that accompanies it. Those drugs considered milder serotonin uptake blockers are drugs such as Elavil (amitriptyline), Tofranil (imipramine), etc. As we have already discussed, though, any drug which affects any of the other neurotransmitters will also indirectly affect serotonin because of the domino effect and can therefore, also inhibit REM.

Another factor to be considered is that serotonin is the primary neurotransmitter in the raphe system within the brain. The raphe system has been found to be

187

very closely connected to sleep (Jouvet & Renault, 1966; Zernicki, Gandolfo, Glin, & Gottesmann, 1984). Balanced levels of serotonin would be essential for proper function of the raphe system and therefore, proper sleep. After the depletion of serotonin levels several studies have noted marked decrease in the duration of sleep (Laguzzi & Adrien, 1980; Pujol, Buguet, Froment, Jones, & Jouvet, 1971).

When we realize that in the REM sleep state the brain creates a complete hallucinatory world and that research has shown that with REM sleep deprivation the REM sleep state will intrude into periods of wakefulness, we should be able to see that REM sleep debt is very dangerous. Bringing that complete hallucinatory world into a period of wakefulness is beyond what most of us could even begin to imagine. Prozac patients report interruptions in sleep brought on by the drug-induced nightmares, muscle contractions and jerking, the striking out and kicking during sleep. This shows us that very little REM sleep is being experienced by the patient and they are making themselves susceptible to an experience with REM sleep intruding into wakefulness.

REM is essential for proper perceptions and memory. We store many, many memories throughout the day, distributing them in many areas of the brain, and layering them upon other memories already stored there. Many new memories are nothing more than insignificant input into our minds and of no benefit to us. It is now becoming apparent that REM sleep is our dejunking time for this useless baggage our brains have acquired throughout the day. Without the opportunity to go through this process of sorting and organizing these thoughts and memories, our perceptions and memories can be altered and distorted leading to misunderstandings and to false memories as we discuss in the PATIENT REPORTS chapter. There is much evidence to indicate that suppression of REM jeopardizes both the learning and memory functions of the brain. Loss of memory and learning difficulties are the two most noticeable side effects reported by the Prozac patient himself.

Remember that any type of disruption of serotonin levels can disrupt REM. Prozac and other serotonergic drugs are "designed" to specifically and powerfully affect serotonin levels. Now compare the Prozac patient's experience with experiences reported by those who are deprived of REM sleep. This includes: personality changes, increased anxiety, irritability, impaired concentration, increased appetite and weight gain, memory and consolidation of memory is affected, inappropriate associations within the brain are not suppressed as they would be normally, strong motivations are not dampened as they would be with sufficient REM sleep, etc. It appears that overloaded circuits are not cleared as

188

we have just described in the "dejunking" of trivial input the brain processes during REM (Crick & Mitchison, 1986).

Clinicians have long known that seizures are increased following a sleep debt. Disturbed sleep and epileptic seizures aggravate and perpetuate one another. Sleep disturbance which produces an accumulated sleep debt will bring on seizures and the seizures will cause a disturbance in sleep patterns. One can bring on the other. (Shouse & Sterman, 1982; Shouse & Sterman, 1983) Another study, Bowersox et al. 1982, indicates that frequent nighttime generalized seizures may cause additional seizures and increased neuronal excitability because of the chronic REM sleep deprivation it produces. Only mild sleep deprivation (24 hrs.) can cause an incredibly high increase in seizures by 30-50%. It is recommended that those suffering seizures monitor sleep patterns through all-night EEGs and make an effort to restore normal sleep patterns which may help to control the seizures. There is much medical research to indicate that many mental disorders may be a series of small seizures. Many medications also produce seizures as a side effect. Seizures are also a side effect of Prozac and are a risk in the withdrawal from many of these psychoactive drugs. While visiting with a radio producer after doing a show on Prozac he told me that when he was tapering his mother off high doses of Valium she suffered such a severe seizure that the muscle spasms broke her collarbone.

The body and central nervous system rebuild structurally and functionally during REM sleep. When REM is repressed protein synthesis in CNS tissue is disrupted preventing this restorative process. Bowersox and Drucker-Colin conclude in *SLEEP AND EPILEPSY* that this interference in protein metabolic processes very likely could be the cause of the seizure (p. 91 - 101).

Those who sleepwalk have been found to have EEG abnormalities. In addressing that Dr. Jacques Montplaisir says, "Consequently, all adult patients with frequent night terrors or sleepwalking should undergo all-night EEG recording, especially those who report self-injury or aggressive behavior during sleep." (*HANDBOOK OF SLEEP DISORDERS*, p. 654)

A REM sleep study on cats showed that deprivation of REM produces much abnormal behavior. One profoundly abnormal behavior was that of male cats sexually mounting almost anything that moved. (Dement, et al., 1969) The deprivation of REM in this study seemed to enhance drive-oriented behavior and somehow indicated evidence of increased brain excitability. The entire nervous system became more excitable. It is understood in scientific circles that repressing REM can have a very stimulating effect upon the brain as it fights to

189

rebound and recapture the lost sleep. Just as any other stimulant it forces us into a situation where we are running on "nervous energy". We continue to run on that nervous energy by requiring more and more stimulants to fuel the fire under those nerves until we either "crash and burn" or we drop from exhaustion and have the opportunity to rest and rejuvenate. This last option of dropping from exhaustion would certainly be far more preferable than the "crashing" option of pushing ourselves to the point that we begin dreaming on our feet in order to make up that sleep deficit. We must understand the seriousness of this condition where someone who is deprived of REM sleep over a period of time will find their brain's compensating by going into REM during periods of wakefulness (Jacobs et al. 1972). If we are lucky it will be a dream we act out. Although embarrassing ourselves is not an enjoyable experience, at least it would give us the opportunity to change and prevent a similar experience from happening in the future. If we have run out of luck, it will be a nightmare we live out (imbalances in serotonin produce nightmares) which can and often does result in death or injury to ourselves or someone else.

This sleepwalk state has over the last several years helped us to understand conditions previously labeled as hallucinations, mania, delusions, dissociation, depersonalization, paranoia, etc. (Even seizures are appearing to be the brain's attempt to recapture lost REM or REM rebound.) In it's extreme this sleepwalk state is referred to as a REM Sleep Behavior Disorder (RBD) and is often called a drug withdrawal state. All of these conditions, mania, delusions, hallucinations, paranoia, dissociation, depersonalization, REM Sleep Behavior Disorder, etc., are so closely connected that clinical differentiation among them may be impossible (Schenck et al. 1990). *Eighty-five percent of those who experience RBD will cause harm either to themselves or others.* [It is important to note that nightmare activity has been found to be mainly associated with REM sleep, not other stages of sleep (Fisher et al. 1970; Fisher et al. 1973).] Mark W. Mahowald and Carlos H. Schenck describe this dangerous sleep disorder, RBD, "...the concept of dissociation will allow the prediction and understanding of a wide variety of unusual clinical disorders (Table 1)(21). The basic state (wake, REM sleep) from which the dissociation arises will determine the clinical condition; i.e., rapidly oscillating consciousness-*dreaming with the presence of muscle tone occurring from wakefulness may explain a conscious hallucinatory state-from REM sleep will present as lucid dreaming with [muscle] tone. Dreaming with muscle tone from wakefulness results in automatic behavior seen with narcolepsy, states of drug withdrawal, and sleep deprivation - from REM sleep explains RBD."* (HANDBOOK OF SLEEP DISORDERS, p.569) States of drug withdrawal, which a patient can experience while yet using a drug depending upon his body's own rate of metabolism, sleep deprivation and narcolepsy can all produce this dreaming with muscle tone during periods of wakefulness - a sleepwalk nightmare clinically termed the REM Sleep Behavior Disorder.

REM generally occurs in a rhythmic pattern at intervals throughout the night and normally includes muscle paralysis. The three general characteristics of REM sleep are: dreams, muscle weakness (cataplexy), and paralysis (Mahowald & Schenck, 1989). It affects the muscles by producing an almost temporary paralysis so that people cannot act out the dreams they are experiencing. But those who are affected by RBD do not experience this temporary muscle paralysis. They somehow bypass this built-in protective measure which would prevent them from living out the vivid hallucinatory dream state occurring within their minds. Instead, they can move freely and are capable of acting out their dreams or nightmares. Often there is no recall of the experience. A study released in 1989 by Chase, Soja & Morales indicates that this abnormal response during REM is related to the neurotransmitter glycine. Glycine is believed to carry inhibitory messages to the motor neurons during REM. Men and women with RBD, who are typically mild mannered during the daylight hours, have been known to act out violent dreams generally during the night and early morning hours. Through it all they display remarkable strength and agility. They have been known to beat sleeping partners, punch holes in walls, drive many miles, smash windows, vault across rooms and even violently murder others... all the while demonstrating strength far beyond what they would normally possess.

Keep in mind the statements from so many Prozac users reporting that they began "living out their worst fears in life, their "nightmares". Michael J. Thorpy describes in *THE HANDBOOK OF SLEEP DISORDERS* the major features of a sleepwalk state: "mental confusion and disorientation, automatic behavior, relative nonreactivity to external stimuli, poor response to efforts to promote wakefulness, retrograde amnesia for many intercurrent events and only fragmentary or no recall of the sleepwalk experience". And there is evidence to demonstrate that reduced serotonin activity or serotonin turnover (lower 5HIAA serotonin) does produce the REM Sleep Behavior Disorder. We have previously listed how many of these mind-altering drugs reduce 5HIAA (serotonin turnover) levels. In light of the horribly violent and gory nightmares Prozac patients relate, it is frightening to realize that they are being chemically induced into a state where they can act them out. These patients acting out in a sleepwalk state with no memory of their actions is beyond anyone's concept of the word "nightmare".

It is important to remember that RBD in humans may be acute, transient, or chronic. The acute form of RBD is what is induced by medications or by toxic-metabolic conditions brought on by such drugs as tricyclic antidepressants, monoamine oxidase inhibitors (MAOI) or biperiden (check REFERENCES section for a listing of the numerous studies on various drugs). Once the medication is discontinued and flushed from the system or the toxic condition taken care of in the patient the acute form of RBD is stopped. RBD is also noted in states of withdrawal and is often referred to as a "drug withdrawal state", especially withdrawal from alcohol (remember that alcohol also raises serotonin levels. Additionally RBD can be produced by reduced activity of serotonergic and/or noradrenergic populations which inhibit REM (Hishikawa et al. 1981). That is, any drug which inhibits REM sleep can produce this condition known as RBD. We should also note that most who suffer RBD do not have any previous history of sleepwalking or night terrors.

This disorder begins with the patients first noticing changes in their dreams - the dreams become more vivid, they seem so "real", they also become more violent and action packed. (The young man in the Yale study on Prozac which is discussed in the previous chapter complained that his first indication of problems associated with Prozac use was vivid, "very real" dreams which he had much difficulty awakening from and that those dreams were also very violent.) Gradually the patient the patients begins to slide up and down on a scale of consciousness, or in and out of awareness as the dream state begins to occupy the waking hours more and more to compensate for sleep debt. This is a very subtle process for the patient. He generally remains unaware of these effects because first of all most individuals suffering sleep deficit remain unaware of it, but the drug is impairing the patient's awareness and judgement through its mind-altering effects, as well inducing a sleep deficit on top of that. With its strong stimulant effect the patient believes the drug is actually making him more alert and aware, while studies demonstrate that stimulant drugs give the patient this deceptive view of his own performance. These changes in a patient's dreams should be taken far more seriously than most doctors do presently. They should be considered a very strong indication of the possibility of this very serious drug reaction. Many Prozac patients report not being able to detect when or if they even sleep any longer.

Patients experiencing RBD also begin to notice that if they are awakened from a dream they are aware that they have just been dreaming about something which to their amazement, they have just acted out, such as striking out in their sleep, etc. Additionally these dreams they act out are not necessarily connected to past experiences. A 73 year old man jumped four feet over his night table, landed on the floor causing a nosebleed and cut on his cheek. He in another episode leaped from his bed causing a cut behind his ear. In all of these dreams he was defending himself in a combat situation. He was puzzled by all these war dreams since he had never served in the military. It has been well documented that night terrors can be associated with vigorous muscle action or motor activity. (This type of thing is also seen quite often with post traumatic stress - another condition involving sleep deprivation brought on by the body's own adrenalin rush.)

The December 1987 issue of *NATIONAL GEOGRAPHIC* had an extensive and excellent article on REM sleep which discussed RBD. They mentioned several case histories: Donald Dorff, 67, a retired grocery merchandiser from Golden Valley, Minnesota explained how the crowd roared as he dreamed he received the football from his quarterback and ran down the field. Then as he continued to describe his dream, "There was a 280 pound tackle waiting for me, so I decided to give him my shoulder. When I came to, I was on the floor in my bedroom. I had smashed into the dresser and knocked every-thing off it and broke the mirror and just made one heck of a mess. It was 1:30 a.m."; the wife of a 77 year old minister related how she had seen him vault from a reclining position up into the air and across the bedroom; Mel Abel, 73, a former real estate salesman tied himself to his bed to prevent himself from acting out dreams where he thought he was breaking the neck of a wounded deer, yet awoke to find his wife's neck in his arm.

According to the 1990 edition of the *PHYSICIAN'S DESK REFERENCE (PDR)*, p.906, the most commonly observed adverse reactions of nervous system complaints from Prozac patients included: "anxiety, nervousness, insomnia, drowsiness, fatigue or asthenia..." Listed as "frequent" reactions are "abnormal dreams and agitation". In the post introduction reports "confusion" is added to this list. So according to the official information published on the drug by the manufacturer we find patients showing signs of suffering a building sleep deficit: abnormal dreams, insomnia, anxiety, nervousness, confusion, drowsiness, etc. All of which indicates an overwhelmingly profound REM sleep rebound pattern. When the REM sleep deficit is great enough they will be forced into compensating for the lost REM by going into a dream state during wakefulness which is classified as RBD when it presents as a violent nightmare.

The description of RBD is an EXACT CARBON COPY of how patients are describing their experiences on Prozac. It is a common report that someone with RBD can go to sleep in one place and wake up miles away and not remember how they got there. People on Prozac often relate getting into their car and not being able to remember how they got from point A to point B. People on Prozac describe the violent acts committed (if there is any recall) as if waking up in the middle of it and realizing they are actually there and it really isn't a dream after all and are themselves shocked to discover that it is real and they are actually there and living out this experience. Research shows that people with RBD will strike out in their dreams thinking they are protecting a loved one when in fact they are actually attacking their loved one. They frequently display aggressive and violent behavior while sleeping and yet when awake are very sane, calm and collected individuals. Their dreams will correspond to their movements. Many of these dreams are violent. They will dream about punching, kicking or leaping when they are in actuality punching, kicking or leaping. They often damage property and injure themselves or others. Some patients have seriously injured or hurt others in car accidents, etc. while in this state (*BIOLOGICAL PSYCHOLOGY*, p.379). Cats whose brains have been damaged to create this disorder will during REM, walk, chase, attack, and perform other actions as if acting out their dreams (Henley & Morrison, 1974; Jouvet & Delorme, 1965).

Akathisia and the REM Sleep Behavior Disorder are very similar in many aspects. Both are known as drug reactions. Both are intermittent. Both often involve violence or violent thoughts. Both can include an amnesia for the violent reaction. Blank stares are reported with both. In both the individuals report performing physical feats beyond their normal muscle strength or capability. The main difference in the two seems to be the angle from which the symptoms are viewed. Akathisia is viewed from a bio-psychiatric stance in examining the impact being made on various neurotransmitters and adrenal system, which in turn produce the violent and suicidal feelings and the behavioral reactions observed in the patient. The Rem Sleep Behavior Disorder on the other hand is viewed from the direction of a sleep specialist in measuring consciousness, sleep debt, awareness or alertness, inappropriate REM episodes which intrude into wakefulness, also in examining the neurotransmitters involved in producing a condition which includes violent nightmares along with a sleepwalk state.

The view of the sleep specialist helps us to understand the extent of the patient's awareness of reality or full hallucinogenic dream state mentally, while physically appearing functional. It helps us to see the disconnection from reality. On the other hand an understanding of akathisia helps us to see how the patient loses control of his feelings as the normal glandular function and neurotransmitter action becomes severely imbalanced and distorted by the interference of a foreign chemical. As the brain fights to maintain normal levels of each neurotransmitter, various foreign chemicals (caffeine, nicotine, sugar, artificial sweeteners, food additives, environmental pollutants, drug residues in meat and dairy products, and all the various mind altering drugs) constantly interrupt that balance and causes a constant revving up of the adrenal system. This repetitive stimulus conditions an overreaction of the adrenals over time. While one foreign chemical

194

affects one or several transmitters, other neurotransmitters react by raising or lowering their own specific levels, which in turn affects additional neurotransmitters until there is massive disruption in brain function and level of consciousness.

The anesthetic sleep state demonstrated by the brain waves of the patient on Prozac at the end of this chapter indicate a state of mind in which we would expect to find this RBD "sleepwalk" state. In fact, many ex-patients have referred to their experience on the drug as "sleepwalking". Although the patients while using the drug believe they are alert and functioning, as is with so many other mind-altering drugs research has shown that this is not the case. Studies of performance and brain wave patterns would most likely produce similar results with Prozac. Patients often describe their experiences as if "in a dream or a nightmare" and even repeat the statement "It was like I woke up and realized that I was *really* there. It wasn't a dream! It wasn't a nightmare! It was real! I was actually there and doing what I thought I was dreaming." How could I count the number of times I have heard that exact statement over and over again from Prozac patients and ex-Prozac patients describing their experience?

A man calling in on a radio show on KSL radio in Salt Lake City related his experience: "I took Prozac, and probably for about four or five months I thought it took the roller coaster mood swings out. Then all of a sudden in the middle of the night the muscles in my legs would just twitch and wake me up. That went on for a while. I really didn't attribute it to Prozac, but then one night I had a dream and I dreamed that I reached out and swung at somebody and I crashed into my nightstand and I sprained my fingers and bruised my knuckles. I remember thinking that I'd never done that in my entire life. Then about three weeks later the same kind of thing happened. I hit the headboard with my hand. I started thinking, "Boy there is something really crazy going on!" About a month later I had another dream like that and woke up to one of the most horrendous things I've ever experienced...that is that I had hit my wife next to me It was such an emotional trauma for me because I've never touched my wife in my life or ever been abusive or anything like that. I immediately got back with my doctor. He said I should definitely stop taking Prozac. I did. I think that it took a few weeks after that, but since then I've never had the muscle twitching that woke me up, and I've never hit the nightstand or any of those kinds of things, so I attribute it absolutely directly to Prozac. So I would think that people, if they have any of those kind of things ought to consider that Prozac might be one of the reasons. And they should reevaluate whether they ought to be taking it."

One young man on Prozac reported, "I came to and found I was standing in front of a mirror with a knife to my chest and I wondered what I was doing!" A young woman in San Francisco reported that while on Prozac she watched herself "tear out and speed across the Golden Gate Bridge, determined to jump off." All the while a long line of police cars with lights flashing and sirens blaring were in close pursuit. She described this almost as if an out of body experience, what psychiatry would refer to as depersonalization, a listed side-effect of Prozac. "Then I was in my car again wondering what on earth I was doing in a high speed chase with the police?!" She, as so many others, report such confusion over being able to distinguish what was real and what was a dream during their Prozac use. They often worry about what they might have really done and cannot remember doing. (This is often reported as a reaction to Halcion also.) They are anxious and even dread learning what might have been "reality" for them during a period they cannot recall.

An example of this dream like situation, which would be labeled as a "manic reaction" in psychiatric terminology, may give you additional understanding. One man thought (dreamed) while on Prozac that he was a very wealthy business man and spent his entire retirement, a sum of several hundred thousand dollars. He is relieved that a doctor friend of his recognized that this was a drug reaction and insisted he come off Prozac, thus preventing more serious developments. When I asked him if his experience was "like a dream", his response was, *"Exactly! That is exactly what it was like! It was as though I began dreaming and I just could not come out of it no matter how hard I tried."*

What a terribly embarrassing, as well as terribly dangerous, position to be put into, living out ones' dreams! No wonder the patient feels so completely uninhibited. Who isn't uninhibited in their dreams? If an individual believes he is only watching himself do something in a dream, out-of-character behavior becomes almost acceptable. This dream state would describe for us what is generally labeled as "REM Sleep Behavior Disorder," "dissociation," "borderline personality disorders," "mania," "depersonalization," "delusions," "hallucinations," etc. Plato stated, *"In all of us, even in good men, there is a lawless, wild-beast nature which peers out in sleep."*

Another case that in my opinion demonstrates evidence of a classic REM Sleep Behavior Disorder involving Prozac happened in December of 1992 in the Salt Lake City area. Mr. Brian Gibson was a single parent raising four children alone after the death of his wife from cancer seven years earlier. According to his friends he was "a great guy". He was well liked by his co-workers and was a good father. Facing the challenge of raising four children on his own was his doctor's reason for prescribing Prozac. Brian became another one of the continually skyrocketing number of suicides reported to the FDA. He ended his life in a most bizarre fashion. He dressed up like his dead wife, red wig and all, attacked two of his children and then set his house on fire. The children escaped with injuries, but Brian lost his life in the fire.

According to Brian's church leader the two most terrible experiences Brian had faced in life were the death of his wife and fire. In fact, he was so frightened of fire that he would not even allow candles to be lit on birthday cakes. Why such an intense fear of fire? For Brian it was totally justified. As a seven year old child he was in an accident which caused him to be burned over 65% of his body. His doctors did not expect him to live. Brian did live through this terrible trauma in his life, going through years of reconstructive surgery, but reacted to this experience by showing extreme caution in order to prevent anything like that from ever happening in his life again or in the lives of his loved ones. If Brian Gibson were just trying to commit suicide why would he have killed himself in this way? If he *consciously* chose how he was to die, why would he have chosen the one method in life he feared the most - a method he knew was the most painful of all? Why are all of these patients saying they lived out their worst fears on Prozac? What are nightmares composed of if not our "worst fears"?

Although Brian only used Prozac from February through August of 1991 and this incident did not take place until over a year after a prescription was filled, it is my opinion that it was Prozac induced. The reason for this is that Brian had Post Traumatic Stress Syndrome from the trauma produced by his accident as a child which would have been magnified by the excess stress produced by the excess cortisol Prozac causes. Another contributing factor was the scar tissue from his accident as a youth which would have left him no way to sweat any excess of the drug out. In other words, it would have made it much easier for him to become toxic and remain toxic because of his weakened condition. To demonstrate the toxic condition he suffered, after his Prozac use he became so bloated that his scar tissue tore open, leaving him with open wounds. As we move into the next chapter we will discuss many more Prozac cases that have symptoms of RBD.

In August, 1992 the Canadian Supreme Court upheld the acquittal of Kenneth James Parks. In 1987, Kenneth drove his car 14 miles to his in-laws home, stabbed to death his mother-in-law and seriously wounded his father-in-law while in a sleepwalk state (RBD). His case is far from the first of this nature. Doctors testifying in his behalf referred to medical literature which contains other cases of sleepwalkers who have killed people. RBD is an unconscious state. The individual has no control over his actions. Reality to him *is* his hallucinatory dream state. What a terribly tragic reality for those patients to have to face upon awakening - that they have taken someone's life while sleeping. Yet even more tragic is the fact that we are chemically inducing this condition with a conscious choice of using the mind-altering drugs.

Generally a sleepwalk experience manifests itself by a blank facial expression, an indication that the level of awareness is greatly reduced. It also includes some indifference to objects or individuals in the immediate vicinity - a dissociative state. The individual may go into various automatic behaviors he usually engages in upon rising, readjust his pillow, etc. before he arises and walks around the room or out of the room. Many movements appear to be purposeless and motor activity is usually somewhat clumsy. Individuals exhibit complex behaviors as well, such as eating, drinking, driving, talking on the phone, playing a musical instrument, etc. *Attempts to awaken the individual or make them aware of reality is often met with resistance since their "reality" is a vivid dream state, not what is happening around them.* (Attempts to awaken someone to reality who is suffering a manic phase [a reaction repeatedly reported in connection with Prozac - see Appendix B] will be met with a similar resistance.) The individual is usually able to negotiate around objects without difficulty, but once in a while will knock over a piece of furniture or break an object. Injuries and dangerous activities with no apparent thought of consequences are commonplace. People have fallen from buildings, smashed through glass doors, been involved in automobile accidents, climbed out onto fire escapes, etc. On occasion persistent aggressive behavior is directed towards specific individuals (such as seen in stalking, another report from friends and families of Prozac patients). Various violent activities exhibited by sleepwalkers have been noted and reported: attempted strangling of a spouse and repeated stabbing of a five year old cousin by a 14 year old boy were both attributed to sleepwalking episodes (Oswald and Evans, 1985). In the forties Schmidt coined the term "schlaftrunkenkeit" for these confused states of sleep arousal. The first recorded report of violence associated with RBD was made by Yellowlees in 1878.

To help me to gain a greater understanding of sleepwalking a friend shared her experience as a young child. She grew up in the countryside in Greece in the early 40's. She and her sisters would often beg to sleep outside to avoid the hot summer nights. On one of these occasions she began to have a pleasant dream about gathering wild spinach. In the middle of the night five year old Valentina found her basket and headed out for their own private wild spinach patch. A family friend on his way to work at 4:00 A.M. that morning spotted her in his headlights as she walked along the road. He stopped her and asked where she was going at such an hour. She explained that she was going to gather wild spinach. Realizing that her parents most likely were not aware of her whereabouts he admonished her to return home and return later to gather spinach. She headed homeward until he started to leave. She then turned back in the direction of her spinach patch, determined to finish out her dream. Her parents friend drove back to her home and awakened the parents. They knew immediately from past experience that she was sleepwalking and rushed to bring her safely home. My friend went on to explain that she had such a seriously persistent problem with sleepwalking that her parents had to lock her in her room at night. One night her sister who shared the room with her knocked to get out in order to use the bathroom. She forgot to lock the door behind her and when she returned little Valentina was already gone. Another set of parents facing the same type of situation in desperation pinned a tag on their daughter stating where she was to be returned when found wandering at night.

What stands out in these instances is that there is such an amazing determination to live out what is in one's mind in a sleepwalk dream state. As cognitive function is not at peak performance, many perceptions are distorted altering one's judgement. Actions become dangerous. They can also become embarrassing to the individual when he awakens and comes to a realization of his actions.

My most vivid recollection of a sleepwalk experience was with my younger brother (who may never speak to me again once this is published). As a teenager I was watching a late night movie on television, ignorantly accumulating my own sleep deficit as most teenagers do, when my brother walked into the room. We talked for a minute or two and then I pointed out how late it was and asked what he was doing out of bed. He explained that he had gotten up to go to the bathroom. I suggested he do so and go back to bed and he left the room. I thought he appeared to be in somewhat of a stupor as he blankly stared at me and wasn't making a lot of sense, but when you are a teenage girl younger brothers always tend to fit that description, so I thought nothing more of the episode. The following morning we all realized he must have been sleepwalking when we discovered that in the middle of the night someone had urinated in a box of oranges my father had brought in and set in the kitchen the night before. My poor brother was caught red handed and red faced. He could not even blame it on the family pet since our dog was a tea cup Chihuahua and was only one third the height of the box. It took a lot of convincing but he was finally forced to face the evidence that he was actually the guilty party, although he denied any recall of even getting out of bed during the night.

To this day I am still amazed that my brother could have been so sound asleep that he had absolutely no recall of the incident, yet I thought he was awake and functioning. This experience certainly helps me to understand a REM Sleep Behavior Disorder and answers a lot of questions about all these reports of experiences by Prozac patients - the blank staring, total denial of any memory of the incident, completely out-of-character behavior, etc. While those around the patient for only brief periods do not recognize this unconscious state until it reaches a critical stage when it becomes obvious to all through the patient's bizarre or violent behavior. Families, or those who associate with the patient the majority of the time, will generally notice any reaction much sooner than most - even before the doctor or the patient himself. As the evidence begins to mount over time and the Prozac patient is forced to face the fact that what he thought he was dreaming or what he has blamed on someone else to rationalize his inability to recall the incident, which was actually his own doing, shock, horror, confusion and embarrassment surface along with the fear of his own future actions. He becomes frightened to trust his behavior any longer. He believes he must be going crazy.

Michael J. Thorpy in the *HANDBOOK OF SLEEP DISORDERS*, p. 535, states, *"It has been suggested that sleepwalking in these patients may be due to specific abnormalities in the metabolism of the neurotransmitter serotonin. Serotonin is also implicated in the development of migraine episodes, and sleepwalking episodes are reported to be nine times as likely to occur in children with migraine."* Sleepwalk episodes can be provoked by acute stimulation during deep sleep. Standing the individual up can provoke an episode. Pain produced by a migraine headache can initiate a sleepwalk state. This helps us to see why these drugs which stimulate the body's adrenalins can so readily produce these hallucinatory dream states during wakefulness. Alcohol (remember alcohol also raises serotonin levels) and sedative type medications along with the hypnotics and the neuroleptic drugs have all been found to induce sleepwalking episodes. Sleepwalking is also more likely to occur when sleep is deepened by fatigue and exhaustion, or during an illness, or after a prior sleep loss, (all events which stimulate adrenalin rushes). It does not matter whether the sleep loss is brought on by worry, stress, fear, chemically induced by medications, etc. Sleep debt produces periods of dense REM as the brain apparently works to make up the loss. Increase in density of REM is common in drug withdrawal. In abrupt discontinuation of alcohol REM rebound has been demonstrated to compose a full 100% of total sleep. We know that RBD is most likely to be seen during drug withdrawal when this REM density is most prevalent.

Rest and especially REM sleep is so essential for the healing of any health

200

problem. General physical and mental well-being is impossible to attain without proper levels of REM sleep. Insomnia is a very commonly reported side effect of Prozac. Beyond this high incidence rate of insomnia, patients report such drug reactions as disruptive violent and bizarre nightmares, muscle contractions and jerking and striking out and hitting during sleep. They report that when they do get sleep they do not sleep well, nor do they feel rested upon waking. All of these factors would indicate little opportunity to obtain REM sleep. This interference or disruption of REM sleep would help us to understand why the Prozac patient reaches a point of total exhaustion just before serious reactions to the drug become very apparent to him and everyone around him through a violent act or suicide. It would also give us an explanation to why the patient who is discontinuing use of the drug generally complains of complete exhaustion and at times finds it extremely difficult to even get out of bed since his body would naturally fight to compensate for the loss of sleep he has experienced during his period of Prozac use.

How many of these patients suffering disruptive sleep patterns are given sleeping pills which only further complicate and compound this drug-induced insomnia? Sleeping pills, barbiturates and tranquilizers can cause a paradoxical reaction and produce insomnia by causing the patient to experience a withdrawal state which prevents sleep (Kales et al. 1978). Taking additional drugs only worsens the problem by setting up a cycle from which it can be difficult to escape. Insomnia, which causes us to accumulate a sleep debt, can be produced by many things: attempting to fall asleep at the wrong time in one's circadian rhythm, sleeping in an unfamiliar place, excessive noise, worry, stress, uncomfortable temperatures, and *drugs or medications* (Kales & Kales, 1984).

Many individuals are given sleeping pills for insomnia, particularly the elderly, when non-drug approaches might be more effective. Just how effective are sleeping pills? According to research they induce sleep 10 to 20 minutes faster and the patient sleeps a grand total of 20 to 40 minutes longer than the patients who do not use a sleeping pill. Even though the patient using the drugs thinks he slept better, it has been found that the drugs do alter normal sleep patterns. They *reduce* the deep sleep stages (3 & 4) and *significantly reduce* REM. They impact memory, coordination, reaction time, etc. for longer than they induce sleep. The benzodiazepines (Valium, Halcion, Xanex, etc.), generally used as tranquilizers or sleeping pills, are known to alter the memory. Patients develop tolerance and dependence to sleeping agents. Then if that is not enough, they are effective for only two to three weeks and then the patient faces going through withdrawal. This withdrawal causes "rebound insomnia" - insomnia which is as bad or even worse than what the patient had before treatment.

Additionally, because of their suppression of REM sleep, they produce "REM rebound" as well - the intensification of the REM state, often with an abundance of anxiety-filled dreams, numerous awakenings producing a general feeling of a restless night. Alcohol has this same effect. *(THE ENCYCLOPEDIA OF PSYCHOACTIVE DRUGS, DRUGS AND SLEEP*, pgs. 51-55, 65) Over all the benefits of sleeping pills do not appear to outweigh the risks and most experts recommend that they be used only as a last resort, after all other non-drug therapies have been attempted. It is definitely recommended that all possible causes of insomnia be explored and all alternative solutions exhausted before medication is even considered because if the patient is on a drug which produces insomnia additional drugs being added to a drug-induced insomnia could pose additional drug-interaction risks.

Presently the only treatment available for RBD is, Klonopin (clonazepam), a seizure control medication which has an even stronger suppression of REM sleep. I have worked with many patients now who are being prescribed Klonopin after having problems with Prozac. This is further evidence of the drug's ability to induce seizure activity and the REM Sleep Behavior Disorder. An especially provocative viewpoint was expressed by Winters (1972) when he suggested ketamine was actually causing epilepsy instead of anesthesia. Could this be what is happening with Prozac as well when inducing a dissociative anesthetic like state? Klonopin's more powerful effect on REM would make the REM rebound experience equally more profound. In fact relapse upon discontinuation of the drug is immediate and the patient is once again facing the frightening symptoms of RBD. In order to have the symptoms continue to be suppressed the patient would have to continue use of the drug and face a highly possible increase in dose, increasing the likelihood of dependence. It is interesting to note that symptoms of RBD can be controlled by the addition of l-tryptophan, an amino acid removed from the market by the FDA because of one instance of a tainted batch. *(HANDBOOK OF SLEEP DISORDERS*, p. 587) This is the same amino acid which was previously used to fight depression. Tryptophan is the natural substance the brain uses to manufacture its own serotonin.

I personally feel that any type of drug therapy for the REM Sleep Behavior Disorder is clearly not a reasonable option and should be considered contra-productive since all the drugs which could be used to control the disorder would only further impair the patient's ability to obtain the REM sleep he needs. The patient's underlying physical condition would worsen because of this accumulating sleep debt. This is evidenced by an immediate relapse upon discontinuation of the drug therapy with Klonopin and by the fact that RBD itself is described as a "drug withdrawal state". Additional drugs will only add to the withdrawal. There is much evidence to indicate that multiple chemical sensitivity should be considered as a cause in this disorder and additional treatment with chemicals would not cure the disease but may control the symptoms for a period of time. The key to bringing a patient out of a dream state or sleepwalk state such as RBD has to be in the restoration of normal sleep patterns. The sleep deficit must be dealt with by restoring the sleep patterns which have been so profoundly disrupted by either Prozac or any other drug, toxic chemicals in the environment, stress, depriving ourselves of sleep by pushing beyond our limits, etc. Whatever the cause, once the sleep deficit is handled and sleep has been replenished, the patient will once again have the ability to cope with life and function normally. One must consider the extent to which he has depleted his sleep bank account and realize it will take time and focused effort to replenish that account.

When Prozac interferes with sleep patterns and specifically disrupts serotonin turnover, this, in turn, produces nightmares or abnormal dreams and sleepwalk. It is my conclusion that Prozac is producing much abnormal behavior by chemically inducing a REM Sleep Behavior Disorder. And all the other states of consciousness we have labeled as various mental diseases, such as mania, schizophrenia, manic-depression, hallucinations, delusions, borderline personality disorders, confusion, obsessive-compulsive behavior with repetitious actions, etc., etc. are a variation of experiencing the dream state during wakefulness. I feel the medical evidence is now overwhelming.

In checking with Dr. Carlos Schenck, who has done much research in the field of REM Sleep Behavior Disorder, I found that he personally has already documented one case of REM Sleep Behavior Disorder which was induced by Prozac. Considering the rarity of this disorder and the fact that one doctor out of a small handful of doctors worldwide who would know to even consider this as a possibility makes his discovery very significant. Because of Prozac's effect and the many other mind-altering drugs' effects upon REM sleep these disorders can happen while the patient is using the drug or at any time after his use has been discontinued - until his sleep patterns normalize once again and his sleep debt alleviated.

The latest research on sleep disorders, much of it being released in the last few years since Prozac has been on the market, is definitely eye-opening (no pun intended) and should awaken us all to the perilous position we put ourselves into when we take these drugs which alter our states of consciousness, putting us each on various levels of consciousness or alertness. By disrupting sleep patterns they even potentially bring on a sleep state during periods of wakefulness. It is far past time for us to wake up to these dangers! It is critical that we do all in our power to maintain a fully conscious and totally aware state of mind. We then, are the ones in control of our thoughts and actions. When we lose that control, that awareness or consciousness to mind-altering drugs, any type of stimulant - be it chemical, emotional or physical (overwork, insufficient sleep,, etc.), we are setting ourselves up for behavior which will be impulsive, out of character, embarrassing or a danger to ourselves and those around us. We are in fact as it were, living on the very edge of what we call sanity.

Both manic patients and depressed patients experience early onset REM sleep (Hudson, et al. 1988). REM begins quickly after dosing off and may occupy a large portion of sleep time throughout the night. It seems most logical that the brain is taking the opportunity to make up lost REM or a REM deficit as rapidly as possible in both of these conditions. In those who cannot take drugs or those who prefer not to use drugs several ways of adjusting sleep habits are known to alleviate depression (Gillin, 1983). "One promising method is to have the person go to sleep earlier than usual, in phase with his or her temperature cycle. The person goes to sleep at, say, 6 P.M., when the temperature cycle is at about the point it is in undepressed people at 11 P.M.; he or she sleeps 8 hours and awakens at 2 A.M. On each succeeding night the person goes to sleep half an hour later, until the bedtime reaches 11 P.M. or some other satisfactory point. In short, therapists treat the depressed patient like someone who is having trouble adjusting to a change in time zones. The result is a relief from depression that lasts for months (Sack, et al. 1985)." (*BIOLOGICAL PSYCHOLOGY*, p. 566) This would indicate that a valid preventative measure for depression or mania or any other mental disorder where sleep is abnormal would be to attempt to always get to bed at an early hour. We have all heard that we get our best sleep before midnight. This chart indicates that *normal people going to bed several hours later than usual enter REM sleep quickly just as someone suffering depression or mania.* They go into REM much faster than they would in normal sleep. Keep in mind that this is a condition that exists in many various mental disorders - depression, mania, anorexia, obsessive-compulsive disorder, borderline personality disorder, schizophrenia, mania, and subaffective dysthymics.

Normal sleep: . . . . . . enter stage 4 sleep . . . . . . enter REM

Depressed sleep or normal people going to sleep
late at night: . . . enter stage 4 sleep . . . enter REM

The old saying, "Early to bed and early to rise makes a man healthy, wealthy and wise," has certainly stood out in my mind as I have learned more about the importance of sleep and normal sleep patterns. The United States Army uses various means to restore normal sleep patterns. One method they employ is to have the person engage in very vigorous activity during the time period they should be awake and functioning. This helps the body to understand that this is when this person is to be active and adjust its inner clock accordingly. It would also help to burn off excess adrenalin so that it does not interfere with sleep.

Dr. Selye also points out that muscular activity or mental activity "which leads to a definite solution" will prepare us for rest and sleep. Fatigue produced by work well accomplished conditions us for sleep. But he warns that intellectual efforts which set up tensions can keep us awake. Throughout the night, we must protect ourselves against being awakened by stress. We all know the precautions we need to take against noise, light, variations in temperature, or the difficulties of digesting a heavy meal eaten just before bedtime. But how do we regulate psychologic stress so that it will not keep us awake? Dr. Selye makes it clear that our stress has a chemical basis and we must consciously monitor it throughout each day and in each and every reaction to stressors, "If you suffer insomnia, there is no point in telling yourself, 'Forget everything and relax; sleep will come by itself.' It does not...It is during the whole day that you must prepare your dreams; for, whatever you do during the day, your next night's sleep depends largely on how you have spent your previous day...Do not let yourself get carried away and keyed up more than is necessary to acquire the momentum for the best performance of what you want to do in the interest of self-expression. If you get keyed up too much, especially during the later hours of the day, your stress reaction may carry over into the night. (*THE STRESS OF LIFE*, p. 423) Adrenalin is a stimulant which will keep you awake and if your body becomes conditioned to producing excess adrenalin in response to any size stressor you produce chronic insomnia. With conscious effort in retraining your responses to stressors, ridding the body of foreign chemicals, and providing proper nutrition and rest which are designed to rebuild the body's glandular and nervous systems, you will gain control over insomnia and can restore proper sleep patterns.

Another alternative people are turning to is Cranial Electric Stimulation (CES), often referred to as electro-sleep, an extremely low battery operated micro current. It helps to restore sleep patterns as well as fight depression and anxiety. CES is similar in action to Transcutaneous Electrical Nerve Stimulation (TENS) a small battery operated device which is used for relief of pain, with practically none of the side effects or risks associated with painkilling drugs (Pomeranz,

1989). CES is similar to the TENS unit but is used on the head instead of the arms, legs, or back. (*It must be pointed out that CES is not electric shock.* In fact, I was alarmed to learn that this incomprehensibly barbaric treatment of electric shock, commonly referred to as "frying the brain" has become an accepted treatment again. Berkley, California psychiatrist Dr. Lee Colman summed up his views on the effectiveness of electroshock in an April 18, 1990 article in *THE SAN FRANCISCO BAY GUARDIAN*, entitled "Electroshock's Quiet Comeback", (p.17), "What shock does is throw a blanket over people's problems. It would be no different than if you were troubled about something in your life and you got into a car accident and had a concussion. For a while you wouldn't worry about what was bothering you because you would be so disoriented...But in a few weeks when the shock wears off, your problems come back." And Dr. John Friedberg, a neurologist who deals more with the *physical damage* rather than the psychological effects, made this observation about electroshock and how it produces its effects in the March/April 1989 issue of *HIPPOCRATES*, pg. 70, *"All ECT (electroshock) does is produce brain damage...If you want brain damage, it's your prerogative.. there's no more effective way than ECT. It's more effective than a car wreck, or getting hit with a blunt instrument."* We should add here that the method by which ECT works to prevent symptoms is that according to Cohen et al., 1967 it additionally impairs REM rebound activity.)

Ideally we conduct our day in the beta state which allows alertness. Alpha wave state is a slightly decreased mentally active state which promotes relaxation, enhanced learning ability and positive thinking. Theta promotes deep relaxation, meditation, increased memory and focus. The delta wave state conducts deep sleep, lucid dreaming and assists in increasing immune functions. When asleep we have either full blown Delta or full blown Theta waves within the brain and occasionally throughout the night, while in deep sleep, we will have both patterns simultaneously. This occurrence of simultaneous full blown delta and theta can also happen when under anesthesia.

This Prozac patient's brain waves are showing him in full blown Delta and full blown Theta, a total anesthetic sleep pattern, with his eyes wide open on Prozac. After only six months of using this drug his brain waves indicate a deep sleep pattern while he appears alert and functioning - a sleepwalk state. (See brain wave charts.) This lends understanding to the many reports from those around Prozac patients about their blank starring into space, which is common in a sleepwalk state. This patient's brain is most likely attempting to compensate for lost REM sleep and his brain waves indicate that he is experiencing a deep sleep pattern while "awake". Yet this same patient's brain waves read almost normal after using CES for only 30 days. This normalization of the brain wave patterns would indicate a restoration of the neurotransmitter activity within the brain. The only significant abnormality after just thirty days of treatment is continued short term memory loss. (This abnormal pattern is indicated in the circled area.) Short term memory loss is the most commonly reported after effect of Prozac, even by those who thought they had not been adversely affected by its use. The patient would need CES treatment for a longer period than thirty days to assist in restoring this area of brain activity. This new device was at the printing of the first edition of *THE PROZAC PANDORA* going into 73 hospitals on the East coast and is now available in many areas throughout the rest of the country. (Our thanks to Dr. Ray Smith and Life Balances, Inc. for the use of these EEGs.

(Brain wave patterns give us a direct indication of what is happening with the overall neurotransmitter action within the brain. It is unfortunate that it is not a common practice to check brain wave patterns through EEG's to see what might be happening with a Prozac or SSRI patient's neurotransmitter action. Doctors report that the main reason this is not a standard procedure is that insurance companies refuse to pay for this simple procedure and doctors feel that patients would not want to handle the added expense. Surely if a patient was given this information he would want to know how a medication is affecting his brain function. It is a shame that insurance companies do not generally handle this expense. They could find in the long run that this simple and fairly inexpensive procedure would have saved them from paying out huge sums in additional medical expenses for the individual as far more serious problems go undetected. Patients using any mind-altering drug should be advised of this and encouraged to have EEG's taken to see how the drug is affecting the neurotransmitters within the brain.)

Brain Waves, Copyright 1991, LBI, Inc.

EYES OPEN SPECTRAL AVERAGES

. . . 31 yr. old male with memory loss, depression and fatigue, on Prozac medication . . . six months into treatment.

SLOW WAVES/PRE-CES

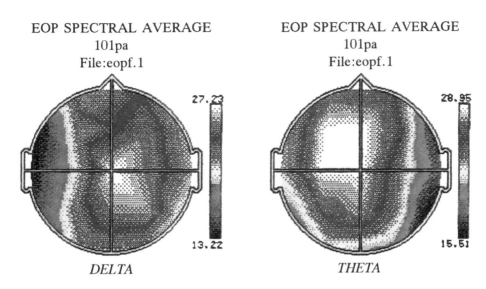

EOP SPECTRAL AVERAGE
101pa
File:eopf.1

27.23

13.22

DELTA

EOP SPECTRAL AVERAGE
101pa
File:eopf.1

28.95

15.51

THETA

SLOW WAVES/POST CES

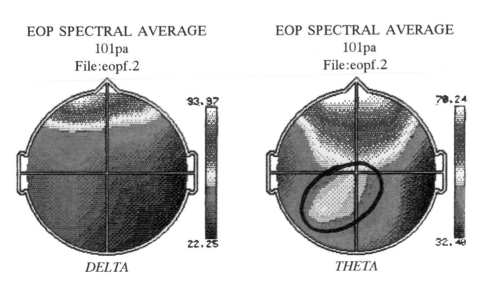

EOP SPECTRAL AVERAGE
101pa
File:eopf.2

93.97

22.25

DELTA

EOP SPECTRAL AVERAGE
101pa
File:eopf.2

78.24

32.48

THETA

CHAPTER 8
THE LEGAL REPERCUSSIONS

It is appalling how very little is known within the entire legal community about the effects of the illegal mind-altering drugs, but even more appalling is the ignorance regarding the legal mind-altering drugs when it comes to their powerful intoxicating affect and the strong impact they have to alter one's behavior. This lack of information is practically turning our courtrooms into three ring circuses and overcrowding our jails and prisons. (Ironically we have judges, prosecutors, law enforcement officials, etc. using these drugs which impair judgement.) Prosecutors, judges, juries and even defense attorneys are generally oblivious to the facts surrounding drug induced behavior in these cases. There are those who have been diligent in educating themselves in this area, but unfortunately they are far too much a rarity. Steven E. Lerner and Richard S. Burns address this issue in an article written for The National Institute on Drug Abuse, Research 64 Monograph Series, 1986, *PHENCYCLIDINE AN UPDATE,* entitled, *Legal Issues Associated With PCP Abuse - The Role of the Forensic Expert.* "It is not uncommon for individuals under the influence of phencyclidine to come to the attention of the criminal justice system. Increasingly, there is a need for forensic experts to advise and testify in cases involving PCP and other psychoactive drugs...Most jurors and many courts have limited knowledge about psychoactive drugs, including PCP. From our experience, it is not uncommon for the average juror to believe that the effects produced by PCP are no different from those produced by other drugs. For this reason, jurors must be educated if they are to be expected to make informed decisions about complex issues with which they have little or no familiarity." Note that this was the situation 30 years after the development of PCP. If this is the case with one of the most dangerous of the drugs which was first used medically, how long might it take for the court system to become informed about the action of Prozac and the other SSRIs? In one of the cases I testified in I approached the prosecutor to inform him that the defendant had experienced a manic reaction to Prozac. He was obviously more informed than most as at the mere mention of the defendant being on Prozac, he threw back his head, rolled his eyes and exclaimed, "No wonder! That explains it all!" He was kind enough to advise me to make sure that the legal defender representing this individual be informed and educated about this important aspect of the defense.

Previously upstanding citizens are experiencing mania as a side effect to these drugs and ending up locked away in mental hospitals or the prison system, gunned down by police at the scene or left with a criminal record. If these individuals who survive are given an opportunity to allow the drug effect to wear off through a drying out period, they are completely appalled, confused and embarrassed about their drug induced actions. Unfortunately many never get a chance to come out of this drug induced semi conscious state because more and more drugs are forced upon them by law enforcement or medical professionals who do not recognize the fact that the condition is drug-induced.

Within our prisons and jails Prozac and other mind-altering drugs are being disbursed in massive quantities to inmates who have been incarcerated for reasons stemming from a variety of addictions, i.e., illegal drugs, alcohol, sex, compulsive spending, etc. Others prisoners who never used illegal drugs before their incarceration are being introduced to these highly addictive psychoactive prescription drugs and finding they are developing addictions to these drugs. We should be greatly concerned over this whole new group of sertonergic drugs as they are affecting the very neurotransmitter which, when disrupted by this chemical interference could be causing or intensifying addictions and compulsions. What will happen to society when these prisoners are released? Why would we want people who have already committed violent crimes given a drug that reportedly produces uncontrollable violent rage as a major side effect? Is it really worth the few weeks or months of control it gives authorities over a prisoner if the end result would produce a raging psychopath with this drug?

Another practice within our criminal system that we should be extremely concerned about is that these prisoners who are being given so many of these mind-altering prescription drugs are subsequently released and instantly withdrawn from the drugs "cold turkey." Keep in mind that this withdrawal period is often the most violent and dangerous period of drug use. The REM Sleep Behavior Disorder we have just learned about is often referred to as a drug withdrawal state. This "cold turkey" withdrawal approach can all too often produce a manic reaction or RBD which can lead to criminal behavior. This is a very dangerous practice, not only posing a danger to the prisoner, but to society as well. If people being withdrawn from these legal drugs even in a supervised situation become so violent and aggressive, so much so, that a large drug withdrawal clinic refuses to take them, what might that imply to innocent bystanders? These prisoners are not being withdrawn gradually in a controlled situation. They are being dropped off cold turkey as they go out the door. And the natural reaction for anyone who has been incarcerated on a drug charge is to go right back to the street to find drugs to alleviate the terrible prescription drug withdrawal he is experiencing. The violence produced by this drug withdrawal state can cause additional, ever more serious crimes to be committed which affect us all. Then the prisoners are returned to their cells defeating any attempt at rehabilitation which our tax dollars already paid for the first time around. This issue of mind-altering drug use in our corrections system must be addressed. It is much too serious an issue and incredibly far reaching.

For an individual to be aware that his conduct is dangerous to another or to himself and in order for him to make a conscious decision to refrain from taking such action or to act without regard to a known danger, he must be able to engage in abstract thinking. Many of these drugs impair the patient's ability to think abstractly. The reason we need to gain an understanding of the action of drugs like PCP and other drugs that cause dissociative states is that most of us still suffer from the delusion that for an individual to be intoxicated, he must also demonstrate a corresponding lack of muscle coordination - the type of intoxication we are most familiar with in alcohol-induced intoxication. With the dissociative state of intoxication, where the patient appears alert and aware, yet is in his own world apart from ours, we all too often continue to use our out of date methods of testing for only alcohol and illegal drugs. Little or no thought of prescription drug reactions are considered when authorities investigate a crime. This negligence in testing leaves the perpetrator of the crime as much a victim as those he or she has victimized in their drug-induced state. When we consider the medical technology now available to us we can see that our whole system of drug testing is archaic. In these situations we need methods to measure the person's level of awareness, alertness, brain function in cognitive reasoning and decision making abilities to determine mental competency at the time of the crime. The degree to which the individual is lacking any of these functions determines the degree to which they were capable of choosing appropriate or inappropriate responses or behaviors in a given situation.

I have already discussed how an electroencephalograph (EEG) is designed to measure all of the above listed brain functions. It is the general consciences of those experts who must testify in these cases that this is a necessary test. If we really want to see true justice done in the future, we need to use this type of testing in our investigation of crimes, especially the more serious crimes. It may cost a little initially to set up this system of testing, but in the long run the huge amounts saved in jailing, prosecuting and imprisoning would stagger our imaginations.

Studies demonstrate that over half of those now imprisoned are there because of behavior produced by their use of illegal drugs. I believe that a very large number of the remainder have found themselves incarcerated because of drug-induced behavior produced by prescription drugs - mind-altering drugs which have not yet been declared illegal. When we begin to see the connection of

212

antidepressants and any other drug which possesses a stimulant profile to mania and then learn of mania's potential for criminal behavior, we should be able to see the problems generated by these drugs within the legal system. These people are being lost in the black hole between the time a drug is released and the time it is declared illegal, but until the court system is educated about the drug. When we consider the fact that with both LSD and PCP it took about twenty years after the drugs were introduced by the pharmaceutical companies who developed them, Sandoz and Parke, Davis, before our government agencies declared them "illegal," we begin to realize the precariousness of our position.

What happens to all the victims caught in this time period when these drugs were considered to have a large margin of safety? Where are these victims? What has happened to them? What we are doing within the legal system to the victims of this process is unconscionable! And the way we are drugging prisoners out of their minds with large amounts of these "legal" drugs is unethical, immoral and self-defeating. It is setting them up and society up for disaster when they are all too often released to go through a "cold turkey" withdrawal from the addictive psychoactive drugs they have been forced to use in prison. We must examine what we are doing to our society as a whole by our open arms to drugs attitude. This examination must be a close and careful one with caution instilled by the terrible mistakes made in the past with these drugs we now class as "illegal".

Mania is one of the side effects produced by the antidepressants. "Schizophrenia is the most common form of psychosis (psychosis is the new technical word for "insanity"). It is a detachment from reality. Paranoid schizophrenia is where the patient may think people are talking about them or are attempting to harm them when it is not real. Manic-depressive psychosis is a swing from depression to mania. In the manic phase they feel elated, nothing seems impossible ['I thought I was Superman!'], and they may commit unlawful acts...Persons who are judged to be mentally ill are not held responsible for their unlawful acts. They are treated in a mental hospital instead of being sent to prison." *(THE NEW BOOK OF KNOWLEDGE*, p. 227) Dr. Dana L. Farnsworth, Former Director of University Health Services, Harvard University discusses a few of the types of psychosis in this quote but leads us to believe that those suffering mania are not imprisoned. He states that they are treated as one who is ill and hospitalized. When the psychosis is drug-induced, this is not always the case. A drug-induced psychosis is often temporary, making it very difficult to understand what has happened.

With memories being impaired or distorted and brain function incapacitated while the patient suffers withdrawal from Prozac (or the other SSRIs), most

213

patients are left with a diminished capacity to fight back by way of filing lawsuits against their doctors or the drug company. All the while Eli Lilly continues to deny allegations while collecting the huge profits from Prozac, their biggest moneymaker ever. Several suits have been settled out of court and "gag orders" placed upon those individuals. Lilly has crossed the line of ethics in these legal battles, offering to defend doctors in malpractice suits and assisting prosecutors in the criminal cases. If you are a large company defending a $100 million per month income, it obviously is worth the expense. So far only two convictions have been handed down "against" Prozac. One was in October, 1990 in Marion, Illinois. Circuit Court Judge William A. Lewis sentenced a man who killed his father to four years probation because *as the judge listened to the evidence he "became convinced that the Defendant was probably innocent as he was merely defending himself from a drug induced attack by his father."* The second was 75 year old Mildred Johnson, who shot her husband while on Prozac. In April she was put on probation after being convicted of the lesser offense of manslaughter.

The attorney involved in the majority of the lawsuits, Hon. Leonard L. Finz, is a conservative ex-New York Supreme Court Justice whose firm specializes in medical litigation. He feels he has hard evidence against Eli Lilly and Prozac. He has sued Lilly in the past for failing to properly test the drug DES (diethylstilbestrol), a synthetic estrogen prescribed to prevent miscarriage. Presently there are 250 ongoing lawsuits filed by the children and grand children of those who used DES. (Check in the chapter LILLY AND POLITICS to see why decades later lawsuits are still being filed against Lilly for damages involving the use of DES.)

Finz points out that Lilly conducted inadequate clinical trials on Prozac lasting only five and six weeks, thus indicating that we do not have positive proof of what could happen to a patient after five or six weeks on the drug. He further alleges that their clinical trials were "whitewashed" and Harvard's Dr. Tiecher has made the same point, explaining this "whitewashing" process as picking and choosing only those patients who would be least likely to experience problems instead of using a broad patient base. Another situation that causes some confusion is the FDA's reporting system for adverse reactions. For example, "suicide attempt" and "intentional overdose" are listed separately. Add those two similar reactions together and you have a high incidence of intentional self-inflicted death attempts. "Depression" is listed as one reaction and "psychotic depression" as another. Add them together and you have a very high incidence report for depression produced by a drug that is marketed and touted as a miracle cure for depression. "Hostility", and "agitation" are listed separately. Add these

214

together and you have an *extremely* high incidence of anger in patients on Prozac.

Finz also accuses Lilly of not sufficiently warning of possible adverse effects. Medical experts including those involved in Lily's clinical trials, such as Dr. Fred Reihmerr of the University of Utah Mood Disorder Clinic have publicly criticized the pharmaceutical giant for not being more elaborate in their warnings about the extreme dangers involved in mixing Prozac with alcohol or other drugs and the dangers involved with prescribing high dosages. The package insert warnings also do not stress to the patient the importance of not using alcohol and other drugs upon discontinuation of Prozac. The reason for this is that Prozac remains in the system for a long time after taking the drug. Therefore, the patient would be mixing those substances within his blood for that long after discontinuation of the drug.

In the October 22, 1990, issue of the *NATIONAL LAW JOURNAL* an attorney, who wished to remain anonymous yet was familiar with the cases, was reported as saying, *"Xanax and Halcion, but more so Prozac, have never been really totally evaluated through the FDA drug process, to the extent that until there were two million prescriptions no one realized what they were dealing with."* Others, including Finz, say that the pharmaceutical companies are "using the broad patient base as their human laboratory." This is clearly demonstrated by the Halcion court case in late 1992 surrounding a policeman who was prescribed .5 mg of Halcion on a daily basis for 600 days. He then shot and killed his best friend. Now it is recommended that Halcion be used at a dosage no higher than .25 mg, one half of what he was prescribed, for no more than seven to ten days at a time. That is a far cry from the .5 mg he was prescribed for an almost two year long period. Halcion was introduced in 1963 and this case took place in the 1980's. What good does it do that man and his family and his friend and his friend's family that Upjohn has since changed their recommendations on the amount and time period the drug should be taken? The devastating damage remains and can never be compensated. Finz's observation of using the broad patient base as a human laboratory certainly fits in this instance. We now know that it most definitely fits in association with Prozac. When we have researchers attempting now, over six years after the drug was approved for marketing by the FDA, to discover a therapeutic level for Prozac so that physicians can dose correctly, we know we are in trouble. In these legal battles this information is most critical. It means that those who have been jailed for their actions while under the influence of Prozac were without question suffering involuntary intoxication. Blood levels were checked to determine the influence of the drug upon their behavior, not brain levels. Blood levels are useless with these drugs.

The tests were not the proper type of test to determine the impact of the drug upon behavior. Remember Dr. Karson's words, "Blood levels generically have turned out to be not so great." These patients were reacting to drug levels 100 times greater than what was discovered in their blood levels. As we discuss intoxication in conjunction with Prozac it is imperative to remember that intoxication can be caused by raising our own adrenalin levels, which Prozac doubles with one single dose, and is a symptom of the serotonin syndrome - high levels of serotonin. Legally the term "accidental or unintentional overdose" should apply. Those families who were left not only without their loved ones who committed suicide while in this toxic state, but left also without compensation from life insurance policies because the death was deemed an intentional suicide rather than "drug-induced suicide" from the overdose, should be compensated.

Are these hundreds of lawsuits and pending lawsuits involving Prozac just cases of depressed people who were following the "natural course" of their disease by becoming suicidal as many doctors have claimed? As we review some of the cases yu will become aware that evidence would not indicate this to be the case.

Rhonda Hala's case against Lilly was the first to be filed on July 17, 1990. She lives on Long Island with her husband and two children. In the fall of 1988 her doctor put her on Prozac after becoming naturally discouraged from a seventh hospital stay for a back injury. Her behavior became so bizarre that even with her bad back she jumped a seven foot fence, attacked her doctor, and although having no previous history of depression or suicidal thoughts, she mutilated herself one hundred and fifty times with anything she could get her hands on, over the next year and a half and attempted suicide six times. Throughout her home Rhonda hid shower hooks, hair clips, pieces of glass, etc. for the periods she would "need" something to dig into her flesh to satisfy that uncontrollable urge to destroy herself. Family members had to take turns watching her to prevent her from hurting herself.

Because of her suicidal and self destructive behavior her dosage of Prozac was increased and along with that increase came an increase in suicidal ideation and self mutilation. Finally her doctor read Dr. Tiecher's report, immediately called her and told her he felt her problem was Prozac. She argued that she must "need" this antidepressant because of her odd behavior. Then as the evidence became clear to her, she asked, "You mean to tell me I have gone through this Hell because of an anti-depressant?!!" Rhonda Hala went off Prozac and returned to a normal mental and emotional state.

Kevin Callahan was also put on Prozac because of a back injury and became extremely irritable. His wife and friends complained about the Prozac, feeling this was the cause of his personality change and his doctor doubled the dosage to 40 mg. thinking he just did not have enough of the drug in his system yet.

When Kevin threw a box of French fries at the attendant at McDonald's because he felt it did not contain enough fries he too realized there was something really wrong with the way this medication was affecting him. At that point he and his wife together went to see the doctor. When they tried to tell him that Kevin was having serious problems with this drug and the wife demanded that Kevin be taken off Prozac, the doctor asked her if she had a degree in psychiatry. He then threatened to jeopardize Kevin's disability status, thereby affecting his compensation for the back injury if he discontinued the drug (reports of similar threats made against patients expressing a desire to discontinue the use of Prozac or a desire to not use the drug at all are being made by many other patients). He once again increased Kevin's dose of Prozac to 80 mg. and did something many doctors are doing. He wrote out a prescription for Kevin's wife so that she could cope with Kevin's increasing irritability and rages which all around him felt were his reactions to Prozac.

Three days later, after a pleasant evening with his wife, Kevin ran to the store to pick up a few groceries. The car broke down on the way home. Kevin took a bus home, got ready for bed without saying anything and then stabbed his wife repeatedly with a butcher knife. His wife described him as having no expression at all, just a blank look on his face through the whole ordeal. Kevin has no recall of the violent incident that required 5000 stitches for his wife. Kevin Callahan was convicted in 1991 for attempted murder. This is surprising since psychiatrist, Dr. Walter Afield, stated publicly in a British documentary on Prozac that aired in December 1990 that he was ready to testify that there is absolutely no doubt in his mind after talking to all the physicians involved with Kevin's medical history that Prozac was the cause of Callahan's violent action.

Avis Martin blames Prozac for her suicidal obsession, hostile outbursts, memory lapses and for pain in her wrists and elbows that was the cause for the loss of her job at a food packing plant. Avis did not start out suicidal and is not suicidal now. She was put on Prozac after having an ovary removed. After taking the drug she reached the point that she could no longer do anything but sit on her bed, rocking back and forth and call suicide help lines searching for any reason to continue living. Their reply was always the same, "You must live for your children. They need you."

Her suicidal obsession was so intense that she resolved to put an end what she was being told was her reason for living by loading her children into the car and driving head on into a large semi truck on the freeway. She is not sure why she stopped just short of doing it, but she is certainly grateful that she did. Not long after that she saw the "Geraldo" show on Prozac and realized that the drug was her problem. She took herself off Prozac and is putting her life back together.

Bonnie Leitsch, is the assistant National Director of the Prozac Survivor's Support Group, even though she was pronounced DOA on arrival following a suicide attempt after only seven weeks on Prozac. Doctors were able to revive her and then doubled her dose of Prozac because of the suicide attempt. She then began having audio hallucinations, craving sugar and alcohol (Bonnie had hypoglycemia before being prescribed Prozac and had a bout with hepatitis in her medical history. This would indicate the possibility of a weakness in both of those vital organs, the liver and the pancreas.), lost her short-term memory, suffered excessive weight gain, insomnia, aggressiveness, irritability, loss of interest in her religion, etc.

Why was Bonnie taking Prozac? She had an earache and was also anxious about caring for her mother who had just broken both of her legs. Her doctor suggested a great new "pick-me-up", Prozac. She assumed that because the doctor had referred to Prozac as a "pick-me-up" it must be a type of vitamin. She, as so many others, was given no indication that this was a psychotropic drug. Bonnie felt great about the extra energy she was experiencing. She was three times as productive as she was before Prozac. I became extremely impatient. I thought everyone was 'off the wall' but me. I wondered how I ever survived all these years around these idiots. I thought I was super-special, that no one was as smart as I, nor as strong and certainly no one on the roads could drive as well as I could drive! I really developed a very defiant 'I'll show you!' attitude." (This pompous, arrogant, "I'll show you!" attitude is repeated over and over again by ex-Prozac patients and is very obvious to anyone around the patient. It should be considered a warning.) She as so many others reported feeling as if in a dream state, constantly unable to determine whether she was asleep or awake. Her mind constantly ran. She said she could carry on a rational conversation while she would be thinking self destructive thoughts. She believes that this ability to communicate on what appears to be a rational level while thinking wholly irrational thoughts is why psychiatrists, doctors and psychologists working with those on Prozac are totally oblivious to what is happening to their patients.

But suddenly Bonnie felt so tired, completely worn out and exhausted and within

218

minutes took action on an impulse she felt to end her life. As is generally reported, there were no visible signs of suicidal behavior, it came on suddenly, swiftly, and without warning. What was her reason for committing suicide? "It just seemed like the thing to do, there was no rhyme nor reason to the whole thing. Bonnie attempted suicide while her husband was out mowing the lawn. She decided to take her elderly mother's medications. After one bottle she became upset and impatient that it was not working fast enough so she took more. Luckily she had felt enough rage inside to want to tell her husband off before she left. He saw her stagger and collapse at the door and was able to get help soon enough to save her.

After reading a report in the *AMERICAN JOURNAL OF PSYCHIATRY,* she too took herself off the drug. Bonnie says every birthday has taken on new meaning to her. She now devotes the life she has had restored to her to helping warn others, in an effort to save their lives, and to comforting those who have survived what she calls the "Prozac-induced Hell" that she has lived through.

Gail Ransom was a registered nurse in central California when she decided she had *no choice* but to kill her mother and made that announcement to her friends and family. Thinking she must kidding or "blowing off steam" after a great weekend spent camping, they paid no attention. No one really dreamed of taking her seriously. All were completely unaware of how her use of Prozac over the last seven months had begun to affect her mind and reasoning abilities.

The compulsions felt to act upon the bizarre thoughts one experiences on Prozac are described as *so overwhelming* that the patient feels they no longer have a choice in what they do. Many have expressed to me, "The minute you take the first pill your agency to act on your own is gone." So Gail drove on, in compliance with the excess adrenalin flow, to do what she "had to do", with her bottle of Prozac and her Bible by her side. Totally "out of character" for Gail, she began drinking vodka and Irish whisky (quite a choice for someone who rarely drank) on the 150 mile trip that Sunday evening. It is still not completely clear to her just what happened when she strangled her mother with a venetian blind cord. She describes it as most do, and as those who experience the psychiatric drug side effect of akathisia do, "as if watching herself as if hovering near the ceiling from across the room". The memory is clouded.

A court appointed psychiatrist to this case, Dr. James Missett, soon discovered that Prozac had more to do with Gail's actions than he had felt possible before learning what he learned from this case. As the curiosity set in, Dr. Missett called in the 30 to 40 patients he had on Prozac. Armed with his newly acquired insight into the behaviors induced by the drug, he began interviewing his own patients with more pointed and deeply probing questions. He reportedly quickly discontinued the use of Prozac in two patients who admitted feelings of wanting to hurt or take the life of someone close to them. Then he discovered an additional aspect the patients were sharing with him - he had five patients wanting to ram cars on the freeway and all had been given tickets for irrational driving and speeding. As soon as Dr. Missett was able to meet with Gail's fiance, he questioned him about Gail's driving. Yes, her experience had been identical to that of his patients. In fact, on her way to murder her mother, Gail was stopped and given a ticket for speeding.

The reports from patients and their spouses about weaving in and out of traffic at top speeds in front of semi trucks and blowing out engines traveling at speeds of up to 110 mph and becoming so enraged that they have turned their cars around and driven as fast as they could in the wrong direction down the freeway to "show the world!" should be quite a warning to anyone that there is a problem with the drug. As one ex-patient reported, "You are not advised to fly a plane while using Prozac, but most patients do fly their cars!" Most describe their driving as an "out of body experience" with little or no recall of how they arrived at point B from point A.

(Keep in mind that Dr. Missett found a total of seven out of 30 to 40 patients with serious adverse violent behavior patterns stemming from their use of Prozac.)

Gail Ransom was given a lighter sentence of only three years, but her case is also being appealed - while she waits in prison. As all the others who wait, Gail continues to find those already in prison who have had similar Prozac experiences that *no one even noticed* - others who have awakened from their nightmare and are wondering how these things could have happened to them. Many have viewed made for television movies about these bizarre Prozac stories where no one ever bothered to mention the Prozac connection. Many of these individuals behind bars are still on Prozac, and yet completely unaware of what has happened to them.

The *Doug Cecrle* case was televised on ABC's Prime Time in May of 1991. Doug had noticed that alcohol was affecting him differently after he was prescribed Prozac. He made the decision to not even have an occasional social drink. His resolve lasted two months. No longer able to fight the compulsion he chug-a-lugged two quarts of Colt 45 and beat and strangled his wife to death with a telephone receiver and telephone cord in front of their children.

The psychiatrist and psychologist in the case both diagnosed Doug's mental state as "dissociative". In a dissociative state a person is, for all practical purposes, unconscious. Dissociation is described as "a selective change in consciousness so that ordinary waking awareness is markedly altered," in other words a semi-conscious or unconscious state while possessing a capacity for muscle movement. This can be understood as a sleep-walk state. Prozac as well as the Capozide he was using for high blood pressure, have as a listed side-effect "hyponatremia" ("water drunkenness" or lightheadedness, no energy, thirsty, etc.). This side effect was noticed in conjunction with the use of Prozac as well in 1990 by Gommans, so Doug was using two drugs which both have the potential to produce this adverse effect. Besides the fact that Prozac could likely be greatly increasing the effects of the other drug to produce this side effect. Basically hyponatremia is brought on by a lack of sodium in the blood stream.

If he was in a sense, unconscious, as our brain wave patterns indicated with the patient in the chapter on sleep disorders, isn't that "involuntary intoxication"? We do know that even the mild serotonin enhancing effects of tryptophan produces intoxication (Sternbach, 1991). If one is unconscious, how does one make a conscious decision or choice about anything in life? Unfortunately some state laws do not as yet allow for this condition of involuntary intoxication through a dissociative state - a sleepwalk type state, still requiring the accused to be physically incapacitated, lacking muscle or motor activity, as well as being mentally incapacitated. This would also not allow for the involuntary intoxication plea in the condition of the REM Sleep Behavior Disorder. Ronald K. Siegel discusses this issue of intoxication, "...Although the definition of the word intoxication (which comes from the Latin *intoxicatio*, meaning poisoning or inebriation) is far from precise, one that is generally accepted in pharmacology and medicine is 'the abnormal state induced by a chemical agent....excitement or exhilaration beyond self-control.' Pollack (1976) defines such intoxication for legal purposes as: 'a temporary state of mental impairment due to drugs or alcohol in which the alcohol or drug influence creates a mental impairment that makes the person unable to form the specific intent for the crime charged against him, although the defendant committed an illegal act at the time....Intoxication is thus a clinical condition that is defined by clinical signs and symptoms, ranging from mild, moderate, to severe, with coma and eventual death...intoxication can produce frustration by interfering with a person's ongoing goal-directed activity, arousing anger, and thus leading to aggressive reactions if suitable aggression cues (stimuli associated with the frustrater) are present. Even if such cues are not present in reality but simply inferred by the user to be present due to hallucinations and/or thought disorders (e.g., paranoia state), the individuals may display relatively uncontrolled, intense emotional responses. These intense reactions to real or imagined frustrations predispose him/her to extremely hostile behavior." *(PCP PHENCYCLIDINE ABUSE: AN APPRAISAL*, p. 258, 284)

Chronic use of mind altering drugs may induce what is referred to as a "poor judgement syndrome" which could be a factor in nonviolent criminal acts such as perjury, shoplifting, embezzlement and theft. This is most likely directly linked to the effect of these drugs upon perception. The hypersexuality sometimes reported during some psychotic stages such as mania may influence motivation involved in assault and rape situations as well. Keep in mind that criminal behavior is often associated with mania. The patient's judgement is distorted by his perception of what is real. Although he may be making proper choices for his perception of reality, it becomes an improper choice when viewed from a correct perspective of reality. How do we judge someone for the choices they made given incorrect feedback from their distorted perceptions?

Prozac's ability to induce psychosis or intoxication demonstrates all the essential ingredients for such a diminished capacity defense: altered consciousness wherein the defendant's attention, awareness, and ability to respond meaningfully to the environment and situation are disturbed; mental confusion regarding the meaning of the act or its consequences; involuntary behavior which can prevent optional courses of action; and interference with goal-directed behavior so as to prevent organizing and directing physical movements. Therefore Prozac or any drug which alters perceptions and behavior through its impact upon serotonin and subsequent impact upon consciousness and perception can diminish the capacity to form or to harbor criminal intent. They do so by interfering with the mental functions which are essential to the mental process of forming intent for an act.

Donald Sokol, Doug's attorney states, *"...I am convinced the tragedy would not have happened but for the ingestion of Prozac. There are just too many similarities* between the story that Douglas related to me after we discovered the Prozac paradoxical reaction syndrome and the stories told to me by Prozac survivors whom I interviewed. They all used the same language, such as 'I had no alternative'. When Douglas first used this phrase in a conversation I was having with him in jail, I was struck by the insanity of it. He not only had other alternatives but the one he chose was the worst possible alternative, yet he considered it to be his only alternative and Douglas Cecrle is not a stupid man. His IQ is quite high."

Doug's was the first case tried in the United States in which the court ruled, after two days of evidentiary hearings on the question of Prozac involvement, that *there was a direct causal connection between Prozac and homicide* and the issue went before a jury. Because of the inability of Dr. Martin Teicher to make the court date to testify and the judge's ruling that testimony from Prozac victims with similar reactions and no prior criminal records were inadmissible, the Cecrle conviction is on appeal and the case is still pending.

St. George, Utah, the same city where, in a manner of speaking, Halcion went to trial for chemically inducing murder and was found guilty, is the setting for one of the "Prozac intoxication" murder trials. A returned Mormon missionary, devoted son, "all around nice guy" and a very caring individual, *J.C. Gardner*. J.C. had worked as a medical technician, teacher and a police officer. His mother reminisces about the kind of compassion her son always demonstrated as a young man by relating an experience about him as a teenager. She says he noticed a young lady at a church dance who was in a corner all alone, not exactly a beauty queen, who was being passed up for the prettier girls for all the dances. J.C. asked her to dance and then gathered all the other boys. He explained to them that there was no reason for someone to be humiliated because of being ignored at a dance. He told them that it would not hurt any of them to dance at least one dance with her and in fact, if they would each dance with her twice, she would dance every dance and leave that evening feeling much better about herself and so would each of the boys. She then explained that he had throughout his life displayed this same compassionate and caring attitude toward others.

J.C. had a very close and loving relationship with his father throughout his childhood. His father was a clinical psychologist who worked with delinquent boys in New Mexico, California and Nevada for thirty years and excelled in his profession. He twice headed the National Counsel on Crime and Delinquency. This was only one of many positions he held as he represented North America on juvenile delinquency, including serving as a representative on juvenile delinquency for North America at the United Nations. Because of their close relationship J.C. became very troubled and concerned by his father's deteriorating health and then devastated by his impending death. His doctor prescribed Prozac to deal with his depression. He and his father noticed problems immediately. Twelve days later they returned to the doctor and were reassured that Prozac was not the problem. They hospitalized him and released him within weeks with an additional prescription of Halcion. Six weeks later J.C.and his father returned. This time J.C. was hospitalized for a two week period. It did J.C. no good to return to his doctor. He and another patient complaining of the headaches they were experiencing from Prozac were laughed out of the doctor's office. Both were intimidatingly assured once again that Prozac has no side-effects. He had begun to go through major personality changes after being put on Prozac. No one noticed the subtle changes in J.C. as they focused on his father and concerned themselves with assisting him in his terminal illness.

Soon, acting very much "out of character" for him, J.C. who had never had a history of drinking began to drink alcohol. He made two very serious suicide attempts even though he had no history of suicidal behavior. These additional warning signals went unnoticed by all involved. J.C. then focused the Prozac-induced rage he was feeling on his ex-wife's best friend and shot and killed her. As with the majority of the cases there is little memory of the murder. What vague memory he has of it is almost unbearable for him with the intense compassion he holds for others.

His attorney, Alan Boyack, says that "what one becomes on Prozac is a psychopath and his client is not, in the classic sense, a murderer". Mixing alcohol and Prozac is a perfect formula for creating a psychopath. This combination insures that one will suffer the most severe Prozac related side-effects. Reading what patients report having felt on Prozac indicates a classic psychopathic pattern. [See the chapter PATIENT REPORTS.] When we have a drug that is, according to the patients themselves, causing an obsession to drink, thereby forcing the patient to mix these substances, how tragic might the outcome be?

The question being raised by most on the issue of "Prozac intoxication" is, "Even if Prozac is causing intoxication, shouldn't these people be accountable for their acts? Someone who is intoxicated because of alcohol is held responsible for their actions, so why not someone who is intoxicated because of Prozac?" The answer to this is that as a society we have been educated to the fact that alcohol causes intoxication, it is common knowledge. But those on Prozac have not been warned nor educated to the possibility that this substance can cause intoxication. Furthermore they have not been given *any indication* of the emotional side effects. Few understand the intoxication produced through what is being called The Serotonin Syndrome - the toxic condition produced through the excess serotonin. These patients' only crime was to have trusted the advice of their physician when they were told they needed this drug to restore their health and their doctors assured them that there was no cause for concern as this drug has little or no side effects. Theirs was not a conscious or educated choice to be "under the influence" of an intoxicating substance. (See brain wave chart of patient on Prozac for six months, whose brain waves indicate a total anesthetic sleep pattern even though the patient "appears" to be awake and functioning. Also check Dr. Janiak's statement on how mixing medications can cause intoxication.)

Yet another case, one of the most heart-breaking, yet the most heartwarming of all the cases is that of **Billy Ernst** in Santa Rosa, California. Billy was given Prozac in 1989, long before the public became aware that there were any questions about Prozac. His doctor had included other medications along with the prescription for Prozac. After having a couple of beers with his friends after a football game Billy rammed his vehicle into another car killing a young couple. There was no indication that Billy had even attempted to stop the car.

During Billy's trial Winifred Potenza, a famous artist and the mother of one of the victims, Jonathan Potenza, was very vocal in her demands for justice in the death of her son. Now Winifred Potenza is very vocal as she fights for the life and the freedom of Billy Ernst. Why? She now realizes that Billy is as much a victim of this drug as her own son. Because of the circumstances involving the death of her son, her stand is the most powerfully moving and most convincing that the Prozac patient in Billy's situation is truly a victim. She knows that Prozac murdered her son, not Billy Ernst.

There has not been a week that has gone by that Winifred is not at the prison visiting Billy. She has nothing but praise for the fine young man which she feels has been so unjustly imprisoned. The Potenza Family and the Ernst Family have become the dearest of friends through their trials. The Ernst's refer to Winifred as an "angel of mercy". Both families are full of hope and pray that Billy's burden will soon be lightened and the opportunity to go on with his life restored to him as his appeal goes before the court.

A report made to the FDA investigating panel on Prozac is one of the most moving and a story that needs to be heard. It will help us to see how Europe is responding to the problems being produced worldwide by the use of Prozac. Kevin's mother stood in dignity and nobility before the FDA panel to bear witness of her son's goodness and honor throughout his life, and of the horrifyingly tragic way his life ended. She is left alone to fight her son's battle for justice - to right the wrongs that cut his bright and promising future far too short.

She testified, "Kevin's student years were happy years. He was a great source of joy to his parents. He had a thirst for life. His life is remembered as a series of vignettes - Kevin climbing the Great Wall of China; riding a camel to the Pyramids of Giza; watching with eager fascination the animals of the Serengetti; he skied during winter month vacations. He spent his summer months with his parents in a private hotel on the French Riviera. For Kevin it was like a summer home. Everyone remembers how popular he was with the staff; how disarming his irresistible love of life."

"His curiosity and enthusiasm, the ease with which he made friends was always taking him off the beaten path. Once his parents took him with them to a Chamber of Commerce trip to the Soviet Union at a time when stringent security measures were still in force, Kevin went off on his own, met young people, enjoyed the amenities of Russian home life; all this to the amazement of nervous security people." After graduating from Wharton he spent a year in Paris before he was diagnosed with Chronic Fatigue Syndrome. He was upbeat about his situation over the next two years..."he never gave up planning his future, nor was he wasteful of time. He worked on a book, composed music, read a lot, played piano. He spoke of his new life to come. He said he wanted to marry and have a large family. He promised his parents many grandchildren."

"Kevin cherished his father. As an example of his love, he wrote in one of his letters to him, 'Dad, you are a masterpiece of a father'. When his father died Kevin was a great comfort in pulling his mother through her sudden loss."

The summer of 1990 Kevin felt much better, enough so that he was able to join his parents at their summer home in France and spend several months there. He returned home for Christmas. During that visit he had an appointment with his doctor and was given Prozac for the occasional headaches which lingered from his CFS. He had no idea that he had been given a mind-altering drug, an antidepressant. He had a fear of sedatives and did not like taking chances of toxic reactions from drugs. A few months after his return to France, his mother voiced concern over his use of Prozac. Kevin replied, "Mom, don't worry about what depressed people do. Not only do I not feel violent, to the contrary I have never felt happier. I am full of love. I love you, I love the world, don't worry about me."

It was not long before his mother received the call from a friend explaining that Kevin "had not been himself" lately and that Kevin and a friend visiting him from Germany, had just been found dead in his apartment. The investigators were baffled. Kevin's past was exemplary. All were instantly enamored by his love for others. They were captivated by his deeply caring personality. His doctor shocked by the news of his death, declared, "I know Kevin, he wouldn't harm anyone, nor would he take his life, it must be the work of a third party."

As they pieced the evidence together they found that Kevin's friend had died instantly from one stab wound in the back. *But Kevin had not died quickly. For several hours he butchered and mutilated his own body and recorded it all on an audio tape. Although right handed, his right hand was entirely severed and left on the bed.* Blood in the shower indicated he had stopped to shower. Even though there were cuts all over his body and stab wound to the Thorax, Kevin did not bleed to death. The wound that finally took his life was the one through the eye, which pierced his brain. By his side laid the weapon, *a dull kitchen knife.*

There were no cigarettes, alcohol or drugs. Kevin did not use them. It became apparent that the only drug involved was Prozac. After the French equivalent of our FBI finished an in depth eight month long investigation, which extended into our country as they investigated our Prozac murder/suicide cases, all doubt had fled. The French papers reported, "A crime was not committed, both Kevin and his friend were victims of an American drug".

Kevin's mother has devoted her life to filling Kevin's dreams of doing great things to be of service to his fellowman. She is currently building a large orphanage in his memory; the one he never had the opportunity to build himself. She wants others to understand, *"He was happy about his success; happy about his good health when he reached for the knife."*

The evidence of a REM Sleep Behavior Disorder was very evident in Kevin's case. Many paintings Kevin had done those last few days were found in his apartment. All were filled with grotesque, nightmarish subjects as Kevin apparently slipped out of consciousness and into his living nightmare. Chronic Fatigue Syndrome would have set him up to be one who would rapidly succumb to a toxic reaction.

Another report the FDA listened to during the September hearings was given by a young woman and her small niece. It is easy to understand why the child had a terrible fear of her aunt (who is her new adoptive mother) leaving her alone. The aunt, speaking on behalf of the little girl, explained how her sister, the child's mother, had violently taken her own life in front of her daughter while on Prozac. A year after that the same little girl's father also under the influence of Prozac killed his girlfriend and then himself. *Another child orphaned by Prozac - how many will we have before we realize what is happening?*

A lawsuit filed in early 1991 that has caught the public eye was filed by LeAnne Westover, the widow of 60's rock star, *Del Shannon* (Charles Westover).

227

(Although Prozac has also been indicated in the death of Abbie Hoffman, no suits have yet been filed.) According to Shannon's widow's attorney, Leonard Finz, "We are charging Eli Lilly with the same culpability as if it was Eli Lilly's finger around the trigger of the weapon that shot the bullet that ultimately took Del Shannon's life."

Del Shannon was one who never would have put Prozac in his mouth had he known it was a mind altering drug. He was very vocal in anti-drug, anti-alcohol, anti-cigarette, anti-suicide causes. He was actively involved in suicide prevention and was the first to step in and help someone reaching out for reasons to go on with their lives. Del was an avid exerciser, walking two to five miles daily and swimming or exercising was his way of ending his morning hike. His body was literally his "temple". He watched his diet closely and would often lovingly scold his wife when he felt she was jeopardizing her healthy heart by putting too much mayonnaise on her sandwich. He leaned more toward the natural way of life - diet, herbs and exercise.

The side of Del his fans never had a chance to see was the kind, loving, empathetic man who was totally devoted to his wife and family. All who knew him were shocked and amazed at his actions. Everyone felt that his actions were just so completely "out of character" for him. Del had been a recovering alcoholic for twelve years when Prozac was prescribed to help him deal with the loss of his energy, brought on by the pressures of his civic responsibilities and a rapid surge in his career. Within days personality changes were evident. He could not think clearly. The family could not understand what was wrong. As so many other families have said, "He was gone. The Del we knew was no longer there." He could not understand what was happening to him.

Two weeks after starting on Prozac Del kissed his wife as she left for the market, asked her to pick up a few things for him, walked back into his home and ended his life with a self-inflicted gunshot wound. His was another classic example of suicide with no warning signs. The personality changes in loved ones might have been a warning if that had been mentioned to the families. These people are committing suicide at exactly the point psychiatrists would not expect it at all...they appear happy, are making plans for the future, etc. Del was in good spirits when his family left, yet within minutes he had taken a violent action that destroyed his life and devastated his family. Another family had become forever affected by this Prozac pandora.

Might a portion of the inner turmoil Del was feeling be that he began to experience that "uncontrollable drive to drink" while on Prozac? Thinking, as most do, that this is their own feeling and not a feeling being produced by the drug? Could he then not bear to face the thought that he had not really overcome this problem? How does one deal with feelings like that when they think they have already overcome something like this in their life? After years of controlling such a difficult obstacle and then feeling such a "irresistible impulse" to destroy all you had worked so hard to correct would literally crush ones's self-esteem. Or was he just so confused he couldn't stand the mental barrage any longer, as those suffering akathisia relate? Unfortunately Del is not here to tell us what the feelings were that he experienced. But Del did leave us a message within one of his greatest hits from the 60's, "Runaway":

"And as I still walk on, I think of the things we've done together while our hearts were young. I'm a walkin' in the rain. Tears are fallin' and I feel the pain. Wishing you were here by me to end this misery. And I wonder...*why? Why? Why? Why? Why? Why?"*

Del does still walk on, although no longer by our side. Though he no longer suffers physical pain, he is yet capable of feeling the pain of a life cut short for no reason, the pain of being torn from his family he loves dearly and the pain of realizing that his death has *yet* been in vain as society still has not learned from what he suffered. We are continuing to suffer from the pain inflicted upon us by this insidious chemical. *There is no doubt that he cries out to us, as do all the victims of Prozac - those we are aware of and those who went unnoticed - to end this misery. They have no choice now but to rely on us who are left behind. We must, for their sakes, as well as our own, find out why this happened to them and why we are continuing to allow their deaths to go on in vain. Why have we not yet learned the lessons they would have us learn from the gift they gave us...their experience, their lives?*

Maria Malakoff is the pharmacist we mentioned earlier who attempted suicide on Prozac and whose husband Gary, also a pharmacist, did commit suicide violently in front of Maria and their four children. Maria refuses to sell Prozac in their pharmacy and warns others of the dangers of this drug. As one whose career is understanding drugs and their efficacy, her powerfully moving and chilling statement to us all is, *"I am the first pharmacist to take this off. I will no longer sell it! This is not a medicine that has gone through sufficient clinical trials. We are being used as guinea pigs! Don't let this keep going! The day will soon come that every family will be affected by this drug."*

Had we heeded Maria's chilling warning in the summer of 1991 we would not have witnessed the terrible tragedies we have seen since that time. Two occurred on the same day, three days before the FDA met to reassure us that Prozac really isn't soooo...dangerous, at least not enough to require a warning label on the bottle. In the first tragedy the small Colorado community of Steamboat Springs nestled in the tops of the Rockies went into shock as the shots rang out killing Jan Coleman and her friend, Luke McKee. A self-inflicted gunshot wound followed eight hours after holding police at bay to put an end to the Prozac induced nightmare of Jan's estranged husband *Bill Coleman.*

Bill had been using Prozac for a year. Only the week before his psychiatrist gave everyone what should have been a *big* clue that trouble was soon on its way - he doubled Bill's dosage. What a horrible shame that no one had warned any of the victims of the danger doubling his dose could pose. Bill's sister had learned only the night before that her brother was using Prozac and had instantly made plans to rush to Colorado to discuss with him the dangers of the drug. But she had learned too late to be able to deliver her warning.

Had anyone been willing to discuss the pattern that all these victims fit into so that others could be warned in advance, in Bill Coleman's case three lives would have been spared.. If they knew to look for the personality changes, the out of control behavior, the gradual pulling away from friends and family - leading to filing for divorce, the blank staring into space - the confusion, the restlessness, the total exhaustion, the desperation as the patient strives so hard to understand why he is becoming "someone he is not", etc., this tragedy would not have occurred.

Bill Coleman perfectly fit the "Prozac profile". Once again, no one who knew Bill could believe any of what they saw now as reality. The Bill they knew would do anything for anyone. This just couldn't happen. The Bill they knew *could not and would not* have done this. And they were right. As so many other friends and loved ones have described their experiences, the person they knew and loved was "gone, just gone". The Bill they knew disappeared as soon as Prozac chemically altered his brain. The Bill Coleman they knew did not do this, nor would it ever even have entered his mind to do such a thing. It was not a choice he would have made.

One of the most bizarre and repulsive of all the cases happened in San Francisco last November 6, 1991, just a little more than a month after the FDA met concerning Prozac. Police responded to a report of a fight at approximately 1:00 A.M. The officer wrote in his report that Barbara Mortenson answered the door with "dried blood covering her face and was wearing a nightgown which was completely soaked with blood in the front." She turned and ran to the bedroom where they found her 87 year old mother Mildred Mortenson "lying on the blood soaked carpet with bruises on her face, arms, legs and stomach." She "had approximately 20 human bites on her face and arms. Several bites on her arm were chewed down to the bone and pieces of raw flesh were left on the carpet." One policeman described the bites like "shark bites".

This case helps us to see the amazing strength of someone going "off the deep end" on Prozac. The patient was obviously experiencing an adrenalin rush which we are accustomed to hearing about with other stimulants such as PCP and cocaine. Remember Kevin completely severed his right hand with a dull kitchen knife even though Kevin was right handed, not left handed. Then there is the one hundred forty-three pound man who had no trouble at all breaking through his ex-wife's front door. He felt as if he were superman. In the very first case we mentioned in Marion, Illinois, the son, Larry Walters, who was a male nurse accused of killing his father who attacked him while on Prozac had to hit his dad seven times. Each one of those blows would have been enough to render a normal human being unconscious. His father was only angered by the blows, continued his attack and reached for a gun, forcing the son to stop the father by stabbing him three times with a butcher knife which he had managed to grab during the struggle. Then there is the 83 year old woman who had to be put in restraints after only three weeks on Prozac and the 12 year old Texas girl who picked up her 225 pound mother and threw her across the room and then attacked her uncle with a screwdriver. The "urban cowboy," who used twenty-eight thousand dollars in city funds to buy a whole herd of longhorn cattle during a manic reaction lasting for quite some time after months of high daily doses (60 mg.) of Prozac, describes the extra strength he felt: "When I was buying these cattle, I would go into a pen (now these are Texas Longhorns that are not really used to being handled). I would go into the pens by myself, I'm not a young man and I am over weight, but I would go in there and take hold of the catch pull (that is a noose we use to put around a dog's neck, like a stiff leash). and before I knew it I'd have those things cornered. I drug them across the pen and into a trailer by myself without any help. And loading a ton of hay was nothing to me then. Now I would probably faint. No one could believe I could do this so quickly and all by myself. These cattle were not tame and weighed five or six hundred pounds. How I got them in there I still can't tell you. Now that I look back on things I certainly did have the ability to do some really stupid things on Prozac! I didn't have any fear. I could load a ton of hay in minutes, just seconds! Today I'd have a heart attack after four bails!"

Law enforcement officials continue to be shocked and alarmed by this. They report "that's really weird stuff" or "when I meet someone on Prozac I take several steps back because their behavior is so bizarre and unpredictable that I never know what to expect." One police officer even made the statement that Prozac was "job insurance" for him and that he rarely investigated a suicide where he didn't find the drug in the victims' medicine cabinet. Government drug and alcohol abuse divisions and law enforcement officials are beside themselves to know how to handle the problem of doctors prescribing so many addictive and dangerous prescription drugs. If you want to gain better insight into the safety of Prozac or any other mind altering drug, don't ask those who are making money from the drug. Ask someone who is in drug enforcement or law enforcement. They are the ones who are left to pick up the pieces and assist these people in putting their lives back together again.

Barbara Mortenson was a college professor. We are not talking about these horribly violent and bizarre actions being taken by hard core criminals. We are talking about people we all associate with on a daily basis in every walk of life. While being taken into custody she blurted out, "...she made me mad, so mad!", indicating once again the *overwhelming rage* patients report that they experience - the side-effect of akathisia.

Alcohol had also played a part in Barbara Mortenson's case. She too could no longer fight that overwhelming compulsion to drink and consumed an incredible mount of alcohol - a half of a fifth of gin before her attack upon her mother. Mildred Mortenson did not live, she died just less than a week after the attack. Her daughter Barbara, even months later, had not been able to remember the attack and swears she did not do it. There is absolutely no recall. Months down the road, as the memory slowly begins to return, she may begin to recall it as a fuzzy nightmare. The memory is so strongly affected it takes almost forever to regain.

Within weeks after the FDA tried to convince us that all is well and that we should all bury our heads in the sand so that we would not see the evidence against Prozac mount before our very eyes, a young mother called 911, and as the police arrived stepped out on her porch, trembling, with blood trickling down the right side of her face and said, "I'm crazy! I shot my daughters."

The *Kristine Cushing case* in Laguna Niguel, California is regrettably becoming a more and more common occurrence. Four months after her psychiatrist prescribed Prozac because of her despondency over a slowly deteriorating physical condition, she shot and killed her little girls, Amy Elizabeth, 8, and Stephanie Marie, 4, and (as most do when Prozac is involved) then made an attempt to take her own life by a gunshot wound to the head.

Kristine was known as a very devoted and loving mother. Everything she did seemed centered around her role as a mother who showed her love and concern for her beautiful little girls in every thought and action. She was very actively involved in their dance classes, soccer team, church, school and other extra curricular activities. When other mothers could not be counted on Kristine was always there, even with her failing health. Her neighbors and friends admired her diligence, her concern and her compassion. She was a Brownie leader, Sunday School teacher, and was generally there to greet her new neighbors with a batch of freshly baked cookies.

In spite of all the good Kristine Cushing had been noted for throughout her life, Lt. Col. John Cushing returned from his fishing trip the next morning to a yellow ribbon no soldier or anyone else wants to greet him on his return home. With terror shooting through him he viewed the bright yellow ribbon draped around his home indicating a crime scene. Cries of pain and anguish rang out as he heard how Prozac had forever affected the lives of those he loved. And one of Amy's classmates voiced the sentiments of all who knew Kristine as she boldly crossed her arms and declared, "I've known Mrs. Cushing a long time, and she would not do that. I don't care what the newspapers said. Newspapers can lie."

Only a short distance away and within just weeks, another Prozac consumer, Stacy Phan shot her little girl in the head and laid down on a freeway with her to die. Devoted mothers killing their own children. Not even the strongest bonds of love and caring - a mother's love for her child nor a child's love for a parent - are strong enough to withstand the powerful effects of this chemical attack upon the brain. This chemical attack which, in turn, alters one's normal actions and behavior.

REDBOOK ran an article on Kristine Cushing in their February, 1992 issue. It probed deeply into Kristine's life and past, **looking beyond the mark** for other reasons for this chemically induced insanity.

If someone had slipped LSD, PCP, cocaine or a similar "street drug" into her food and she then had a "bad trip" during which she shot her little girls, no one would search her life and past to find the "reason" for her bizarre behavior. It would have been obvious to everyone that it was a reaction to the drug. Why is it so difficult to understand that a drug is a drug and an individual could have a similar reaction to a prescription drug? Chemical substances do not go through a type of miraculous metamorphosis to change them into a substance "guaranteed safe or harmless" just because a doctor or pharmaceutical company, rather than a "pusher" is the one marketing it.

If anyone is still suffering from the delusion that the FDA or the government are our great protectors, they should *seriously rethink* that position in light of the recent silicon breast implant scandal and radiation scandal, government chemical mind control experimentation, not to mention the long list of deadly drugs which have been removed from the market over the years - all those which, in spite of the FDA's stamp of approval, time and experience have proven to be not only unsafe and harmful, but even fatal. In light of the disclosure of financial interests held by FDA panel members who voted on Prozac warning labels, those still believing in the infallibility of the FDA should study the details mentioned in the chapter LILLY AND POLITICS. Beyond that, most of the general public still mistakenly believe that the FDA is the organization that actually tests all the drugs, instead of understanding that the testing is done by the drug companies manufacturing and marketing it...*those who have a vested interest.*

We sit in our living rooms and watch news coverage of a major drug ring being arrested and we cheer. We con ourselves into believing that great strides are being made in the drug war while we ignore the overwhelming problems involving prescription drug use and abuse. Yet drug enforcement officials and detoxification unit workers admit these drugs have worse withdrawal and are more dangerous to handle in detoxification and police report their concern over what they see associated with these drugs. When the "pusher" cloaks himself in the robes of sophistication, political manipulation and a marvelously professional advertising campaign to convince us that "bad is good and good is bad" we even find ourselves fighting to protect the interests of this large pharmaceutical company who would have us believe that they have our interests at heart as they turn a deaf ear to the rapidly rising number of suffering victims and rake in their profits. Then the pharmaceutical company, in it's effort to appear respectable and acceptable, either cons or buys out the one person we trust with our very lives, our family doctor. We sit back and call this capitalism, "the American way" or just "business as usual" and wonder what has gone wrong with our country's health care!

Dr. Julian Whitaker in the January, 1992 issue of *WELLNESS TODAY* says of his fellow physicians, "On television, doctors like Marcus Welby and Trapper John, M.D. are angels of mercy. They are motivated only by a desire to make people well. These modern-day saints are above the temptations of status, prestige, money and personal pleasure.

"But that's on television. It's quite different in the real world. *Most people would*

234

be shocked to discover that their doctor's advice could be colored by less than virtuous motives. You're supposed to believe that everyone in the medical community is in it purely for humanitarian reasons. If you believe that, just try to see a doctor or check into a hospital without flashing your insurance card!..Did you know that some hospitals offer special incentive deals that give doctors valuable gifts like fax machines and car phones if they schedule surgeries when the hospitals are hurting for business?..If your doctor is prescribing a certain drug for you, wouldn't it bother you to know that the makers of the drug may have offered him a free trip to New Orleans in return for his patronage? Drug companies regularly bribe doctors with free drugs, dinners, trips and even cash."

A similar article with the same accusations ran on the front page of the *SALT LAKE TRIBUNE* on April 3, 1992. It was an Associated Press article entitled, "80% of Doctors Say Drug Firms Try to 'Buy' Business". It quoted Richard P. Kusserow, inspector general of the Department of Health and Human Services, "Some of these offers, in addition to being inappropriate, may be illegal." But the pharmaceutical firms don't stop with doctors, they include your pharmacist in bribing you to use their drugs too. *THE SEATTLE TIMES*, April 5, 1994, ran an article on the pharmaceutical firm Miles Inc. who market Adalat CC, a drug identical in content to Procardia XL, which is sold by Pfizer, the makers of Zoloft. They were given a $605,000 penalty for paying out $358,415 over a four month period to pharmacists to who encouraged patients to switch to their product. It is clear that drug companies have no qualms about "buying business."

How can we be so sure that our system is so infallible and not blinded to the all too plausible possibility that this violence is being chemically induced by Prozac? According to personal interviews with the large and growing number of ex-Prozac patients, *excess adrenalin* **chemically demands** *"fight or flight" action, and one needs no logical reason to commit murder while on Prozac.* As the level of excess adrenalin rises, the rage that builds up inside is described by them as "so totally overwhelming, unlike anything ever experienced before". [This rage is the most common report that patients notice in themselves next to memory loss.] Because they cannot understand where this rage within them is coming from, they often assume that those closest to them must be "the cause" for the upsetting roller coaster feelings they are experiencing. These people were always the ones who caused feelings to run deep enough to inflict such pain before so that must be the case now. They then often focus that rage on those they care about the most. So because of these confused thought processes and misplaced blame for deeply disturbing feelings, it is often someone close to the person on

Prozac whose life is in danger.

When that chemically-induced rage is coupled with reports of feeling no concern for the consequence of any act, feeling no guilt, feeling no ability to care about others, coupled with chemically-induced confusion, and "irresistible impulse" which the medical reports repeat over and over, what inhibitions are left to stop them from acting upon the rage that they find so overwhelming? How often they repeat the words, "I found myself doing things I didn't...I didn't want to do."

Although Kristine Cushing appears very much alone as she sits silently in her jail cell trying to sort out what has happened to her and her family, she is far from alone and her precious daughters are not either. Tucker Moneymaker's wife shot both of their young sons before turning the gun on herself. She had only been on Prozac for three weeks. We already mentioned the case of Kenneth Seguin who killed his two children and his wife. The reader must be made aware of the seriousness and magnitude of this problem nationwide. We have many patients who have now been on Prozac *far longer* than they can safely stay on such a powerful drug and many at high doses who are literally "living on the very edge" of their own Prozac Pandora. The "explosive nightmare" Judge Leonard Finz speaks of is at our doors. A few weeks ago I contacted someone about a mortgage on my home. When it was mentioned that I was just finishing the writing of a book on Prozac, he said, "My wife was on that when it first came out and attempted suicide." As we finished our conversation I told him I was glad to learn that his wife was one of "the lucky ones" who survived her Prozac experience. He replied, "Well she has a couple of friends who were not so lucky. One is in trouble now and she is trying to help her. The other is in prison in another state after killing her little girl while on Prozac." In my own neighborhood there are at least three Prozac patients within one block in each direction who are all showing definite signs of being on the verge of "going off the deep end on Prozac," not counting the four who are disabled, almost completely unable to read or write or work after at least two years on Prozac. They report an inability to focus or concentrate long enough to comprehend what they are reading and creative thought becomes almost impossible to engage in. This is only one neighborhood. How many others are there similar to this one? What about your own? Since doctors have been telling their patients that they should tell no one they are using Prozac, you may have difficulty even finding out who is on it.

Many groups are beginning to voice concern over the problems arising from the use of Prozac. The National Firearms Association has run a long series of articles to inform their members of the problem. They are especially concerned because of the obsession Prozac patients have with guns. Just yesterday another family called to report concern over an elderly aunt who is playing with a gun. She was rolling the barrel of the loaded gun back and forth in her mouth. These stories never cease to amaze even those who think they have "heard it all"! There are more and more patients admitting the obsession they develop with guns and knives. Mothers are coming forward and admitting that while on Prozac they began visualizing either stabbing or shooting their children and even after discontinuing the drug have homicidal flashbacks. They refuse to watch violent or gory television shows or movies because of the feelings they are reminded of having experienced while on Prozac.

Because these thoughts are so foreign and repulsive to them it is difficult for these mothers to admit to ever having such thoughts cross their minds, they want Kristine Cushing and other mothers experiencing this to know that they are not alone. They hope that by coming forward they can help a mother who may be having these feelings understand that it is the drug. Those feelings are chemically induced and the Prozac patient can have control over thoughts and feelings again as the drug leaves the body and mind. This is the hope they wish to share as they courageously come forward with their "unspeakable" experiences...those thoughts and experiences which they can barely tolerate relating in tones above a whisper.

Prozac survivors groups are still continuing to take reports of mothers who jump in their cars and drive three to four hours away in order to be far enough away from their children so as not to give in to the sudden powerful urges they are feeling to hurt them. These mothers are puzzled by their own feelings and behavior and do not trust themselves. It is heart rending to hear how their little children cling to them as they are ready to leave for school, crying, "Mommy are you going to be here when we come home from school today? Please Mommy, we miss you so much!"

The older children, who are more aware of the seriousness of their parent's situation, report flushing the prescription of Prozac down the toilet whenever they get a chance. In this way they voice their own unique statement of concern, or they make comments to their grandparents, such as, "Mom takes those pills and they make her crazy!" Then they try *so hard* to find a way to adjust to the *bizarre dysfunctional behavior* they see in their family as it falls apart slowly. And the children themselves become even more dysfunctional as they attempt to adjust to the insanity, while holding onto the memory of the parent they have loved. The parent they have loved who is disappearing before their eyes or is described as being "gone, just gone" or "no longer there". It is a far too common practic among the parent on Prozac to share their prescription with their children. They also often take them to a physician to get their own bottle of Prozac, until the whole family is on the drug, including small children. (Why do doctors go along with this insanity?)

Divorce is something the children generally have to deal with as the Prozac parent goes through the drastic personality changes and begins withdrawing from their mates. They blame their mates for the rage they feel. They can no longer feel the deep love or compassion they had for them. They have distorted memories of reality and have trouble sorting out what is real in their relationships. Divorce is one of the most common experiences. Then as the members of the extended family are pushed away by the Prozac patient, the children don't even have them to turn to for the help they so desperately need as they seek to understand the nightmare that is tearing their family apart.

The children are also confused by the barriers produced by the drug which are blocking them from the love and concern their parent can no longer feel for them. All across the nation children are being put in an extremely perilous position as they are being left alone with mothers on Prozac. The fathers who have become unable to tolerate watching as their families are falling apart or their wives on Prozac become someone they no longer know are leaving home and leaving the children behind. Or the husbands are being driven out of the home by their wives on Prozac who begin demonstrating violent, cold and abusive behavior. The children in these instances are left to fend for themselves. And fathers on Prozac are becoming so violent that wives and children are in constant fear for their lives, not knowing where to turn for help or what to do.

Mothers report that they have even picked their children up and thrown them across the room. Then as they wait for reactions of shock and disbelief to be expressed at their disclosure because these behaviors are out of character and shocking to them. They confess that they no longer have any feelings of love or concern for their children, even for newborn babies. They are hesitant to admit this. The whole situation is so foreign to them and contrary to anything they have ever felt before. They understand *intellectually* that this absence of feeling is not right, yet they become completely incapable of accessing those feelings.

How much pain and suffering will it take before someone hears the cries of the children and does something? If you are using Prozac now and experiencing any of these feelings toward your children, or you know of someone in this situation, please contact either the national Prozac Survivors Support Group listed in the back of this book. Please do not try to continue to control the thoughts and feelings you are experiencing without support. These are *powerful chemically induced compulsions* which can overwhelm the patient. Please do not take the chance. There are those who understand. You need the support and understanding of someone who has already "walked in your moccasins". It is up to you how many more children will suffer such terribly violent deaths and abuse.

Many of those who sense they are in trouble on Prozac give their children away. Betty Broderick is one who did this. Betty was a wealthy La Jolla, California divorcee' who in November of 1989, one month after the Wesbecker massacre in Kentucky, before dawn broke into her ex-husband's bedroom and shot and killed him and his new wife. I am appalled that little to almost nothing has ever been mentioned during her court case or any interviews about how her use of Prozac could have played a major part in this murder. A *TV GUIDE* article from February 29, 1992 pointed out a woman's magazine with the cover reading, "Why did Betty Broderick wait so long to kill her husband?" Has anyone ever even mentioned that one of the more recent changes in her life was that she had begun to use Prozac? All around her seem oblivious to what has happened to her except for those who have been personally affected by Prozac in their own lives.

Oprah did a two day interview in the fall of 1992 with Betty and her family. Not one word was said about her use of Prozac even though she has been using the drug since almost the introduction of Prozac to the market. Oprah's interview brought out all the classic Prozac-induced symptoms reported by other Prozac patients: refers to herself as "evil"; intended to kill herself after the murder, but had no bullets left in the gun; no one believed she was capable of murder - her children, her friends, even the victims themselves; the murder happened in the early morning hours (A large number of Prozac murders happen at night or in the early morning when sleepwalk would generally be expected to happen displaying further evidence of a chemically induced RBD.); she was calm before the murder indicating the impulsiveness of the violent behavior; she feels no remorse indicating the inability to feel emotions or guilt. Her uncontrolled swearing is typical. She left her children on her husband's porch one at a time and then in her confused state thought he had kidnapped them (we will discuss in more detail the False Memory Syndrome or false accusations in the following chapter). Other types of paranoia appeared evidenced in her belief that her husband was trying to destroy her and believing that she was the victim in the situation. She also was described by her attorney as having a "narcisstic" personality (self-centered, blaming others for everything and taking no responsibility for actions). All these reactions demonstrate an all too typical pattern of someone in trouble on Prozac. These indications should not necessarily be expected to be drug related. There are other factors in life which lead to these behaviors, but when someone is using a mind-altering substance which can cause these reactions, a drug relationship should be the *first* possibility considered. If Betty was found to be legally drunk we would have no problem understanding such behavior. We need to begin to look at mind-altering drug use with this same type of understanding because *their mind-altering effects are far more powerful than alcohol.*

It is true that Betty was having problems with violent outbursts and suicidal thoughts before her use of Prozac. In 1986 she kept a butcher knife under her car seat, tried to shoot her governess and ran ranting and raving down the street. If we knew her psychiatric drug use history it would help us to understand more about the role any of these drugs had to play in her behavior. Prozac is not the only one that has been implicated in violent and bizarre behaviors by inducing akathisia reactions. The fact still remains that she never reached the point of actually losing enough control to commit murder before Prozac and her previous behavior was not any indication to her family or even to her victims that this would have been a possibility.

In Tacoma, Washington, Fran Turner worked as a paramedic. She was one of the best until a nearly naked woman ran screaming into the emergency room one evening with 23 stab wounds and the knife still imbedded in her chest. In an attempt to help her onto a gurney, Fran ruptured a disc in her back. With the first surgery Fran, in her early thirties, no one asked her before administering anesthesia if she was smoking and taking birth control pills. The combination caused a stroke. Her drug induced nightmare had begun. After several years of relearning how to do many things and continuing back pain, she began to see psychiatrist Jessy Ang. Dr. Ang prescribed Prozac. Fran experienced several grand mal seizures. (Her mother's demands for answers were never even acknowledged.) She listed the drug side effects as: total deprivation of sleep, radical rise in depression, increase in muscle spasms (severe and prolonged) in L4-5 back, increase in spasms in left hip, increase in pain in both legs, decreased sensation in both feet, increase in (severe and prolonged) headaches, diarrhea, dehydration, total loss of appetite and alternating chills and sweating. [How many symptoms of the toxic condition, the serotonin syndrome, did you count?]

The list of drugs grew as she experienced more and more side effects. Amazingly, even under the influence of such an unbelievable array of drugs, Fran had the where with all to continue to demand that she be taken off the drugs, Dr. Ang refused. He felt she needed to stay on Prozac longer. He argued with her GP that the GP should be the one to take her off the drugs he had prescribed to her. Fran wrote to Dr. Ang just before she died. "I was depressed so you fed me Prozac. I couldn't sleep so you gave me Halcion and Sinequan. Whenever I was pushed beyond my limits you ordered Serax. These drugs were *your* choice of treatment, not mine. If anybody is responsible for me staying on them for too long it's you not me. Your course of treatment was to deal with the symptoms - not the underlying causes...The next time you order your favorite drugs for someone, think of me and be aware that patients need the *counseling* skills you've learned far more than the drugs your 'MD' allows you to cop-out with."

Only days before and on her own she discontinued Prozac, Halcion, Serax, Dilantin, Midrin, Lasix and Vistaril. She continued to take Darvocet, Soma, Lioresal and Deseryl until a few days later she pulled a gun in Dr. Ang's office and shot herself.

Fran's 71 year old handicapped mother placed a memorial to her in the Tacoma paper. One reference was made to Dr. Ang. "My days and nights are filled with sorrow and sadness for you Honey, all because your doctor kept you on Prozac too long. It was your doctor and Prozac that took you away from me." She also mailed him two photographs of Fran - one in her wedding dress and one in her coffin. She also continued to call to get some answers about her daughter's death. This prompted legal action by Dr. Ang. The news article caption read, "Psychiatrist complains mother blames him for daughter's death." He filed charges for harassment and sought legal assistance in stopping her. Personally I have about as much sympathy for him as I do the doctor who has a friend's father on 23 pills daily, six of them are Prozac.

This chapter represents a very small sampling of many, many, many cases taken from volumes of material. These we have related are not even among the most tragic of the stories. Many of the worst are still under investigation with little information yet available to the public. Others have been settled out of court and gag orders placed upon those involved. We do not have time or space to relate the stories behind all of the lawsuits. According to Michael O'Brien of the Citizen's Commission on Human Rights, "The majority of people [who suffer the adverse effects of Prozac] will either kill themselves, be unable to find a lawyer, never find out the drug caused it or be so shattered by the destructive effects of the drug that they will never be able to secure their rights."

Dr. Janiak, who explained to us about drug interactions, refers to those who have adverse reactions brought on by a combination of drugs as "victims." These

241

people are literally victims of adverse drug-reactions, drug-interaction and drug overdose. Those facing legal proceedings have suffered a chemically-induced "Hell" to which the court system could not and *should not* add. Any punishment the court system might impose upon the victims of Prozac would not even begin to compare with what they have already suffered as a result of the effects of the drug. As I look out across the Utah State Prison from the mountain above my thoughts turn to J. C. Gardner who now waits there for his appeal to be heard. His was an exemplary life before Prozac. Now it is shattered. How does one who has always had such high morals and values cope with such devastating chemically induced actions taken on their part? Many now understand that the person who took those actions was not them, but a chemically created and controlled being they never knew and never want to see again. My heart cries out to those who never had a chance to know that these were not choices made on their own, but actions which were drug-induced, chemically-induced...those victims who still wonder why or how such things could have happened in their lives.

J. C. is now physically imprisoned - restrained from outside physical activities, but at least he has been set free from the far more terrible drug-induced mental prison he has experienced for three years out of his life while on Prozac and recovering from Prozac. His mind is now his once again. Isn't he better off than the individual still continuing to suffer this *prison of the mind* produced by continued Prozac use? There is no doubt in my mind which would be easier for me to handle. Funny, I've never thought of prison as a haven from a fate far worse. Perhaps it is what Winston Smith alluded to in George Orwell's book *NINETEEN EIGHTY FOUR*, "'They can't do that,' she said...'they can't get inside you.' 'No,' he said a little more hopefully, 'no; that's quite true. *They can't get inside you. If you can feel that staying human is worth while, even when it can't have any result whatever, you've beaten them.'"* Remember that with a drug they can get inside you.

We must keep in mind that one does not have to be classified as a "basket case" or labeled with a serious mental condition to be given a prescription for Prozac, as we have seen, a headache or a case of the flu is all that is necessary. It can happen and could have happened to any of us. Many of the victims were extremely careful about anything they put into their bodies. The fact remains that the truth was not told to them about the drug they were prescribed. They believed in their fellowman enough to trust what was told to them. How terrible to add legal complications to the pain of these experiences...experiences which will follow them...experiences which will haunt them throughout their lives.

Who is the responsible party in all these cases? The *NATIONAL LAW JOURNAL* summed up the legal aspect of the Prozac controversy in October, 1990 saying, "Prozac's safety ultimately may be decided by the civil litigation surrounding its use." This appears to be the case. It serves as a sad commentary on what is the motivating force behind consumer protection in our country today. We can be sure that profits will cover the business losses even after the lawsuits for damages are settled. After all that is the bottom line in business.

CHAPTER 9

PATIENT REPORTS
LISTENING TO PATIENTS, NOT PROZAC

If someone is contemplating buying a product, how often does he just take the word of the salesman and the manufacturer about it? One generally goes to previous customers of that particular product to see if those consumers were "satisfied customers". Eli Lilly did not miss a trick in their marketing strategy though. They made their previous customers out to be "depressed", "crazy", "mentally incompetent", "a nut case", or someone with "mental" problems who would not have been on a psychiatric drug if they were "okay" or "normal". Who would want to listen to what these patients, who are obviously "not competent" anyway, would have to say about their experience with this miracle cure?

In reality, the ones who are unaware of what they are experiencing are those who are still under the influence of this mind-altering substance which affects one's reasoning and judgement. Dr. Breggin addresses this issue also, "In their mild delirium, patients themselves will say they are improved, due to the temporary high or euphoria associated with the initial stages of brain dysfunction and delirium. This is a familiar phenomenon that occurs frequently during the early stage of alcoholic intoxication. As in intoxication with alcohol, mild degrees of drug-induced delirium may be undetected by the patient or other observers and yet impair the individual's capacity to feel anything, including depression." (*TOXIC PSYCHIATRY*, p. 170) How many would believe a drunk when he tells us how great he is or how much he can do in his drunken stupor? How many reporters would in all seriousness interview a drunk and ask him to expound upon the "marvelous benefits of alcohol"? Yet reporters around the world are doing exactly that with those using Prozac. It's amazing, just amazing that someone who is now "sober" (no longer using the mind-altering substance, Prozac) is considered less credible than someone who is "drunk" (still on the drug and telling everyone how great it is).

If anyone would like to interview a long list of unhappy Prozac consumers or their widows or widowers or fatherless, motherless, childless survivors - those given the drug for post-operative pain, yeast infections, Chronic Fatigue Syndrome, back pain or many other conditions - non-mentally related conditions, contact the National Director of the Prozac Survivor's Support Group listed at the end of this chapter who can refer you to as many individuals as you would like. There is so much insight to be gained from those who have experienced these things that it is important to relate their experiences to help others understand. To give the reader an idea of what living in this Prozac pandora has been like for these patients, we will discuss some of their stories in detail and then let them in their own words describe their own experiences.

Let's begin by discussing a personal interview with a woman who had called to defend her use of Prozac, or give a "testimonial" for the drug. She works as a government office employee with government insurance funds covering her prescription costs. She has always been very religious and has a daughter who has always meant very much to her, particularly so because of the difficulty she experienced in conceiving this only child. She had nothing but praise for her daughter. This woman has always been a good mother and an honest law-abiding citizen.

The interview began with her stating that "Prozac had saved her life". She "could not live without Prozac" and she didn't know what she would do without it. She then announced that her use now spanned a period of *four years*. Red flags went up immediately for me. I have found that generally someone who has been on the drug that long has begun to experience reactions from the drug.

Someone in this woman's situation will generally defend the drug for 30 to 40 minutes before they will begin to admit the problems they have begun to notice in their lives. The reason for their defense of the drug appears to be two fold. The first reason being that they have attempted to come off the drug on their own when they first began to notice the drug was producing problems for them, but the attempted withdrawal was *so terrible* that they are frightened to death of ever attempting to go through it again. Most state they know they will be far too ill to hold onto their jobs, if they attempt withdrawal, and they cannot afford to lose the income. They are correct in assuming that the withdrawal could produce such debilitating symptoms that they might lose their jobs because that is often the case. The probability cannot be ignored, especially when someone has been on Prozac for four years. The second reason is that their reactions to the drug usually have to reach *the worst possible* scenario before the patient can even recognize the problems, because their ability to see and reason is so severely impaired. They generally state that everyone around them saw the problems, but they themselves were unaware of their own condition.

This woman laid out a background describing a life of devotion to her church, family and her little daughter, the daughter she had finally been able to conceive after ten long years of waiting. After continuing to defend Prozac for about 35 minutes the woman made this statement: "Well...I must admit that it does really bother me that *I just can't stop shoplifting and I've got my 10 year old daughter helping me!* I always tell her that what we are doing is wrong, but I just can't stop. Last night I even took something from the store where my husband works and he could lose his job! What am I going to do? I don't take anything I need. I don't even understand why I would take the things I take. It's crazy! I even got caught one day trying to put a shopping cart in my trunk at the grocery store! I don't know what I was going to do with it. My daughter was screaming at me not to do it when a man came over and asked me what I was doing. I can't believe he didn't arrest me. I just know I am going to get caught!"

At that point you want to say, "Hello! Is anyone home?" or "Have the lights come on yet?" The thought processes become so confused that the patient can no longer think through a problem to arrive at a reasonable or logical conclusion. The confusion becomes too great. Throughout the conversation her little girl was standing near her mother to monitor the conversation. The children with their amazing sensitivity and intuition generally understand that their parent is in trouble and needs to be protected so the child takes over - just as with an alcoholic parent. The mother then told her daughter, who had been loudly voicing her embarrassment for her mother's confessions and recommending that she say no more, to leave the room. With the daughter out of the room, the mother, hand cupped over the mouthpiece on the phone, said, "I don't want her anymore. Isn't that *terrible* for a mother to say?! I can't feel anything for her anymore. All those years I waited and hoped for a baby and for so many years she was *everything* to me and now *I don't feel* anything for her! What am I going to do? I can't stand feeling like this!!!"

As so many ex-patients have stated, the only thing she can do is stop taking the drug to end the compulsive feelings causing the shoplifting and to regain her feelings of love and concern for her child. I expressed their feelings to her. Her response to any suggestion of getting help to quit using Prozac was, "I can't do that. It's too hard. I know I won't be able to keep my job and we need the money." When asked if the job was worth the possible loss of her life or her daughter's life she ended the conversation.

The next time you hear a patient say, "Prozac has saved my life! I can't live without it." Please consider that if you could probe deeper into their minds and hearts *with love and concern and understanding and a strong belief in who that individual really is and a recognition of each unique strength they possess,* you may find that they will confess to you the same fears, trauma and desperation which they generally find so difficult to admit to those around them. This woman's story is one of *many, many more just like it*. In fact I could easily write an entire book with similar stories.

To give an example of a common call from someone wanting questions answered about what others are experiencing with Prozac, let's refer to a call that came in from a woman visiting Utah from Colorado. She was in town to visit a friend in a psychiatric hospital. When she had been in town visiting this same friend three months earlier she had heard a radio show on Prozac and began to wonder about what she was seeing happening to her friend. She stated the her friend she was visiting had been "the most stable human being I have ever known" before she began taking Prozac *three years* earlier. Now this same friend has been in and out of a psychiatric hospital for the past year, going through a pattern of in two weeks and out one week before she collapses and is readmitted. She uses a razor blade to cut tic-tac-toe games into the flesh of her legs. Just two months before this the friend's doctor diagnosed her friend as having multiple personalities and diabetes. (I am constantly amazed at how often in interviews patients reveal that they never began to "split off" into multiple personalities until *after* a period of mind altering psychiatric drug use.)

When the woman was asked if she was aware or if her friend had been advised by her doctor that diabetes is listed as a possible side-effect of Prozac, she was shocked and said she would immediately discuss it with her friend. She then went on to explain why she personally had begun to suspect that Prozac was causing these problems in her friend's life. First was her own sister's experience with the drug. The sister, after going through a divorce, took the drug for a year and she went through a complete change in personality. After being off Prozac for a year this woman voiced concern that she may never see her sister (the sister she knew before Prozac) again. She felt that her sister had experienced permanent brain damage from the drug use. She was not aware of the *very long period of withdrawal* that patients report. She also pointed out that the sister had remarried during her period of Prozac use and had "totally destroyed" the marriage. She had also become quite hostile and had even accused their father of molesting her. The caller had explained that she knew this was impossible since the father was with her in another state when the sister reported that he had supposedly molested her sister.

Then the caller's voice became very soft, almost a whisper, as if she was giving a confession. "Well I was on it too, very briefly, two years ago. I took it for only five days and I couldn't stand how it made me feel so I went off it. I felt *soooo...tired* on it!"

I explained to her that she was lucky to have come off Prozac so quickly since that feeling of total exhaustion was generally a sign that one is on the verge of having very serious problems with Prozac. She then said, "Well two days after I came off I did commit suicide and was revived. That is the main reason I am in town to review a book that was just released on my near death experience."

Her story gives us an idea of just how far reaching the effect has been in the lives of so many. This one call represented three individual patients whose lives were shattered and nearly destroyed along with all those around them who love and care for them or associate with them. Just how many other lives were affected by their experiences? How far reaching does it have to get before something is done?

Others remain completely unaware of what is happening to their loved ones on Prozac and what is beginning to mount up as a direct threat to their own lives. One wife was still suffering from the delusion that, after three years of use, Prozac was "saving her husband's life". She was totally unaware that the type of marital problems they were experiencing and the bizarre behavior her husband was exhibiting were both commonly reported patterns from people on Prozac. The most critical information of which she was completely unaware was the fact that her husband was playing with and had been carrying a hunting knife for several months. He had frightened their eleven year old son by showing it to him just a few weeks before. The son had not mentioned it to his mother. This man had asked me if I thought his behavior could be related to Prozac, because he has never had such a fascination for knives before. He keeps the knife near him, in his briefcase, as he conducts his business throughout the day. Prozac users want the weapons nearby "in case they need them". It is as if the knives and guns are a comfort to them...giving them security. Perhaps this is the only way they feel they can exert control over their situation because they feel so completely out of control internally. Does it become, in the end their only way of exerting control over their own behavior...the only way they feel they can stop themselves from doing the things they "don't want to do" which they feel so compelled to do?

Another young father whose wife for over a year thought her husband "had really mellowed out and was doing very well on Prozac" was shocked to learn what he was really feeling inside. After going through withdrawal and finally starting to feel like himself again, he broke down and tearfully expressed his gratitude for learning what was happening to him. It was the day before his baby's first birthday (his first child) and he was so excited to be able to share that with her, just to spend time with her, to enjoy sharing this experience with her. He said, "I don't even remember her birth. I have no recall of that most precious event in my life. I feel like I was robbed of the first six months of her life because of my fears of being anywhere near her. While on Prozac the thoughts I kept having about her were so violent that I was afraid I might hurt her, so I stayed away from her." His wife never knew he was going through this or having such thoughts and fears. How do you admit to someone you love, someone you want to continue to have respect for you and to admire you that you are having thoughts and feelings that even you find so repulsive, thoughts and feelings which you believe that no one could understand? If you can't understand them yourself, how do you share them with anyone else? And if you do...will they still love you? It takes very strong, solid loving and caring relationships in order to work through these types of situations.

The thoughts of violence and self destruction are expressed in many ways. One woman went into a terrible rage and took a baseball bat to her husband's antique car collection. Many focus their anger on one person and begin stalking them. A radio producer told me about the woman he had dated just before meeting and marrying his wife who was the talk show host I was about to do a show with. His girlfriend and he were driving down the road about a month after she started on Prozac when she gave him a sharp punch in the jaw. Shocked, he asked why she did it. She replied that she had no idea, no reason, she just felt like doing it. Of course at that point he gave her an ultimatum, "me or Prozac". She made her choice and he married the talk show host instead.

Many reports come in about those on Prozac having quite unnecessary *multiple* plastic surgical procedures. It is almost as if they want to justify their compulsion to cut themselves by having someone else do it for them. One woman's reason for the multiple surgeries was that she wanted the painkillers she was given. It was her way of getting more drugs. So many bizarre behavioral reactions occur in conjunction in this self-destruct mode. The young woman who called in on a radio program and tearfully revealed to all the listeners how she had thrown herself down flights of stairs, cut her arms, etc., etc., during her three months of Prozac use was definitely one of the most bizarre. To finish the list of self-destructive acts she told us that just the week before she had even run over her own arm with her car! I thought I had heard everything. In fact, I actually thought her call must be a prank until a young woman and her husband showed up at a lecture on Prozac the following night. When I noticed the cast on her arm, I thought, "No, it can't really be possible that her story was real!" I recalled that the name she had given was Stacy. As I walked toward the extremely shy couple I said, "You wouldn't be Stacy would you?" It was! After a brief conversation I found that the therapist's solution for *her* problems was for *Stacy's husband* to start on Prozac too so that he could then deal with *her* self-destructive behavior! This was also the case with eighteen year old Cris Reid in Seattle, Washington. Cris's girlfriend was put on Prozac in order to help her deal with his death and she nearly took the life of her family while driving wildly on the drug. Within five short weeks on Prozac Cris's mom was shocked to notice that his arm was only skin and bones as she put her arm in his to walk down the isle at his sister's wedding. The weight loss had happened so quickly his mother had not noticed what was happening until then. She immediately made a mental note to call his doctor the following day, but never got the chance. Later that same night Cris, who had always been the one so full of life, took his own life. A short time later another friend was reminded by Cris's father, who was yet unaware of the Prozac connection in Cris's death, that he should be sure to take his medication so that he did not end up like Cris. The young man took his Prozac and committed suicide by ramming his car head on into another car on the freeway on his way home. So many cases are complicated by these multiple Prozac situations as loved ones are given the drug to cope with another's tragic death or psychotic reaction. Cris's mother has been shocked by the fact that almost 100% of those who have committed suicide in the suicide support group for family members that she attends were on the "antidepressant" Prozac at the time of their suicide and so many surviving family members have been given the drug to help them "cope" with the deaths. She asks, "If this drug is such an effective antidepressant, why do so many commit suicide while on it? Where were the antidepressant effects of the drug when these people needed them?" The sister of the sixteen year old on Prozac, who hung herself with her tennis shoe strings from a tree in the church yard, made identical comments about the suicide survivors group she attends in Virginia. From coast to coast these are the reports.

Another woman who was prescribed Prozac for an eating disorder became so obsessed about cleaning her house that she worked herself to the point of complete exhaustion. Feeling too tired to continue living she climbed to her roof to put an end to her misery by jumping off. Even in her confused and desperate state she determined that the fall would not be far enough to accomplish a successful suicide and gave up the idea, but she did notice how filthy the roof was and busily cleaned until it was spotless. When her poor husband arrived home and was not observant enough to comment on her spotless and sparkling roof, she "hit the ceiling" and flew into a rage telling him he never noticed anything she does for him. These are perfect examples of the total lack of logical reasoning the patients are experiencing as a result of Prozac toxicity. Is it any wonder why we are seeing *so many* divorces?

Patient after patient is developing what is referred to as a narcissistic personality.

This is a complicated mental state. Briefly, as they and those around them explain this state is that the patient began to feel that he was infallible and began blaming everyone else for his problems. With the memory so commonly affected and strongly affected, this becomes an understandable occurrence.

FALSE MEMORY SYNDROME, OUR 1990'S DRUG-INDUCED WITCH HUNT One of the most priceless of all our possessions is our memory. Most of us rarely ponder the critical role memory plays in our lives. We receive and transmit information within our brain via messages delivered by the chemicals in the brain. Anything we gather through all of our senses is recorded through this process. Emotional responses are also produced through these brain chemicals. In fact, the greater the emotion connected to an event the greater is our ability to remember the event. Perhaps Prozac's disruption of the chemical processes affecting emotion plays a significant role in memory impairment. Does blocking emotions block the memory process to some extent as well?

Philip G. Zimbardo explains the importance of memory in an article entitled, Mind Control: Political Fiction and Psychological Reality, from the book *ON NINETEEN EIGHTY-FOUR*, "...vital...is the individual's development of a balanced temporal perspective of the past, the present, and the future. Central to human nature, then, is a mental facility for becoming involved in what was, what is now, and what will be. When a moral-ethical system is added to this temporal trilogy, human behavior is guided by an awareness of what could have been and what ought to be.

"Memory establishes the continuity of self over time and thereby a sense of personality. The past provides the present with standards, criteria for comparison, the wellsprings of tradition, and the stable references for the transient flux of immediate experience. Feelings connect us to other people through our passions and compassion for them -- and theirs for us. Strong affect engages us fully in the expanded moment of the present, giving a vibrancy to our experience that intellect alone cannot. Through affectionate relationships, love and trust replace instrumental utility of others as the basis for bonds of attachment and empathy..." (p. 198)

Sir John Eccles, an Australian who has won the Nobel Prize in Medicine confirms this, "If you have no memory, you do not know how to exist; memory is everything." In the March 1992 issue of *WORLD PRESS REVIEW* the case of a Dutchman, Theo Goossens is discussed. Mr. Goossens suffered from migraine headaches. As a cure for the headaches he underwent a type of surgery which, along with the pain from the migraines, wiped out all his memory. He became totally paralyzed because he could not even remember how to move any of his body parts. True his headaches were gone, but what a terrible price he had paid. With additional medical intervention Mr. Goossens' headaches were restored along with a portion of his memory. His response to the outcome was, "I can call myself a happy man. The pain is still tremendous, but it disappears before the fact that I am no longer unable to do anything. There is nothing worse than being nobody."

According to Dr. Peter Breggin the heaviest concentration of Prozac lodges in the memory centers of the brain. He worries that long term memory problems may result in connection with the damage he feels Prozac is doing to the brain's ability to produce and maintain normal serotonin balance. Amnesia or confusion surrounding events during and after the use of many of the newest psychoactive drugs is a common occurrence. Short term memory impairment is about the most common complaint I hear from patients on Prozac. Short-term memory is critical for piecing together our concept of reality. It provides what is termed "contextual" information, the information we would find necessary in putting together the thoughts necessary for recalling where we have parked our car, left our shoes, etc. One ex-Prozac patient from California who testified at the FDA hearings was out on her own for the first time in two years after her Prozac use. Because of the strong effect Prozac had upon her memory her family would not allow her to go anywhere on her own because she could not remember how to return to her own home.

Those Prozac patients or ex-Prozac patients who lack any recall of an event that has happened in their lives will often totally deny ever having taken part in that event. They must be shown through evidence that this happened and that they were involved. Even after they become convinced by the evidence that they were responsible, they express shock and disbelief that such a thing could possibly have happened without them having any recall. One young woman, a counselor herself, had to have her best friend sit her down and prove to her with solid evidence, the type which she could not dispute, that she had actually done the things she did while under the influence of Prozac. Now, 10 months after coming off the drug, she has just accepted the reality of what she has done and is in shock at her own behavior and her lack of memory of it. She still asks in disbelief how and why she would do something to destroy all she had worked for and devoted her efforts toward throughout her life - her career, her family, her circle of friends, etc. Everything has been lost because of her own actions while under the influence of Prozac - actions which she still has no recall of ever happening.

A young man reported experiencing one of these memory blackouts. He says that after 20 mg. of Prozac for three months. He experienced several blackouts. He described the last blackout: "All I remember is that I came to with no realization that I had lost any time at all. The next thing I became aware of was a friend of mine doubled over in pain in front of me. Shocked and concerned I asked her what was wrong and reached out my hand to help her. She pulled back and screamed at me to go away. She then explained that I had just beat her up! I could not believe it I had done such a thing!"

Hope Livingston, reported one of the blackouts she experienced during her Prozac use. The last she remembers she was sitting in her hot tub, but her next conscious memory was "waking up" to find herself in her garage with a crowbar in one hand and her leg laid open and bleeding.

Heidi Kelly went through drastic personality changes within the first month on Prozac. She continued to experience the persistent thoughts of hurting herself. She would often put an unloaded gun to her head and pull the trigger just to get the feel of it. These feelings would come on suddenly along with the rush of energy to accomplish the thoughts. One day at work the feelings came rushing in and she grabbed the gun, jumped in her car and drove off. Anything that happened after that she knows only because others have told her. She has no memory of driving her car into a tree and rolling the windows *up* rather than down when her car burst into flames. Luckily for Heidi a passerby ran to the car, broke a window and pulled her out.

A dear elderly friend of mine, an old neighbor from another city, suffered the experience of losing five close friends and family members in one month. He is someone who has a very big heart and feels deeply the pain of others. Because of the depression (definitely a "normal" reaction for someone who has just lost five loved ones) he felt because of this situation a doctor put him on Prozac. By the end of the week he could not write his name. In fact, by the end of the week he didn't even know who he was. The diagnosis was "rapid onset Alzheimer's disease" and it was recommended that he be placed into a nursing home or psychiatric hospital permanently. His family suspected Prozac, took him off the drug and his "rapid onset Alzheimer's disease" disappeared. He is fine and has had no relapses although he has little recall of the experience.

This phenomenon of drug induced altering of perceptions leading to false accusations is not new to any of us. All are aware of the Salem Village witch hunts in the 1600's where women were falsely accused of witchcraft. What happened in Salem is now considered in scientific circles to be false accusations brought on by the accusers' LSD induced hallucinogenic state. Two separate studies, Linda Caporael (1976) and Mary Matossian (1982), have postulated that this hallucinogenic state was caused by ergot poisoning. Ergot is a fungus which grows mainly on rye. Ergot is also a serotonergic agent, the natural source of LSD. Ergotism, or the long-term ergot poisoning (it is accumulative), was once a fairly common occurrence. It was life threatening and the result of eating contaminated rye.

Those making the accusations in Salem, mostly children and teenagers, who would have been more strongly affected by the poisoning, reported symptoms, mental as well as physical, which are identical to ergot poisoning: pricking sensations on the skin or crawling sensations in the skin, vertigo, visual hallucinations, pain, nausea, diarrhea, painful muscular contractions and convulsions, periods of blindness and deafness, etc. The psychiatric symptoms were mania, melancholia, psychosis and delirium. At least three of the accusers died of the various symptoms. Those suffering the symptoms accused others of being witches who had invoked a witch's curse upon them to cause these symptoms. Approximately twenty people were convicted of witchcraft and were executed. Nineteen were sent to the gallows and one pressed to death in an attempt to force him to make a plea so that he could be tried.

Three hundred years later we are still suffering in our own society from these false accusations brought about through toxic conditions of the brain. We have pointed out the similarities between the action of LSD and the SSRIs upon serotonin. Yet one of the most potent pharmacological agents in ergot fungus has only one tenth the activity of the synthetic version of LSD. With these far more potent synthetic pharmacological agents which enhance serotonin, our current Salem experience could prove to be far worse in the end. The Salem experience was accidental. We are deliberately and voluntarily ingesting serotonergic drugs and encouraging others to do so.

James Kalat explains that serotonin receptors affect perceptions and abnormal stimulation of these receptors leads to abnormal perceptions (BIOLOGICAL PSYCHOLOGY, p. 88). Ex-Prozac patients will attest to the fact that their perceptions became distorted in varying degrees and in various ways during their use of the drug. Yet they relate being unaware of the effects the drug itself was having upon them during the period they were using it. They relate the strong impact it had upon their memories causing them much mental confusion. They relate extreme difficulty in detecting a dream state from reality, which led them to draw strange conclusions from these abnormal perceptions they developed. Many go on to report that these abnormal perceptions were formed by vivid nightmares of violence, sexual abuse, etc. These drug induced nightmares were such a *vivid* hallucinatory state, mimicking reality to such an extent that the patients assumed that they must actually have been sexually molested, or abused in other ways. They could not see any other reason for their dreams being so vivid than a "remembering" of past abuse, because no one had discussed with them the effect of these drugs upon their dreams. They and their therapists (who should know better because they should be aware of this side effect of Prozac and other psychoactive drugs) assume that these dreams are the patient's way of "remembering" what has happened to them earlier in life. (Recall from the chapter on REM sleep that the patients related that they not only dreamed of things they had never experienced in life, but even acted out those things they were dreaming about in a sleepwalk state.)

Dr. Peter Kramer in his zeal for remaking our personalities with the use of drugs states that the antidepressants actually allow the patient to reinterpret history. Or as he puts it the "Medication rewrites history." He points out, using one of his patients as an example, that the injuries he experienced in his past were made more "real" in his mind and even became exaggerated in his mind. A perfect example I have of a case which clearly demonstrates this is a young mother who actually did suffer sexual abuse by her father as a child. After being prescribed Prozac her history of abuse grew greatly exaggerated through this rewriting process brought on by the drug. Now she is convinced that her mother was also involved in the abuse she suffered and she has come to the "realization" that she also had a twin sister that was murdered by her father. This has become so "real" for her that she even tells her own small children about the twin sister she use to have that Grandpa killed. There is no record of a twin sister ever existing, but Prozac has done such a great job of "remaking history" for her that she is positive that this is what actually happened in her past. Her small children are growing up believing these terrible nightmares of their mother are what really happened in their family. How tragic for her and all involved to have to deal with far more than what she actually experienced! Wasn't the original pain enough to bear?

If there are those who are thinking that it serves her parents right to have this additional trauma in their lives to suffer for what actually happened to their daughter, their desire to condemn is clouding the real issue at hand. The severity of her father's terrible indiscretion against his daughter should not be belittled or ignored. Child abuse is a very terrible thing that needs to be understood and corrected in our society. It causes much pain and suffering to those who are the most innocent members of our society. Yet what needs to be understood in this case is that the abuse caused by the father was actually less than the abuse created in her own mind for her by Prozac. Added to the initial pain of her real past she now has to deal with far more trauma and abuse and the loss of yet another parent, her mother, who has become an enemy through her imagined suffering caused by this parent. She is dealing with all the feelings produced by this chemically created history of abuse and it is being related to her children as well. This is her new reality. She has lost her mother through something far worse than death. At least with death there are memories to keep love alive. With a mother she now believes has abused her, there is nothing left but additional pain and suffering to deal with. She also feels the pain of a sister's loss - a sister who never existed. Her small children are growing up believing that this warped, delusional past was reality for their family. Without drug therapy, she would have only had to deal with the hurt which was a result of her father's abuse. Now she has a multitude of pain and suffering from her "new past" to work through. She also no longer has a mother left to turn to for the support she needs to deal with that pain. Is one type of abuse any worse than the other? Was the original abuse worse than what she has suffered through what has been chemically created in her mind? Abuse may be a hell on earth to go through, but why add to it?

Inappropriate serotonin and dopamine neuronal functioning is thought to render one incapable of sorting through thoughts and perceptions, producing an inability to determine which of them are real and which are imaginary. Prozac and the other SSRIs affect both the serotonergic and dopaminergic systems. This hypothesis that the dopamine system sorts out our perceptions fits with what is known about the mental state of psychiatric patients experiencing acute schizophrenic decompensation. Psychosis enters in when patients resolve the discrepancies between illusion and reality by adopting a new set of concepts - their delusions are then accepted as reality.

In this confused state the Prozac user becomes very easily controlled or open to suggestion. The patient, in the very vulnerable position of not knowing what has actually happened in a situation because of the drugs' impact upon their memory, becomes an easy target for control and/or suggestion. And as we see the total anesthetic sleep state produced in the Prozac patient whose brain waves are in this text, we can see that this state appears to be an even deeper hypnotic state than that brought about through hypnosis. Dr. Sidney Cohen points out that this is also the case with LSD, "The fact is that LSD produces an intensely hypersuggestible state." *(THE BEYOND WITHIN, p. 251)*

It takes very little to create a "new reality" for the patient whose memory is so profoundly affected in this toxic state. Whether it be a therapy session, through also affects serotonin and we are aware of the delusions it can produce, we can more easily grasp what is happening in this situation.) I am convinced that this is the reason why many involved in therapy are being led to falsely believe they have been sexually abused. Many are being convinced that the very vivid nightmares they are experiencing through the disruption of serotonin levels are "repressed memories" coming back to reveal their hidden past. This situation of false accusations of abuse, sexual or otherwise, has become so common now that it has been given the title, False Memory Syndrome. A national organization has been formed with over 10,000 members to date in order to deal with the issue (1-215-387-1865 or 1-800-568-8882) and several studies are under way. Although Prozac with its strong impact upon memory and its altering affect upon serotonin which can, in turn, alter perceptions is not always the drug involved, it is proving to be a common denominator in the *large majority* of these cases. For instance out of the twenty-five calls coming in during a one month period the summer of 1992 to the Salt Lake City group 100% of those making the false accusations of sexual abuse were Prozac patients. Here where the use of Prozac is so incredibly high one of the most prominent attorneys in town, who has become very interested in the false memory - Prozac connection, told me that if there was as much sexual and ritual abuse going on as people report to him in an attempt to file suit, no one would have time to get anything else done in life.

Roseanne Barr Arnold has made her accusations of parental abuse a public matter. She has also made her almost four year use of Prozac and the fact that she is using two other antidepressants in combination with Prozac a public matter. It is unfortunate that few have connected Roseanne's Prozac use and her accusations of abuse against her parents even though her entire family has continued to deny the alligations. It is my opinion that Prozac has made Roseanne, as well as her family, victims, by way of altering or rewriting her history. Her family cries out as so many others in lamenting the loss of one they love so deeply as they hope and pray for the return of the person they once knew. This drug induced nightmare is tragic and embarrassing enough for patients and their families to go though privately. How terrible it must be to have the whole world watching you go through it.

My hope is that Roseanne will be able to physically, mentally and emotionally survive and recover from this ordeal. I could make a list several columns long of very serious adverse side effects manifested in her life over the last several years - adverse side effects which are clearly associated with Prozac use. The reactions she has been experiencing seem to be getting worse very quickly now - most likely brought on by the toxic condition of combining the other drugs. Her

257

long and extended use of Prozac and then mixing it with two additional antidepressants is a perfect formula for very serious drug-induced mental and physical problems. The toxic condition would clearly produce the multiple personalities she has now been told she has. New York Supreme Court Justice Wachtler experienced this same type of drug-induced multiple personalities through a combination of several psychiatric drugs and went on 20/20 to talk about his experience.

Roseanne is being pressured far too much at this point. Reporters need to back off and give her a break. It is beyond me that no one seems to be able to notice the seriousness of her condition when there are so many obvious physical side effects she is experiencing in association with this drug. Apparently not even money can insure good mental or physical health care in this country today. Look back on how many great actors and actresses we have lost in the past to prescription drugs. My heart goes out to Roseanne and her family, along with all the others who suffer such tragedies stemming from these chemically induced false memories.

These false perceptions of abuse are so common among Prozac patients that for two and a half years now I have made it a standard procedure to ask patient's and their families if there have been "recovered memories" of abuse which were not evident before the use of the drug. Let me give you an example of how often I run into this. We just had new neighbors move in. When they discovered I was writing a book on Prozac, I very quickly heard how Prozac had affected their lives via his sister who has been on the drug for three years. They report her behavior as becoming increasingly bizarre. She now believes she has multiple personalities. And when I asked about false accusations of abuse they stated that she has accused two individuals already. These false accusations of abuse or offenses toward the patient are not limited to parents. They are often aimed at mates, sisters, brothers, children, friends, etc. It causes much strife in families and is often the cause for divorce and severing of relationships and friendships as well. While I was acting as a witness in a case a police woman checking me into the courtroom related how her mother on Prozac began to accusing her of many things. Although none of this had any basis in reality, her mother became quite hostile about the accusations. The woman stated what I often hear, "had I not seen it myself, I would never have believed this could happen."

Ex-Prozac patients are reporting that they do eventually realize that these perceptions they developed while on Prozac were false, but the process was generally a very long. One woman said that by the time she realized that all those perceptions she had developed about her husband were distorted it was too perceptions they developed while on Prozac were false, but the process was generally a very long. One woman said that by the time she realized that all those perceptions she had developed about her husband were distorted it was too late. She had already divorced him while still on Prozac and he had gone on with his life.

Reality and imagination become so scrambled in patients' minds that they either cannot remember anything they have done and deny everything they that has happened while in this semiconscious state or they cannot distinguish between an incident as something they have dreamed or reality. This inability to detect dreams from reality is a listed side-effect which is labeled "depersonalization", a state of "dissociation". (Check in Appendix A to read the medical definition.) "Almost all the stimulant-type drugs are dangerous as far as memory and brain integrity are concerned, both functionally and structurally" *(REVERSING MEMORY LOSS*, p. 79). When we understand that memory is an electro-chemical process, it is easy to see how chemicals can so effectively disrupt the process. This scrambling of memory can obviously cause very devastating problems within a family as the innocent are accused. Families are torn apart and the innocent wrongfully prosecuted for an act that took place only within the Prozac user's mind.

The families of these patients, many who live in constant fear of their loved one, the accused, who now find that they themselves are victims of this drug-induced nightmare also, ask: "How will this end? Where will it all lead? What will happen to our loved ones when this is over? Will their memories be restored to them so that they can see reality again, and if so, how long will it take? Will they be able to recognize what they have done to us through their false accusations, and if so, will they be able to deal with it? Will they even make it out of this drug induced nightmare alive? How will we find ways to welcome them back and make the process as simple as possible for them and for us? Will we ever be able to understand their experience and forgive them for the pain they have caused us because of this drug-reaction? Will they ever be able to comprehend that their behaviors and thoughts were produced by the drug and *not by an informed choice made by them,* so that they can then forgive themselves, pick up the pieces and go on with their lives? Will they ever again be themselves - the people we knew and loved before we all stumbled into this real life nightmare?

When one is taking a drug that alters the mind and, therefore, alters ones behavior, it is very hard *emotionally* for the patient and his family to comprehend that a pill has brought about these terrible situations in their lives. It was not the patient making the decision to do the things they have done or say the things they have said. That is very difficult to sort out in one's mind emotionally. It can be comprehended on an intellectual level, but emotions run deep, making this a very difficult situation to handle. We have been conditioned to take these things personally. How do we resolve that these behaviors by one who means so much to us have been drug induced?

The patient begins to act completely "out of character". We have Prozac patients who were considered to be stalwart citizens of the community gradually feeling less and less guilt. They begin shoplifting, robbing or embezzling, or becoming obsessed with sex, alcohol or money. They push those they care about the most out of their lives, their family and friends, and have little or nothing to do with them. They feel they can no longer trust themselves and often form co-dependent relationships by turning that trust over to a strong authority figure, i.e., business acquaintance, doctor, therapist, etc. They become so impulsive that they are unsure of what they might do next. They feel totally out of control. They leave their religions because they can no longer *feel* the spiritual feelings they had previously. They feel a rage unlike anything they have ever felt before and assume it must be brought on by the person closest to them as they begin to turn against those they care about the most. They become very arrogant and critical of those around them. They either become oversexed or do not want to be touched at all and report no longer being able to actually *feel* love. They often begin drinking alcohol, whether they ever have in the past or not. They begin experiencing homicidal and suicidal compulsions, even to the point of stalking those they loved the most before using Prozac. All of this "out of character" behavior calls for a very large degree of understanding and forgiveness, not only by the family and friends, but by the patient as well on his or her own behalf. *The task of rebuilding one's life and self-esteem after this type of reaction is overwhelming.*

It takes a very strong and loving mate or parent to hold on to the person they instinctively sense is still there...somewhere...buried under this other chemically-induced personality who they do not know. The insult and injury brought on by the patient's abnormal behavior makes one want to just react by striking back. What must be kept in mind is that the Prozac victim's injury is not visible as it would be if they had a broken arm, a cut, a burn, a bruise, etc. The injury is internal. The brain has been chemically altered (experiencing chemical interference). As Dr. Breggin explains, the brain is actually malfunctioning because of organic changes and damage brought about by a toxic condition, which then alters the patient's behavior and personality. The patient is reacting to toxins built up within the brain which is causing interference in thought processes. No one should take offense or react to a chemically induced behavior. This injury, perhaps not as visible, but just as real as a cut, broken bone, etc., needs the opportunity and time to heal.

Loved ones need to understand that those feelings of love the patient once had for them are still there and *if* the patient *could* access those feelings they *would*. It is not their "fault" that they cannot feel love, compassion, sympathy, etc. They have been chemically cut off from those feelings. The family, with that understanding, can continue to express unconditional love until their loved one "returns".

It is the patient who is unhealthy, who is not strong and needs help. The healthy individual in the relationship, who is still capable of feeling love, should realize that it is their responsibility to stand by their loved one and help them to heal. This is not easy. But, if the tables were turned and they had been the one who was unwittingly duped into taking a drug which caused a similar reaction, how would they want their spouse, child, parent, etc. to react toward them? When we begin to delve into the realm of chemically induced feelings and emotions, the whole issue becomes clouded, very confusing and frightening. How many relationships have the capability or willpower to survive this Prozac pandora is yet to be seen. The number of severed relationships at this point is overwhelming.

The big promotional thrust of the pharmaceutical reps is the claim that Prozac has no side effects or fewer side effects than other antidepressants and each succeeding SSRI supposedly has even fewer than the last one. Patients have been so unaware of the effects because of these claims and so confused, shocked and embarrassed through suffering those adverse effects that they have been unable to make their doctors aware. Also, because they assume, from what they have been led to believe about the side-effects, that all those strange and foreign feelings, thoughts and actions must be the *proof* that they really are going crazy.

Generally those around the patient are the first to become aware of the effects of Prozac upon their loved one. It is imperative that they point these out to the patient. The mind altering effect of this drug is so powerful that generally the effects must become *very serious* before the patient is capable of being aware of them himself, if he can at all. The patients who come forward to warn others by sharing their experience in order to spare others the pain are the true heros. It takes amazing strength and courage and is very humiliating to come forward and admit such "out of character" behavior. It also takes a lot of faith in oneself and one's personal integrity to do so.

261

Perhaps even more devastating than the physical side effects are the emotional side effects reported by past Prozac patients. After coming off the drug they describe their experiences with Prozac as "crazy" or "insane" and relate the following feelings. Although I have worked with several hundred patients, I will include the only the most commonly repeated statements. Keep in mind that this is only a sampling. As some of these quotes have been used elsewhere throughout the text to emphasize specific points, you will find repetition.

"I always had a mask on that was smiling, but what was going on inside of me was indescribably horrifying!"

"The anger I felt was so intense!"

"Prozac rips your very soul out!!!"

"Prozac actually made me do things against my own will...Things I would not have done even under hypnosis."

"On Prozac it became impossible to cry. It feels so good to have that natural release process [crying] again. The ability to cry is so important for emotional healing! Now that I can cry again I feel I can work through my problems."

"I was too embarrassed to tell my doctor the thoughts and feelings I was having while on Prozac because I was afraid he would think I was crazy."

"I thought the entire world was out of line and I was the only one who was okay. I really thought I was Superman!"

"I thought everyone was talking about me. I knew it was not good things they were saying. I felt that everyone was out to hurt me."

"I'll just be happy to have the 'old me' back again! Even with my imperfections and no matter how rough life might become, I would rather face reality and solve my problems than to ever go through anything like this again!"

"Prozac starts out doing you good and then the next thing you know it turns on you. It flips like that in your head. Doctors must get perks. There must be something about this whole medical establishment that has gone totally wrong."

"It took me almost one year to regain my health after a toxic reaction to Prozac known as the serotonin syndrome."

"After two months on Prozac I had a terrible nightmare that involved me dismembering someone! Never have I experienced anything like that before! That was enough for me! I told my doctor I wasn't about to put up with that kind of side effect and I was getting off the stuff. His solution was that he wanted me to double my dose of Prozac!!!! Can you believe it? I am so glad I got off it when I did!"

"If I go just one day without Prozac I can really feel it. It's horrible!"

"As skeptical as I was about the bad things I heard about Prozac because I it seemed to be helping me, I now see that Prozac was the problem. I was getting worse, not better, physically as well as mentally."

"If I could go back now and be given the choice between someone putting a gun to my head and pulling the trigger or taking Prozac, without question I would choose the gun. You could never offer enough money to pay me to go through what I have gone through because of only five months use of this drug."

"I would wake up each morning thinking, 'Oh God, I'm still alive! I have to live another day of this hell of wanting to die!' I thought of running into trees at a high rate of speed."

"Everyone accused me of being pregnant when I stopped taking Prozac because of the bloating and weight gain I experienced. Even the men I know look pregnant when they come off this drug."

"I traveled across the country to visit my family then spent all three days I had planned to visit barricaded in the basement. I told the whole family that if any one of them came near me I knew I would kill them. I couldn't stand having those feelings!"

"Before I was prescribed Prozac, I thought all these people were just making excuses for their behavior. After using the drug and experiencing what I have, I now know for myself that these are not excuses!!"

"I have started smoking and using marijuana again since beginning on Prozac. Although I was baptized a Christian two years ago I feel I cannot turn to my church for help. I had given those things up with promises to no longer use them. I am too embarrassed now to tell them I no longer have that control."

"Behaviors I abhorred before my use of Prozac, I became obsessed with doing!

My values changed completely. Everything I had felt was 'wrong' before was now 'okay'."

"During the month I spent on Prozac I could think of nothing but various ways of killing those closest to me - my family, my mom, my dad and my brothers and sisters." (A very sweet and sensitive 14 year old girl who took herself off Prozac because of these thoughts it was causing her)

"I found that I was blaming the person I loved the most, my husband, for this terrible upheaval of emotions. I took everything out on him. How could I have ever treated him the way I did?!"

"My mother used to be a good mother. She used to care about us kids and take care of us. After three years on Prozac she never does anything for us. She just doesn't care anymore!"

"When my wife reached the point where she was sitting in our front window trying to decide which passerby to shoot, she finally realized that she had to get off Prozac. Being frightened by the drug-induced rage she was feeling, she dropped off the drug 'cold turkey' and two weeks into withdrawal she committed suicide."

"On Prozac, my whole personality did a complete change. I started becoming intentionally self-destructive although I didn't know why and I didn't care. As my behavior got stranger and more destructive, the doctor didn't see that the behavior changes were due to the drug, and he increased the dosage from one to two and then to an occasional third a day."

"I had constantly recurring throat infections which interfered with my employment."

"Everything that I built for the first 36 years of my life was thrown away in a one hour Prozac induced manic reaction."

"I look at him and there is nothing left of him anymore. He is a shell with no soul."

"I became incapable of learning because I could not retain what I read nor recall what I had been told. It all became scrambled in my brain."

"I felt I had to kill myself but I could not leave my family alone. I planned how

I would accomplish the deaths of my husband and children in detail. How could I ever have had such thoughts?!"

"Although I have never been one to use foul language, I swore like a sailor when coming off Prozac. I couldn't stop shaking or crying. I talked non-stop. Being around me was really a chore!"

"I had an overwhelming compulsion to spend. I went heavily into debt. I couldn't stop."

"When I started taking this drug I felt that something inside of me wanted to get out, something evil, and the only way to get it out was to cut myself."

"After the things I did, I just thought I must have gone crazy. I felt I was really certifiably 'nuts'. I was ready to say, 'okay, take me away and lock me up.'"

"It was almost as if my body was acting on its own apart from me."

"I thought that everything that happened in my life had nothing to do with me. It certainly wasn't my fault, it was all someone else's fault."

"My vision was very much affected and now I need glasses."

"I began to question all decisions I had made throughout my life. I began to think that all I had felt was right in the past was actually wrong and all that was wrong before was right."

"I was furious all the time!"

"Prozac made me trust people I never would have trusted with anything before."

"I did not like, in fact I could not stand the person I had become. I began to assume that this 'new me' must be the 'real me' with all my brain chemicals balanced. I didn't know how I was going to live with this person!"

"I was sure that it was my husband who was causing all of these awful feelings I began to have after beginning to use Prozac, so I divorced him. Now that I am off Prozac I can see it was not him after all. The feelings were produced by the drug and now my husband is gone and my family torn apart."

"I had to hit the same telephone pole three times with my car before I finally

figured out it was the Prozac screwing up my driving! I got off it!"

"Not many weeks after starting on Prozac, I was visiting with a neighbor and I thought, 'I wonder what it would be like to pick up that yardstick and hit her up the side of the head'. My thoughts were just so odd!!!"

"Everything felt like a personal attack!"

"I was happy one minute, horribly depressed the next minute and very angry the next, with no apparent reason for any of these feelings."

"I thought all the kind and loving things those around me were doing for me were only being done out of spite or that they had some sinister or ulterior motive, not because they cared about me".

"I can't believe that the government, who we trust to protect us, has such a callous attitude toward the lives of our children."

"I felt there was something bad inside of me and cutting myself with razor blades would let it out. So instead of me doing the cutting myself I became heavily involved in plastic surgery so someone else would cut me up."

"After only two weeks on Prozac I wanted to run away from myself. I couldn't stand myself and I couldn't stand my husband either."

"I noticed my behavior and thoughts were so strange. I would be talking to someone and think, 'Well, I've talked to this person as long as I am going to and I really don't feel like talking any longer.' And I would get up and walk away in the middle of a conversation!"

"I became obsessed with death, with my sickness. I became obsessed with the idea that I was a sick person who would have to be on antidepressants all my life. I became obsessed with dying. I thought dying was the only way out, and I had never contemplated suicide before that time."

"Throughout my life I have always been known as 'Mr. Mello,' but the rage I felt on Prozac helped me to understand how someone could murder another."

"My doctor neglected to tell me that I would no longer be able to find a job because most companies will not hire someone who has used a psychiatric drug and most insurance companies will no longer insure you."

"I would fall into the wall, bounce off and just laugh about it."

"After taking only one pill I sat with my arms wrapped around me the rest of the day to stop myself from doing anything to my children! Needless to say, I never ever took a second pill!"

"I thought and acted just like a teenager again. At forty-five I grew my hair long and put psychedelic designs all over my car! I was very defiant about everything with everyone. No one could get anywhere with me. You couldn't tell me anything because I knew it all!!!"

"Wicked! That's exactly how you feel on Prozac, wicked, just plain wicked!"

"I wanted to hide. I felt so drained. I didn't want to be around anyone, especially someone who might require something of me. That could have been enough to push me over the edge and set me off."

"Prozac caused me to lose all logic and reason."

"It worked okay at first. I seemed to have more energy and felt okay but after about six weeks it turned on me. I was mad but I didn't know why! It was like a monkey on my back! I felt a rage unlike anything I have ever felt before or since."

"I reached a point where I had no feelings whatsoever. I had a new baby and could feel nothing - no feelings at all for my baby! Isn't that terrible?! To this day I feel so guilty about not having feelings for my child. I began taking other drugs just to be able to feel something again and developed a problem with prescription drug addiction."

"The doctor prescribed Prozac to me for anxiety attacks. It seemed to work at first, then the anxiety became far more intense than it was before I began to use the drug."

"I continued to take the Prozac, because I felt like a Dr. Jekyll and Mr. Hyde. I thought it was me. I didn't think it was the drug. And my doctor was perplexed. He also thought it was me, and he just continued to prescribe it."

"I threw all caution to the wind. I started doing many life threatening things, i.e., driving at high speeds, participating in life-threatening sports, exposing myself to aids, etc. I thought I was invincible!"

"I felt so completely alone for no reason. My husband and family lovingly stood by me, but I felt so alone!"

"I had weird thoughts with no rhyme or reason."

"Nothing mattered to me, especially my life or anyone else's. I didn't care about anyone or anything!"

"You saved my life. If I had not flipped on my radio and heard your show on Prozac, I would not have realized the serious reactions I was having to the drug. My doctor informed me that if I had not come right in, I would have lost my lungs. I already have diabetes after using Prozac for a year and a half."

"I've been a reformed alcoholic for twelve years, but while on Prozac I started craving alcohol again!"

"Someone snoring was reason enough to commit murder when I was on Prozac!"

"The things that mattered most to me when I was on Prozac, you know, the kinds of things you would be willing to die for, mean absolutely nothing to me now. None of those things matter in the least to me now that I have been off Prozac or anything else for a year."

"I became a habitual pathological liar during the time I was using Prozac."

"I love my husband dearly, but while on Prozac I could have cared less if he dropped dead any minute! I actually became incapable of loving!"

"I felt possessed!"

"The entire time I was on Prozac was like an out of body experience! I watched myself do things I would never ever dream of doing and say to myself, 'Oh my gosh, that can't be me! I would never do such a thing!' But another part of me would say, 'Of course it's you. It must be you, look. You're really doing it!' I would argue again, 'But it couldn't be me! Yet it must be me, I see myself doing these things.'"

"My short-term memory is gone."

"After attempting to take my life in a car accident, I have been in a back brace for a year in terrible pain. My sister committed suicide on Prozac and my other

sister's marriage was destroyed as a direct result of her use of Prozac. It has taken such a toll on my life and the lives of my family that I cannot even say Prozac! I want this stuff off the market, but want nothing more to do with it myself. When enough lives are affected they will remove it. I refuse to give it any more power in my life by even discussing it!"

"My behavior was completely irrational!"

"I have been off Prozac for three years and still have thoughts of stabbing and slashing when I see a sharp object! Never in my life have I had such disturbing thoughts! Today I was dicing potatoes while my little boy was playing with blocks on the floor nearby. The picture of stabbing him in the back over and over again kept flashing through my mind. The feelings were so intense I had to throw down the knife and leave the room. This was the third such incidence today and its been three long years!! How long can this go on?!!!"

"I craved alcohol and sugar."

"I would lay in bed and think of things I could do to hurt myself. I hurled myself down stairs, poured boiling water on myself and beat myself in the face and blamed it on someone else. I cut myself, and then last week I even ran over my own arm with my car!" (Unbelievable? I thought so too, until I saw the arm and documented it.)

"As a child I suffered terrible abuse that caused life-long bouts with depression and extremely low self-esteem. After years of counseling and growth, Prozac destroyed my self esteem overnight! My actions were totally out of character, causing me much grief and embarrassment."

"I thought I had someone else's brain in my body!"

"I had more energy and then after about six months, I became very compulsive over food, money, sex, and alcohol."

"I felt no guilt. There is healthy guilt (feeling badly because of unethical practices or for causing pain to others) and unhealthy guilt (accepting responsibility for things for which you are not responsible) but I felt neither."

"Do I have any rights? What about redress? Can I sue my doctor? How does anyone pay me back for years missing out of my life, physical, mental, emotional, and spiritual health and my self-respect?"

"After using LSD in my past, I can tell you that taking Prozac is like taking half a hit of LSD, except that it also made me angry and aggressive."

"I feel like I'm under anesthesia after coming off Prozac. I feel retarded."

"Although it was completely out of character for me, the compulsion to drink was so strong after starting on Prozac that it became impossible for me to drive past a bar."

"I am a good Christian, yet I could no longer feel the influence of the Holy Spirit upon me. I could not pray. I was no longer me!"

"I wanted to stop using Prozac, but I was addicted. How could I be addicted to a drug that my family practitioner gave me?"

"I was so out of control, yet convincing to all around me as to how 'well' I was doing on Prozac. How I wish someone would have kidnapped me to take me off this highly addictive substance!"

"I felt completely out of control! And because I felt so vulnerable I became almost paranoid about others trying to control my life."

"I used to be a brilliant and articulate woman. I am very well educated, but after using Prozac I noticed that I reached a point where I could no longer concentrate; reading and assimilating thoughts became an impossible task! I could not hold thoughts in my mind long enough to form a logical sequence of thoughts to arrive at a conclusion. My mind just raced!"

"I never dreamed these thoughts and feelings were being produced by the drug. I thought I was going crazy!"

"I don't need to go to hell. I can tell you all about it because I've been to hell and back on Prozac."

"What will I ever do to put my life back together again? I have done things on this drug that I could never tell my husband about, it is difficult to admit it all to myself!"

"Ever so often my legs would just go weak and give out, right from under me."

"After being on Prozac for one week I had an argument with another motorist

and attempted to run over him with my car!"

"After my wife shooting and killing our only two children while on Prozac and then turning the gun on herself, I want to know when murder and suicide are going to be listed as side-effects on the label of this drug?"

"I got to the point that I was mad, but I didn't know who I was mad at, and I took a ballpoint pen and tried to stab my wife. I was not aware that there was anything wrong with me, only those living in my house could see it."

"On Prozac my life became an 'open book'. I divulged things about myself I never before would have discussed and did so with individuals I never before would have trusted."

"How anyone on Prozac can hold a marriage together is a mystery to me! I became so rude, distant, arrogant, aggressive, so easily offended by what I interpreted as personal attacks, etc., that I lost or cut off most of my friends, family and husband."

"My hair started coming out by the handfuls! I hadn't realized it was caused by Prozac. I thought I had done well on the drug."

"I had hypoglycemia when my doctor put me on Prozac. Now it has progressed to diabetes."

"I have a coffin without a body to put in it. The person I knew and loved for a lifetime is dead. This other person he has become - the person I never knew before Prozac - is out there somewhere walking around now hating all of us who he loved so much before."

"Withdrawal is where the hell started for me with this drug. Coming off and getting your mind back is not a simple task!"

"How do I go on with my life? I've lost several years out of my life! They're gone. No one can bring them back. These years of Prozac use are such a blur - 'like a dream', that I don't know what I actually did do or didn't do, what was a dream and what was real!"

"My own doctor was on vacation and the one I saw instead recognized my symptoms as serotonin syndrome. His insight saved my life. I had spasms from my mouth through my intestinal tract."

271

"I gained 60 pounds on Prozac as did three of my friends, while another gained 75 pounds!"

"I was embezzling money from my employer. I had no conscious. I knew it was wrong, but there were no feelings of guilt. I continued buying the most outrageous things you could dream of and cannot even recall many of the purchases I made with the money."

"I felt as though I was on a combination of speed and cocaine."

"After starting on Prozac I developed migraine headaches. After nine months of brain scans and every other medical test known to man at the cost of around eighty thousand dollars, I came off Prozac and the headaches disappeared!"

"The withdrawal was terrible! The suicidal tendency became more intense, I had the shakes, single words would pop into my mind and then race out, my ability to concentrate was almost nil and all this lasted for four months. Why don't they warn you about this terrible withdrawal?"

"I became enraged and despondent. I was hostile and aggressive toward my family and friends. I was obsessed with killing myself. The muscle spasms and suicidal despair continue. As each day goes by, I seem to be relieved of some symptoms and bothered by others. My primary concern is the hostility, because that's not my nature and I don't like having it in my life. The joint pain is still intermittent and that's a real problem in getting around."

"I feel this drug was pushed on me. What upsets me so much is that since I've had this [adverse] reaction, I've seen this drug treated as a wonder drug on the covers of magazines and on television. It seems like someone has been pushing this on the public and not talking about the side effects." (A nurse in Fairfax, California)

Three detailed case histories: Case #1 *"I'm through the whole ordeal now and I just don't want old wounds opened up because I do have a family. It all happened when I had a hysterectomy and my doctor immediately put me on* **Prozac.** *I kept getting worse and having more headaches and things like that. He kept just giving me more and more until finally it was full blown into a drug addiction. I was taking three Prozac a day! It was awful, because I got caught shoplifting, then I got caught for prescription fraud. I then went through drug rehabilitation which encouraged me to stay on Prozac! People who were not on Prozac there were put on Prozac!*

Right after I got out of the drug rehabilitation, which lasted four months, I was caught again for shoplifting. What I had were these incredible obsessions and compulsive behavior! I had never done anything wrong in my whole life before this, ever! It totally devastated me! I've got four kids. Luckily my husband stayed with me through this whole thing. I'm just trying to stay out of jail now because of the amount I had taken it was considered a felony that I committed. Then I heard this woman on Joan Rivers' show. Thank Goodness!!! I'd been praying my heart out to try and find a solution to what was going on in my life, because even after I was caught I still wanted to go out and shoplift again. I mean normally you would think you would just stop! Anyway this woman's story was my exact story to a T. I just immediately stopped taking Prozac. I was already suicidal. I thought, "If this is what is causing all this to happen, I don't want it in my body anymore!" I just came right off of it. I felt like I was having an out of body experience. I knew they were withdrawal symptoms because this was the third time I'd gone through withdrawal during this ordeal, not only from Prozac, but the other drugs too.

Luckily my defense attorney for the second shoplifting charge was compassionate enough to say that he believed me about Prozac causing all this. He had me go to a doctor and the state had me go to another doctor. Both doctors really believed I had a problem with this. I ended up with 150 hours of community service and a $750 fine. I've already been on probation for six months and paid off the fine.

I'm not telling this story for my own benefit. I am really truly over the pain of it all even though I still wish it had never happened. The main reason I want people to know what I went through is so that no one has to go through this ever again! I want them to stay away from Prozac. You see my uncle killed himself on Prozac. My sister was on it and she committed adultery. You not only lose your religion on Prozac, you lose your family. I had a baby and could feel no emotions toward him whatsoever! It's taken this long to get my emotions back! It's been a year and a half since I came off Prozac.

What's crazy is that they wanted to put me on different anti-depressants because I was depressed over what I went through on Prozac. The trial was horrible. I live in a middle-class neighborhood and I've been arrested three times! I have friends who are on it and I see their abnormal behavior too. I've spent thousands of dollars on counseling now. It's just been incredible. But I now have two years of sobriety from my narcotics use - the prescription drugs I became addicted to after using Prozac, and a year and a half from my Prozac use. Can you imagine trying to get over that? It affected more than one store owner too.

273

My church knows now that I've had a drug problem but they don't know anything about the Prozac and shoplifting or anything like that. It is so embarrassing! Those who have no compassion just look at you and say, "Oh?!"

I also have a basement full of cross stitch I don't know why I bought or what to do with it. It's totally weird! You can ask my poor husband. I have been truly insane! What's sad is that I chose things I enjoyed when I was not on the drug and made it to where now I am even afraid to pick it up out of fear that somehow that could possibly start the whole thing up again. So I started my own little therapy group with just me. I tell myself that I can do a little bit and I won't go crazy. I may as well open a shop. I have so much of the stuff! My boys' room is completely filled to the brim with toys! That was just guilt buying on my part. Crazy.

My poor husband thought I was having an affair because I was gone so much (this is often what mates begin to think). *I didn't want to take any responsibility at home and was trying to hold on to what was left of it. I cut my arm. I broke my foot on purpose. I hit myself in the face with a rock to make myself look like a battered wife. It's almost like you are trying to get a demon out of your body. You reach the point where the pain felt so good because you were actually finally feeling something, anything. You find out that there really is blood inside of you. No one could possibly understand that.*

My sister did the exact same thing on Prozac. She rolled her car. She threw herself down stairs. She broke her elbow. She hurt her knee so badly that she had to have surgery. She had a baby. She went through two divorces. She found the guy she is living with now at a alcohol recovery center that she was attending. She had begun drinking. This is how crazy it got for her. She set up someone who supposedly came into her house and accosted her. She made up this big scenario for the police and reported it twice. She said it happened and then it happened again where these guys came in and hurt her. She actually threw boiling water on herself. It really got crazy! She was doing theses like that to get more Valium and other painkillers. She just wasn't able to function and did not want to be in reality. Luckily the investigating officer realized she was lying and confronted her about all the drugs. He was able to talk her into getting into a recovery program and she got off everything.

There were so many just completely insane things. Believe me, you just lay in bed or sit there and think, "Oh I could do this or I could do that." You think of all these terrible things. It's so awful! You are in a totally different dimension or dementia is more like it. *You go insane on this drug. Then you* become addicted to other drugs because you are trying to feel any type of emotion, so you take more drugs in search of emotions. Then you take drugs to sleep because you can't sleep. All the while your whole life is falling apart all around you. It's like when you become emotionally drained, adding one more thing to what is expected of you is impossible. You just can't do it. I used to be a real estate agent but I just couldn't do it anymore. I was making good money, but I am grateful I am staying home now with my kids. That's what I'd rather do now. I couldn't even keep a thought pattern long enough to make a sell after using Prozac. I think there's more than just getting off a drug in this case. I think you are really messing up your brain chemically and it has long term effects.

It has been an incredible ordeal! My relationship with my parents is totally messed up. They could not understand how their daughter who had lived such a noteworthy life and had been married in the Mormon temple could have been doing such incredibly horrible things. My daughters are at ages where it is going to take a lot to pick up the pieces and help them to understand what happened. It has been really hard on them. I'm sure it will still take a long time. The Prozac aftermath is incredible!

You have to realize that I was on it for two years. I told my husband that I just want to get back to where I care. Its like Satan is finding ways to get moral people to be immoral. Even though I have always been very religious, I could not feel the Spirit. Then finally a month ago I felt a witness of the Holy Ghost. It has been five long years since I have felt that! It was so wonderful to finally have such sensitivity back again! Then is when I realized that everything was going to be okay. It was possible to overcome the effects of the drug. I knew that I could forgive myself for all the crazy things I had done on the drug and it really would be okay now. I knew I could make it.

These stupid doctors. I have a neighbor who is on Prozac and I see her going through some of the same things I did. She's getting into Ativan and all these addictive type things. It's because you can't sleep, you know. You just can't sleep on this stuff so you take a bunch of pills so you can sleep. I took so much medication the I pinched a nerve in my arm and had no use of my right arm for two months.

You get into this self destructive mode and there is nothing anyone can say to you because the drug has such a strong effect upon you. It does rip your soul out. I stopped going to church and it was awful. When you are going through that much pain and not realizing that this is not your fault it is terrible! I mean you get night sweats just thinking about what you've done. I don't know who that *person was. And I am not yet the same person I was before. I don't know how long before I will be. It seems to take a part of you that you can never regain.*

It has given me a deeper compassion for everyone. Now that I have spiritually grown again I have a totally different outlook on life, a better quality look."

Case #2: "I started taking Prozac last December on a Tuesday. The prescribed dose was 20 mg. in the morning, once a day. I began feeling the effects that same night. *It was just like 'bing' - something hit me. By Friday afternoon I knew I was having a drug reaction. I ended up at an emergency center because my knees got really shaky and my skin was kind of tingly, hot on the surface of the skin. It felt like I had a rash, but there was no rash there. I felt really jittery, like my nervous system was just, well, at the surface. I got the shakes. I would hold my hand out and it would just shake. Luckily my husband was home at the time and took me in. When I told them I was taking Prozac it was amazing to me that they didn't know much about it. They got their big thick medical book out. In fact he checked two medical books. He said it might be and might not be a drug reaction. He said I might just be coming down with the flu. But his recommendation was to stop taking it. So I stopped taking it Saturday. Monday I felt fine again so I took Prozac again. I tried one pill every other day and after three weeks of that I seemed fine. I thought I just had to get used to it. Looking back I can see that was really dumb on my part.*

After the fourth week I got really weak again and started getting twitches. I felt like my arm couldn't hold still. *My muscle would just kind of go into little spasms...I didn't know where to turn. I felt kind of like a tree twisting in the wind. At that point I called my gynecologist and told him what was happening. He said that we would have to find something else similar to Prozac to try me on. I gradually went off and a week later I was just really, really low. I couldn't even get a thought into my head. I was so down that I thought, "I need this stuff to get back to where I was feeling good again." I talked to my pharmacist and he said that some people break it in half because 20 mg. is more than you need anyway. That way they would take just 10 mg. That sounded okay to me so I tried that for a while. Then I just started gradually decreasing my dose because I decided that using it and going through all this was ridiculous.* **I came off really gradually and I haven't felt down from it. I don't need any drugs because now I am running every morning and I am very much aware of my diet and physical condition.**

When I started on Prozac it was like having to get to know someone else. I knew the person I call me and I knew how to self talk. I didn't need my thoughts screwed up. I just want my own thoughts back. Like I told my husband, I just want to get back to where I care again. I would be talking to someone and it wouldn't bother me at all to think, 'I don't want to hear anymore of this. I can just get up and walk away and be through with you.' It's awful. And the other day I was talking to my neighbor and this weird thought came into my head. There was a yard stick sitting on my counter and I had never though anything like this before. She was talking and I wondered what would happen if I just picked up this yardstick and whacked her on the head.

I have five children. I used to be right on top of things. *I reached a point after a very short time on Prozac that I would be thinking about fixing dinner and think, 'Oh well, if you don't fix dinner they can just do it themselves.' That type of irresponsibility is not like me at all. I didn't like it...When I first started taking it I recall my husband and I discussing how I felt I had lost my edge and I asked him if that was the way 'normal' people really are. I thought maybe I was just too on top of things. I mean I was just different. My driving habits changed. It was like well they just changed. I want to live my life the way it was and deal with my own self, on my terms rather than a drug's terms! Forget it! Three months was too long! It's like a pit bull...you don't know when it's going to go off!...When I went off it for that week the first time I felt so down. I bet a lot of people are just afraid to go off it. They are afraid of what they will feel like because it does make them feel better even though they might not realize what's going on inside their heads nor the potential dangers. I learned to just go off gradually. If that could just be stressed to people they could probably get off it...It is so deceptive! After I had been on it for a couple of weeks I felt like my mind had opened up. I remember thinking, 'Oh, this must be what normal people feel like.' I wondered what decisions I had made in the past...decisions made when I was abnormal...over the last seventeen years that were all screwed up. Your thinking processes change. You begin to wonder if you would have done this differently or that differently in your past because now you feel like you are smarter and can just do anything. You wonder if choices you have made in the past when you were abnormal were wrong decisions. I didn't think that way about everything in the past, just some things. I thought, 'If I had been normal, would I have gone on to graduate school? (It's like all of a sudden your brain is having all of these thoughts.) If I would have thought this way sixteen years ago, where would I have been today? I'm so motivated now. I have spent all these years being abnormal, so how many things did I get all wrong?' I don't want to go back to that way of thinking. I look back at that and I just have to laugh at myself.*

It was such a good feeling to begin with that you just wanted to stay on it

forever. *You know it almost helped me because it was so awful that I realized that I've got to handle life on my terms and that is just the way it is. You analyze your situation and ask yourself why you are feeling what you are feeling. You deal with your problems rather than thinking that a pill has to fix you. It was enough for me to realize that this isn't the way I want to go. I tried it and it is certainly no longer an option!*

It is almost like it is cocaine or something, but it is legal. *My doctor didn't seem to have much background of the drug and yet, it was kind of like he was pushing it. He didn't say check back with me in six weeks or anything. He just gave me a year's supply and said, "Happy sailing!" I'm sure my doctor is not the only one...I don't spank my kids. If fact, I don't like physical violence at all. I don't generally yell at them either, but I found myself one day going on and on at my 13 year old after becoming upset with him. I was leaning over him and my tone of voice was just not like me. I remember thinking, 'I don't act this way.' After my doctor said I needed this chemical to balance my brain and no amount of counseling was going to help me. Then I started thinking, 'Well, this must be what I am really like with all of my brain chemicals balanced. So now I'm normal? This is the person I really am and this is the person I have to get to know.' But it was Prozac that was making me act that way and feel the way I did. It wasn't the real me. That is what I have found out since I stopped taking it and started learning more about the drug. I know I really don't want to be on this. I've been on both sides of it now and I just hope and pray that I can get my old self back. I like my old self better even through the down times."*

Case #3: *"Two days ago I read an article in the February issue of RED BOOK about the woman who shot her two little children. I must have read that at least half a dozen times and I thought it was so sad. As I was reading the article I kept waiting for them to say she was on Prozac. Finally, there it was, BINGO! They just danced all around the whole topic of her being on Prozac. I couldn't help but think that these people have no idea what they are even talking about. They haven't lived through this.*

I was on Prozac for only a year three years ago. Even today I took some scissors out to cut some cellophane bags open and the thoughts came to me and I just threw the scissors down on the grass. *The way I have controlled this is the same way alcoholics do. I went to my higher power and said, 'I surrender this. I cannot hurt my children and I surrender this feeling because I have no control over it.' Since then it has been a lot better...For me these effects did not come while I was still on the drug, it was after I came off. I'm not a depressed person by nature anyway. They gave me Prozac to deal with my ex-husband and what* *he was going through. Now I am married to a good man and I have good kids. I have a pretty relaxed life, so I don't have a lot of anxiety. If someone were in a situation where there was a lot of anxiety, it could trigger it. I couldn't help thinking how terrible it was that someone wasn't there to tell this woman what the drug does. If you are aware of it, you can have a lot more power over your life. It helps if you know what to watch for versus it just coming up and grabbing you. Without any doubt. Every time I read an article about something like this, I just watch for that word Prozac to come into it and it never fails. It is always part of it."*

If you have suffered any of these adverse reactions or have a loved one using Prozac who fits into any one of the following categories: #1 was previously suffering from a serious or debilitating illness; #2 has experienced a drastic and rapid weight loss on the drug; #3 is often staring blankly into space as if "no one is home"; #4 working long, long hours and, or odd hours, basically "driven" and unable to rest, or whose biological clock seems confused to the point that they are up all night and sleeping during the day; #5 has reached a point of total exhaustion or is sleeping excessively on Prozac; #6 has developed a rash; #7 demonstrates that an uncontrollable rage is building within; #7 mixing alcohol and/or other drugs with Prozac; #8 is using high doses of Prozac (many practitioners feel that the smallest dose (20 mg.) is too high so over one pill per day should fall into this high dose category) or increasing their own dosage; you need additional information and support. Please contact your local Prozac Survivor's Support Group by calling one of the following.

PROZAC SURVIVOR'S SUPPORT GROUP:

U.S. NATIONAL DIRECTOR:

Bonnie Leitsch
2212 Woodbourne
Louisville, Kentucky   40205
1-502-459-2086

CHAPTER 10

COSMETIC PSYCHOPHARMACOLOGY, PERSONALITY IN A PILL?

"How could the same drug be hailed as an unparalleled avenue to transcendental or visionary experiences and denounced as an agent of psychotic interludes? Originally researchers viewed LSD solely in terms of its ability to create an experimental toxic psychosis..."good trips" were no exception...Tripping and psychosis are one in the same. Tripping can be an awful schizoid feeling. Also there are hebephrenics - happy schizos. Their experience is similar to a good trip." (ACID DREAMS, p. 54)

Crazy faith in better living through chemistry? Aldous Huxley said, "The urge to transcend self-conscious selfhood is...a principal appetite of the soul. When, for whatever reason, men and women fail to transcend themselves by means of worship, godly works and spiritual exercises, they are apt to resort to religion's chemical surrogates." A massive advertising campaign to promote chemically inducing a complete change of personality to overcome depression is an intriguing proposal. In theory, if an individual is originally suffering depression and goes through a complete personality change it should follow that he will become a "new person" and that this other personality will be a "happy and carefree" personality, right? The theory was intriguing enough that Dr. Peter Kramer wrote an entire book on just that. He asks, "How is it that taking a capsule for depression can so alter a person's sense of self?" He goes on to say that, "Alternatively, we can say that they are normal people, and that if they ask for Prozac they are requesting, according to our point of view, legitimate enhancement, legalized cocaine, or a neurochemical nose job. If I am right, we are entering an era in which medication can be used to enhance the functioning of the normal mind. The complexities of that era await us."

The complexities of that era do not await us. Dr. Kramer's theory of a personality pill is nothing new. The theory came long, long ago and has been repeated over, and over again throughout history. For many years there have been advocates for chemically inducing changes in personality. If you will recall I mentioned in the chapter on legal and illegal drugs that in 1990 at the Annual Meeting of the American Academy of Neurology Drs. Robert F. Ulrich and Bernard M. Patten referred to the potential uses of LSD as a wonder drug by stating, *"We now know that will never happen. LSD was part of an era of crazy faith in better living through chemistry."* Hofmann, the drug's developer, felt that the materialistic American life-style and resultant feelings of alienation from nature and lack of a meaningful philosophy of life is what drew people to LSD. Although there is a lot of truth in what Hofmann had to say, part of what drew people to LSD could have been that they were told in *TIME* magazine that this drug would clear up mental illness. Here we are again only three years after hearing that this "crazy faith in better living through chemistry" would never return facing it again. Dr. Kramer is rehashing the theory for us. His suggestion is that we create a better living by remaking our personalities through the chemistry of Lilly's latest "wonder drug," Prozac. He calls it "cosmetic psychopharmacology" - creating the personality you want through various chemicals. Yet in association with the use of LSD Huxley described a *loss of self*. "A loss of ego boundaries is one of the hallmarks of psychotic disintegration, according to psychiatric dogma. In my own case, the powerful feeling of oneness with the universe was followed by a loss of awareness of just who I was. I began to call out, 'Who am I? Where is the world?' At the height of this disintegration, I was terrified.I tried frantically to remember my name - hoping thus to recapture reality - but it eluded me. In the end, I grasped at the one name I could think of: 'San Francisco, San Francisco, San Francisco.' It seemed to be a clue to where I was and *who I might be*."

Just how far into 1984 are we in the year 1994? George Orwell addressed this issue of changing the personality in the name of politics in his classic *NINETEEN EIGHTY-FOUR*:

"The Party is not interested in the overt act: the *thought is all we care about. We do not merely destroy our enemies; we change them.*" This chemical erosion of our identities and its far-reaching impact upon society is covered extensively in a book published by Stanford University in 1983, *ON NINETEEN EIGHTY-FOUR*: "The nineteenth and twentieth centuries have amply documented man's insouciant betrayal of his own personhood in exchange for technological efficiency and expedience. Depersonalization in its many forms is indeed the central problem in our society, and its link to technology seems indissoluble, despite our best efforts to understand it...*Clearly, the joke is on us. We embrace our new technologies enthusiastically, and with ample justification, as a great boon, only to find that there is a price to be paid that was not in the original contract. Invariably some part of the price is a further diminution of our sense of personal autonomy.* In the revolution in biology and medicine, technological depersonalization has the most far-reaching implications. Biomedical technologies have an impact far more direct and profound than that of any other technology because they are applied to man himself. The person has become the machine, to be repaired or even modified, like any other - a chemical machine nonetheless...Equally with the body, the mind loses its autonomy as all aspects of experience and emotion are dissected through the chemical and anatomical analysis of the brain by ingenious new techniques.

"The depersonalization that results from these extraordinary biomedical advances is subtle and pervasive. There is scant resemblance between our traditional view of man and the 'molecular man' of modern medical science. It is a great irony that our traditional concept of man, with his 'right' to the dignity of good physical and mental health, is leading us toward *a medical millennium in which the person, as once understood, will disappear* ...The problem, not surprisingly, greatly perplexes theologian, one of whom, according to a recent *NEW YORK TIMES* report, asks plaintively: 'Might we do things in genetic engineering that muck about in the soul?'...*Our sense of moral responsibility is being steadily eroded by depersonalizing forces that are far beyond our control. Most potent among these forces are our technologies, and in particular those that are being developed in the context of medicine...*In the long run, this century's great biomedical achievements may well increase the vulnerability of our descendants to totalitarian control. Developing biomedical technologies, for all their benefits, could be perverted to control people whose very familiarity with them had enfeebled their will to resist...*We must on no account forget what can happen when Big Brother tells us who is 'human' and who is not."* ("The Biomedical Revolution and Totalitarian Control," Raymond B. Clayton, pp. 78-84)

"In *NINETEEN EIGHTY-FOUR,* we are cast as observers of an unnatural experiment in the negation of human nature. One by one, each of the qualities at the core of that elusive construct called human nature are stripped away. *The System's goals are proclaimed clearly and coldly: 'To extinguish once and for all the possibility of independent thought'; to eliminate conditions that enable even one 'erroneous thought [to] exist anywhere in the world, however secret and powerless it may be'; to crush the core of humaneness so that no person is 'capable of ordinary human feeling'; and to enforce such total behavioral obedience to its authority that everyone is 'prepared to commit suicide, if and when we order you to do so.' Its mission is to be supreme authority over every individual's thoughts, feelings, and actions.*

"Winston Smith is the reluctant hero because he is the last person capable of independent thoughts, self-contained secrets, passionate feelings, and occasionally rebellious deeds. He is the enemy of the System, who represents the only principle that can still defeat its brutal omnipotence -- 'the spirit of his free will, maintaining his autonomy, and sustaining a sense of compassion for his fellows. The absolute power of the oppressive System is threatened by the presence of even a single dissident who can laugh at its pretentiousness by remembering when life was different, and by imagining future realities with meaningful options and choices: 'You are a flaw in the system, Winston. You are a stain that must be wiped out.'" (*"Mind Control: Political Fiction and Psychological Reality,"* Philip G. Zimbardo, p. 197)

The November 1, 1993 issue of *TIME* magazine printed a couple of letters in response to an article they ran on Prozac and personality in their October 11, 1993 issue. They echo the pleas for reasoning we have just quoted. Horst Barwinek of Grathorn, Austria wrote, "Reading your article, I could not help thinking of Aldous Huxley's 1932 novel *BRAVE NEW WORLD*, in which he describes a Utopian system that controls almost all human beings in all matters. People are satisfied with this situation, however, mainly because of the use of a stimulating drug called Soma. There are similarities between Prozac and Soma. Depressives who take Prozac change into socialites. Huxley's exhausted men and women of the future swallow their Soma and have orgies. Huxley's Soma makes people happy with things they formerly felt unbearable. It is sad that at the end of a century that has brought prosperity to much of the industrialized world those leading a normal, even successful life cannot resist the need to banish their bad moods by swallowing a pill." And Bruce W. Chambers of Hamden, Connecticut asks the most poignant question of all, "In a society where everyone is upbeat, even-tempered and socially skilled, does anything get accomplished?"

Personality, this sense of identity we all experience which actually gives us our foundation for life, is generally associated with memory and memory is strongly affected by these drugs. Serotonin is intricately linked to the memory process and each of these psychoactive drugs that profoundly affect personality have a strong direct effect upon serotonin. Memory is critical for personality and all these drugs impair memory. Even those who feel Prozac has helped them will generally notice memory problems. We just discussed in the last chapter the great importance of the memory/personality connection, "Memory establishes the continuity of self over time and thereby a sense of personality. The past provides the present with standards, criteria for comparison, the wellsprings of tradition, and the stable references for the transient flux of immediate experience." Most patients report that Prozac has caused an identity crisis for them. Patients begin to realize that they can no longer remember who they are. They use phrases like, "Until I could remember who I was before my use of Prozac, I did not know I could get well." Or "I am no longer the same person I was before I used Prozac. I don't know if it is possible to ever be me again." Or "I'll just be grateful to have the old me back with all of my problems." This loss of identity is what is termed mental illness, insanity, etc. A loss of identity would be even more damaging both to those young people at an age where they are just beginning to learn who they are and also to those with Borderline Personality Disorder (generally anyone who has suffered any physical, emotional or sexual abuse, which covers many of those who are being given the SSRIs). Those attending the annual convention of the American Association of Psychologists in 1992 were warned not to use Prozac because of this factor in those with this disorder. In spite of this warning there was a book written on Borderline Personality Disorder last year which promoted the use of Prozac for these individuals. And Soloff et al. 1986 reported a paradoxical *increase* in suicidal threats or behavior after antidepressant treatment in those suffering from Borderline Personality Disorder.

The CIA, obsessed with mind control, had emulated the Russians in their mode of accomplishing this control of the mind. They felt that eradicating the personality and then rebuilding it to their specifications was how it was to be done. *"A seminar was devoted to the deliberate and active steps required to strip an individual of his selfhood, and how to build up something new from the bare psychic foundation that remained. In this assault upon identity a key factor was to create a state of infantile dependency, so that a person became disorientated until finally, like a young postulant entering a religious order, he 'dies to the world.'...Faculty doctors explained how the process could be accelerated by the use of drugs to create rapid disorientation, induce fear, produce confusing stimuli, and cause fatigue and physical debility...*Considerable time was devoted to probing the mechanism of personality, not only to understand it as the meeting place of all relationships, but to learn that it could be dramatically affected by drugs that, for example, altered the function of the thyroid, reducing a person to near imbecility,...Dr. al-Abub was initiated into how many of the discoveries of the major pharmaceutical laboratories in the West, like Sandoz and Eli Lilly, could be adapted to assist in mind control." (*JOURNEY INTO MADNESS*, p. 69, 70, 74)

LSD was an excellent means of stripping someone of their personality and making them believe that they were going insane. Self identity is completely lost. Cleon Skousen an ex-Salt Lake City Police Chief made a tape in the late sixties entitled "Instant Insanity Drugs" and reports "medical authorities tell us that the LSD user degenerates *gradually* into a mental vegetable, without ambition, without goals and without the will to struggle. Gradually the user withdraws more and more from social contact as the inner core of his entire personality seems to wither away."

White, the agent in charge of Midnight Climax for the CIA said, "Clear thinking was non-existent while under the influence of any of these drugs. I did feel at times like I was having a 'mind-expanding experience' but this vanished like a dream immediately after the session." *(ACID DREAMS*, p. 33) Only about 5% had "bad trips" or adverse psychotic reactions in early use. An eighteen year old who had taken LSD speaks of his loss of identity, "After LSD I felt I didn't exist anymore. I was nothing. I shouldn't be alive. I had no feeling of who I was. That so depressed me that I started on Heroin and then I didn't feel anything anymore." His experience helps us to clearly see the uncanny ability of LSD to strip one of their personality or identity. L. A. County General Hospital during the sixties noted that 66% of those brought in after a reaction to LSD were classified as extended psychosis patients, meaning they required immediate commitment to a mental institution for prolonged treatment. Sandoz proved to be correct in their suggestion that LSD could induce insanity in "normal subjects" thereby assisting scientists in determining how this process develops. Do not lose sight of the fact that those researchers believe that LSD and the other psychedelics have their effect through their effect upon serotonin - the same type of effect upon serotonin as the SSRIs have.

Depersonalization is a listed side effect of Prozac and the SSRIs. Remember the quote from *ON NINETEEN EIGHTY-FOUR,* "The depersonalization that results from these extraordinary biomedical advances is subtle and pervasive...Our sense of moral responsibility is being steadily eroded by depersonalizing forces that are far beyond our control. Most potent among these forces are our technologies, and in particular those that are being developed in the context of medicine." Sharon DiGeronimo's experience with Prozac helps us to see how Prozac strips the personality and feelings of value also, "It was as if I had been demonically possessed. My personality went through a complete reversal. At times I had feelings of invincibility...and then I felt I was the dirt on the bottom of mankind's shoe. I felt like God's biggest mistake. I was sure the world be better off without me." LSD and Prozac both strip the personality, act as serotonin enhancing agents in the brain and were both promoted as a way to help "clear up mental illness."

If someone refused to cooperate with the KGB, they would threaten to keep them forever in a state of chemically induced insanity with one of these instant insanity drugs. LSD became the drug of choice for some time for the CIA. Curiously enough Eli Lilly, the makers of our latest "personality pill," Prozac, were the manufacturers and suppliers of LSD for the CIA. PCP also alters the personality, as does alcohol. Changes in personality were also noted with one of the earliest antidepressants, imipramine, which has approximately half the potency for serotonin uptake as Prozac and less than one third of the potency of Paxil. It was often prescribed for what was first referred to as a character disorder and later a personality disorder. Changes in personality are one of the first symptoms families are told to look for as an indicator that a family member is beginning to have drug abuse problems. Drugs and personality changes have always gone hand in hand. Yet there are psychiatrists who are suggesting doing away altogether with the distinction between "personality disorder" and "mental illness," believing they are the same. Dr. Kramer points out just how far reaching this "defective labeling" process is becoming, "If other doctors are tempted to use medicines to treat vagueness of thought in patients...then in time as a society we will find ways to understand this practice as acceptable. Perhaps we will expand the definition of disease, so that patients...are considered ill, even in the absence of depression." It was this very mind set which became the setting to pave the way for the holocaust of World War II Germany.

All mind-altering chemicals interfere with the neurotransmitters which regulate thoughts, feelings, emotions and actions. A few drinks of alcohol may *temporarily* lift loneliness, but many drinks may greatly intensify those same feelings. A few drinks may produce euphoria or tranquillity, while continued drinking may progress into moodiness and eventually into deep depression or intense violence. "Long and hard drinking invariably leads to emotional upsets, erratic behavior and personality deterioration, all caused by the action of alcohol on the body and brain." (*EATING RIGHT TO LIVE SOBER*, p. 29.) We know that alcohol also has a profound effect upon the hormones. That hormonal malfunction has recently been found to be the key to alcohol's ability to induce cancer and destroy the immune system.

This depersonalization or the eradicating of personality is an accurate description of the "personality changes" brought about by chemicals. These changes are actually a *deterioration* of personality. This change in personality is produced by the patient's actual loss of his identity. He no longer is in touch with who he is because of the intoxicating effects of the drugs. In fact psychosis, which all of these drugs produce is described as "personality disintegration and loss of contact with reality." Kramer mentions psychologist Paul Meehl's assertion that there are people at all levels on a scale of ability to experience pleasure, from those who are "born three drinks behind" to those who are "born three drinks ahead." Their solution for those "born three drinks behind" is to give them those three drinks in a pill. We all have a good understanding of what three drinks will do, but we have little or no understanding that those three drinks may be subtly slipped into a psychoactive tablet or capsule prescribed by a physician who believes his patent might be "three drinks behind." With statements like this being made by professionals, why would any state not have laws which include these psychoactive drugs under an involuntary intoxication clause?

Dr. Robert K. Siegal explains, "...the changes in perception, mood, and thinking are perhaps the least understood but also among the most important in determining the precise nature and form of...intoxication." (*PCP PHENCYCLIDINE ABUSE: AN APPRAISAL*, p. 132.) In other words this personality change is an indicator for the degree of intoxication brought about by the drug. The strong impact of the SSRIs upon the personality should be a clear indication of the intoxicating effect of this new class of drugs. We also know that elevating serotonin has an intoxicating effect through increasing the flow of the body's own amphetamines - the adrenalins. The brain waves in the chapter on sleep disorders would also back up this evidence that Prozac is producing a strong intoxicating effect as well. We have also learned that the mixing of drugs can cause this intoxicating effect. When we add to that the fact that Prozac is multiplying the effects of most other drugs by 1000%, we have an incredible formula for intoxication. Blunting someone's consciousness is not a cure.

Dr. Solomon Snyder of Johns Hopkins gives us a physiological explanation or why these serotonergic agents cause a blurring of the concept of self, "Very recent research in numerous laboratories has revealed that psychedelic agents do exert potent effects on a serotonin receptor subtype...psychedelic drugs mimic the effects of serotonin. The relative strengths with which psychedelic drugs influence...receptors parallel the drugs' relative psychedelic potencies in humans. By influencing neurons with...receptors, which have connections to the locus ceruleus, psychedelic drugs may indirectly change the firing of cells in the locus ceruleus. [accelerated firing is produced by LSD]...the research into the actions of psychedelic drugs has already enriched our understanding of how the brain regulates behavior...*The research on psychedelic drugs also suggests that the amazing sense of oneness with the universe produced by psychedelic drugs might reflect an extreme activation of the locus ceruleus which causes a breakdown of the barriers between self and the nonself.*" (*DRUGS AND THE BRAIN*, p. 205)

Dr. Kramer reports that "'Obsessionality' and 'compulsiveness' are now used by those who treat illness with medication to encompass what in earlier days would have seemed mere personal idiosyncrasy." (LISTENING TO PROZAC, p. 33) He actually advocates using Prozac for those who are shy to bring them out of their shell. He admits treating a case of homesickness with Prozac! He also looks for young people who are "well into the usual age of courtship," who haven't had a romantic relationship or someone stuck in an abusive relationship as candidates for Prozac. To demonstrate how far out of line this labeling of "normal" as "abnormal" has gotten, I refer to an ad in the *SALT LAKE DESERET NEWS* dated December 19, 1993.

**ARE YOU BOTHERED BY
EXCESSIVE SHYNESS OR TIMIDITY?**

Do you avoid situations because:
　　*They involve significant contact with others?
　　*Your fear you may say something inappropriate or foolish?
　　*You might be the focus of attention?

Do you fear:
　　*Being embarrassed by showing signs of anxiety in front of others, crying or blushing?
　　*Public speaking?
　　*Criticism?
　　*Doing something while being watched?

Do social situations cause you to experience:
　　*Blushing, palpitations, trembling, or sweating?

IF YOU HAVE BEEN TROUBLED BY THE ABOVE, YOU MAY HAVE SOCIAL PHOBIA AND COULD BE ELIGIBLE FOR A RESEARCH STUDY INVOLVING FREE PSYCHIATRIC AND MEDICAL ASSESSMENT.

FOR INFORMATION CALL: 581-8806
[UNIVERSITY OF UTAH MOOD DISORDERS CLINIC]

The drug being used in this study is Ondanzatron, a drug generally used for nausea during cancer treatment. Why a drug like this would be used in the treatment of "Social Phobia" remains to be seen. This drug has an antagonist effect upon serotonin. I am sure we will soon hear the rationale behind this one in a whole new advertizing campaign.

Now, I don't know about the rest of you, but I certainly qualify for the fore mentioned study. I have been shy most of my life and most definitely camera shy. In fact I was voted the "Most Bashful" in my senior year of high school. Amazingly though, as I have matured, I have overcome that shyness - without the use of drugs or psychiatric care. This ad describes nearly every human being

I have ever met in my life. What is wrong with people being allowed the time and space to grow at their own pace and through their own experiences? Do we all have to be clones, developing at the exact same pace?

The authors of TRANQUILIZING OF AMERICA as early as 1979 predicted the coming of this drugging of individuals to rid them of idiosyncrasies as leading us to a "loss of the self." We quote, "As we have followed the tranquilizing of America, we have seen the individual - the 'me' in all of us - get swept aside in a heedless rush for the quick and easy chemical way out...*As we approach the day of a drug for every mood, thought, feeling, and deed, we need to ask ourselves whether we want to take the risk of a continual dwarfing of the human spirit by making the 'me' the drug in me."*

Even though Dr. Kramer promotes the use of Prozac for shyness he also refers to this chemical dwarfing of the human spirit as well. He compares Prozac to the drug "Heavy Sodium" from the last novel by the Southern writer Walker Percy, *THE THANATOS SYNDROME*, "...a maverick doctor finds that plotters have introduced an insidious chemical, Heavy Sodium, into the water supply. On Heavy Sodium, shy and anxious women - the first example is 'a housebound Emily Dickinson' - become erotic, bold, competitive, slim, un-self-conscious, and insensitive to the point of perfunctoriness. They shake off 'old terrors, worries, rages, a shedding of guilt like last year's snakeskin.'

"Percy was writing before Prozac was marketed, but *Heavy Sodium is like Prozac in so many respects that we must credit him with creating the art that life imitates.* To Percy, the drug's effects are all to the bad. One Heavy Sodium, people are 'not hurting, they are not worrying the same old bone, but there is something missing, not merely the old terrors but a sense in each of her - her what? her self?' Heavy Sodium *reduces a person to his or her ignoble, animal being*, a point Percy emphasizes by having the book's villains, overdosed on Heavy Sodium, take on the posture and behaviors of apes. *By reducing human self-consciousness, the drug robs individuals of their souls.* What links men and women to God is precisely their guilt, anxiety, and loneliness." (*LISTENING TO PROZAC,* p. 250)

Oh how often have I had an ex-Prozac patient look at the cover of Dr. Kramer's book with the figure of a man lifting his head off and the person remaining has no face, and say, "That's exactly what Prozac does to you! It rips your head right off and there is nothing left of you!" They have told me in almost identical words over the last four years, "Prozac rips your soul right out of you!" Dr. Kramer gives the impression that these feelings of guilt, anxiety and loneliness are detrimental to us, counter-productive, and that they hold us back in life. He argues that by chemically ridding ourselves of these feelings we can press forward in life with nothing holding us back. He contends that Prozac "lends people courage and allows them to choose life's ordinarily risky undertakings." I would describe the same effect as Prozac causing a removal inhibitions and inducing impulsive behavior with no concern for consequences. To me he is saying that with these feelings of guilt, anxiety, etc., removed the patient can get up and kill their kid in the morning and go right on with the day without any remorse for their actions. When one is robbed of his soul - his sense of right and wrong, his inhibitions, why not? Anything is possible, including the terrible nightmarish effects being reported by so many. Kramer's patient Hillary tried to explain these feelings to him, "I don't get hurt. When I break up with a man, I have no bad feelings whatsoever, and I don't worry about whether I am hurting him. Sometimes I wonder whether I haven't suffered a loss of moral sensibility."

Dr. Kramer points to this disappearance of uncomfortable feelings as a question arising now about Prozac and as being the main concern with the "mother's little helpers" back in the fifties and sixties. "This particular contrast - the contented and discontented perfectionist - gives rise to further thoughts about the notion of the 'mother's little helper.' Mother's little helpers were pills - Miltown, amphetamine, barbiturates, Librium, and Valium were the most popular and widely available in the fifties and early sixties - that were *used to keep women in their place, to make them comfortable in a setting that should have been uncomfortable*, to encourage them to focus on tasks that did not matter." (p. 39)

Dr. Breggin explains that the drugs used in psychiatry are designed to chemically interfere with the neurotransmitter action that connects the frontal lobes of the brain with the remainder of the brain, thus creating a lobotomy type effect "...I saw no mystery in how the treatments worked. By damaging the brain and mind, they made the patients docile and passive---suitable for control within these abusive institutions." He additionally explains: "...The frontal lobes are the seat of higher human functions, such as love, concern for others, empathy, self-insight, creativity, initiative, autonomy, rationality, abstract reasoning, judgement, future planning, foresight, willpower, determination, and concentration. The frontal lobes allow us to be 'human' in the full sense of that word; they are required for a civilized, effective, mature life." (*TOXIC PSYCHIATRY*, p. 6, 53)

Listen now to ex-Prozac patients and the families of those still using Prozac - those families who have been left behind, those who have noticed such a drastic change in personality in their loved ones that they refer to them as the "walking dead":

"The thing to me that seemed to be so confusing about this when I talked to my cousin when she was taking Prozac was that she felt she was really doing well. Yet, it was almost like looking at a copy of her. She looked like her, she talked like her, my first impression was, 'Oh, she's so much better, she's not depressed.' But as I lived with her for a few days when she visited with me, I saw that she was not herself. This was not the person I knew. It was somehow like somebody copying her."

"It's like I have two personalities. Actually it's like I am two different people. It seems like I'm not even myself. It seems like something has got control of my body."

"I have these thoughts I can't control. I never thought it could be my medication. Part of me is saying, 'Don't do that, it's irrational. You are wrong to do that.' And another part of me says, 'Do it.' I can't control it. Within a month after taking it I hurt myself several times to where I ended up in the hospital for three weeks and they are still telling me it is not the Prozac! Since that time I've probably hurt myself several times. I don't know what to think. I just keep saying, 'This is not me!' I have no control over this person."

"Prozac seemed to really help me for about the first six months and then it just turned on me. We had a new baby and I began to have such violent feelings toward her that I was afraid to be anywhere near her...Finally I decided that I had to get off the drug. My wife was shocked. She had no idea at all that I had been having trouble with Prozac. She thought that I was doing very well on it and that it had been a life saver for me. I had been afraid to tell her what was happening to me because I thought I was going crazy! There was a smile on my face but no one could describe the horror I felt inside!...I was only on the drug for a year and have been off almost a year. Even after being off Prozac for a long time I still remained convinced that I must really be crazy. The confusion, racing and disconnected thoughts, violent and suicidal thoughts, depression and sleeplessness persisted for so long. It seemed to cycle. There would be a few good days and then a few bad weeks then a few bad days followed by a few good weeks until I finally got through the withdrawal. During the down periods I had no recall of the good days and therefore could feel no hope, only despair. Even though I feel great now, there is still an occasional day when I have kind of a flashback and I'm afraid it is going to start all over again. These are just brief moments though and then they are gone...I remained convinced I was crazy until

I finally reached the point that I could remember who I really was - the type of person I was before taking Prozac. I finally was able to remember that before using Prozac I was the kind of guy who would pick a spider up and carry it out of the house rather than kill it. I really wasn't this terrible person I had become with all these violent thoughts. Once I had memory of who I really was I knew I was going to be okay...The doctors were no help. I became very frustrated. They gave me one antidepressant after another after Prozac. Elavil was one and Zoloft was another. Neither helped. They seemed to only magnify the reactions I was already having to Prozac. Elavil zonked me so badly I was driving into snow banks on it and had to be pulled out...Although I had never tried alternative treatments before I decided to try because so many others were doing so well with them. I stopped eating meat, exercised (slowly working up to a brisk walk for four miles a day) and used Ginkgo. I lost the excess weight I had gained on Prozac and my mind began to clear. My health, physical, mental and emotional seems better than ever, but my doctor just found abnormal enzymes in my liver and I have lost my insurance because of that. So I have just started working to rebuild my liver with another alternative method - barley green. Hopefully it will work as effectively as the other alternatives I have tried and I will be able to get my insurance back."

"The person I knew is gone just gone."

"Behaviors I abhorred before my use of Prozac, I became obsessed with doing! My values changed completely."

"I have a coffin without a body to put in it. The person I knew and loved for a lifetime is dead. This other person he has become - the person I never knew before Prozac - is out there somewhere walking around now hating all of us who he loved so much before."

"I always had a mask on that was smiling, but what was going on inside of me was indescribably horrifying!"

"When I started on Prozac it was like having to get to know someone else."
"Prozac actually made me do things against my own will...Things I would not have done even under hypnosis."

"I'll just be happy to have the 'old me' back again! Even with my imperfections and no matter how rough life might become, I would rather face reality and solve my problems than to ever go through anything like this again!"

293

"Everything I had felt was 'wrong' before was now 'okay'."

"My mother used to be a good mother. She used to care about us kids and take care of us. After three years on prozac she never does anything for us. She just doesn't care anymore!"

"I began to question all decisions I had made throughout my life. I began to think that all I had felt was right in the past was actually wrong and all that was wrong before was right."

"On Prozac, my whole personality did a complete change. I started becoming intentionally self-destructive although I didn't know why and I didn't care. As my behavior got stranger and more destructive, the doctor didn't see that the behavior changes were due to the drug, and he increased the dosage from one to two and then to an occasional third a day."

"Prozac made me trust people I never would have trusted with anything before."

"I did not like, in fact I could not stand the person I had become on Prozac. I began to assume that this 'new me' must be the 'real me' with all my brain chemicals 'balanced'. I didn't know how I was going to live with this new me!"

"After only two weeks on Prozac I wanted to run away from myself. I couldn't stand myself."

"I noticed my behavior and thoughts were so strange. I would be talking to someone and think, 'well, I've talked to this person as long as I am going to and I really don't feel like talking any longer'. And I would get up and walk away in the middle of a conversation! I never would have treated anyone that way before."

"I had never contemplated suicide before that time."

"I thought and acted just like a teenager again. At forty-five I grew my hair long and put psychedelic designs all over my car! I was very defiant about everything with everyone. No one could get anywhere with me. You couldn't tell me anything because I knew it all!"

"I continued to take the Prozac, because I felt like a Dr. Jekyll and Mr. Hyde. I thought it was me. I didn't think it was the drug. And my doctor was perplexed. He also thought it was me, and he just continued to prescribe it."

"The entire time I was on prozac was like an out of body experience! I watched myself do things I would never ever dream of doing and say to myself, 'Oh my gosh, that can't be me! I would never do such a thing!' But another part of me would say, 'Sure it's you. It must be you, look. You're really doing it!' I would argue again, 'But it couldn't be me! Yet it must be me, I see myself doing these things.'"

"I have been off Prozac for three years and still have thoughts of stabbing and slashing when I see a sharp object! Never in my life have I had such violent and disturbing thoughts!"

"I thought I had someone else's brain in my body!"

"Although it was completely out of character for me, the compulsion to drink was so strong after starting on Prozac that it became impossible for me to drive past a bar."

"I am a good Christian, yet I could no longer feel the influence of the Holy Spirit upon me. I could not pray. I was no longer me!"

"I never dreamed these thoughts and feelings were being produced by the drug. I thought I was going crazy!"

"What will I ever do to put my life back together again? I have done things on this drug that I could never tell my husband about, it is difficult to admit it all to myself!"

"On Prozac my life became an 'open book'. I divulged things about myself I never before would have discussed to individuals I never before would have trusted."

"How anyone on Prozac can hold a marriage together is a puzzle to me! I became so rude, distant, arrogant, aggressive, so easily offended by what I interpreted as personal attacks, etc., that I lost or cut off most of my friends, family and husband."

"I became shocked at my own behavior."

"I became enraged and despondent. I was hostile and aggressive toward my family and friends. I was obsessed with killing myself. The muscle spasms and suicidal despair continue. As each day goes by, I seem to be relieved of some

symptoms and bothered by others. My primary concern is the hostility, because that's not my nature and I don't like having it in my life."

Is Prozac a drug which chemically induces psychosis, thereby mimicking the disease state, and classifying Prozac as a psychotomimetic like the other insanity inducing drugs?

*It was "Like I was driving in a dream...I remember hitting another car, someone telling me to get out of the car, and **waking up** at the police station."*

"It was like a dream."

"I was feeling out of my body..."

"It could have been a dream. To be honest, I don't know if I was physically up there or spiritually there."

"Chronic users reported personality change, social withdrawal, social isolation, and divorce...violent behavior was one of the effects." Loss employment and disrupted education and criminal arrests were also reported."

"...chronic...users experienced persistent cognitive and memory problems. Speech difficulties included stuttering, poor speech articulation, and difficulties in expressing themselves to others, effects lasting 6 months to a year following prolonged daily...use. Mood disorders also occurred; viz: depression, anxiety, and violent behavior. Purposive activity became more difficult with resultant loss of employment or impaired school performance."

"There can also be a preoccupation with death or death-related thoughts (meditatio mortis)..."

"Behavior: Agitated, excited, combative, regressive, self-destructive or 'bizarre' behavior, insomnia, anorexia, incontinence, followed by depression, irritability and emotional lability."

"The patients are dangerous to themselves, because of depression and suicidal impulses, and dangerous to others, because of paranoia and strong tendencies toward violence..."

"...In one reported case, loss of pain sensation resulted in an act of self-injury by biting of the forearms almost to the bone (Grove 1979). Irrational acts...may

be manifestations of...toxicity. Other general characteristics include waxing and waning of the mental status or behavior and evidence of increased strength. "

"Patients with...intoxication can have a clear sensorium, or they can be disoriented, confused, stuporous, lethargic, or comatose....Frank psychotic symptoms, including hallucinations, delusions, and paranoid ideation, are not unusual. "

"Some patients with...toxicity display inappropriate behavior. Behavioral effects include muteness, staring, violence, and agitation. Violent behavior occurred in 35 percent of people with...intoxication. "

"Thoughts of...intoxicated subjects are usually short, confused, wandering, rapidly changing, and involutional in nature. The intoxicated individual experiences waves of such thoughts interrupted by waves of blank (amnesic) periods. The rapidly accelerated thinking itself, coupled with the drug-induced hyper-excitability and euphoria, can lead to the clinical condition called 'flight of ideas' or 'mania.'"

"Frequently, the intoxicated individual considers himself/herself endowed with unique and superior abilities (both bodily abilities and mental abilities) as a result of the thought changes. In the extreme cases, this state can be manifested as paranoia, whereby the subject tries to account for these thought disturbances with persecutory or grandiose delusions. "

"The most common thinking disturbances [in association with the use of this drug] have been described in the literature as 'loosening of association,...overinclusive thoughts,' 'concreteness,' 'delusional thinking,' and general 'disorganization.' Associated with these phenomena are 'negativism' and 'hostility.'...The most consistent high point of the EWI [Experiential World Inventory] was the ideation scale, which strongly suggests thought disorder including unbridled fantasy activity, inability to connect experiences purposefully, flights of ideas [mania or hypo-mania], and serious loss in the capacity to select and resist thoughts and to produce and connect new thoughts. Other consistently high scores were seen on both sensory perception, time perception, and body perception scales. "
"Users also experienced a feeling of strength and endurance. They described feeling 'powerful,' 'superior,' 'arrogant,' with 'bursts of energy,' 'like...you could move mountains.' There was also a loss of inhibitions. It was felt to be difficult to do things; one had 'to think about moving or talking.' In addition, they described feeling restless and nervous. "

"...taken in typical...doses was reported to prevent sleep for 8 to 12 hours, decrease appetite, and to cause constipation and urinary hesitancy."

"...users reported persistent problems with memory and speech, and difficulty with thinking following long periods of regular use of the drug. Recent memory capability appears to be primarily affected. Users complain of stuttering, inability to speak or blocking, and difficulty with articulation. Speech and memory difficulties lasted as long as 6 months to 1 year following prolonged daily use of large doses..."

"several chronic users complained of anxiety or nervousness during and following periods of regular...[use and some] became severely depressed, and attempted suicide on repeated occasions."

Under the influence of high doses of the drug, "the patient may keep his eyes open and seems 'disconnected' from the environment. It seems as if higher associational functions of the brain are markedly depressed, a clinical impression for which there is some human and animal physiologic data (Corssen, Miyaska, and Domino 1968; Miyasaka and Domino 1968; Corssen, Domino, and Bree 1969; Winters 1972). During emergence from [the influence of the drug], the patient may go through a phase of vivid dreaming with and without psychomotor activity, manifested by confusion and irrational behavior."

"...users were also found to have a more extensive involvement in the [criminal] system."

"New problems have surfaced in communities in direct proportion to the frequency and regularity of...[use]. Violent and bizarre behavior is seen in the home, in public places, and in schools, often disrupting education...unexplained speech problems, memory loss, thinking disorders, personality changes, anxiety, severe depression, and suicidal and homicidal tendencies."

"An increasing number of young people appearing violent, bizarre, unresponsive, extremely confused, or acutely psychotic are being seen in local emergency rooms. With increased use of..., an upsurge in violent crimes that culminate in homicide is observed.

"Police report erratic driving and inappropriate behavior following automobile accidents in individuals who have no apparent evidence of alcohol or sedative hypnotic ingestion."

*"...The defense attorneys in the majority of cases claim that their clients were not guilty either by reason of diminished capacity or of insanity (**drug-induced psychosis**) [my emphasis]. With defendants showing bizarre and violent behavior and sometimes defendants claiming amnesia to the event, (given the unique properties of [this drug])..."*

Many accidents occurred because the person "could not respond appropriately to imminent danger."

If you have had a personal experience with Prozac (or one of the other SSRIs), you would have sworn that all of the above quotes were made by those on Prozac because of the amazing similarities in experiences with Prozac and the drug above which was introduced in the late 50's. Like Prozac, it too was touted by medical studies to have a large margin of safety. The drug we are talking about is PCP (Angel Dust). (All of the above quotes were taken from the *NATIONAL INSTITUTE ON DRUG ABUSE'S MONOGRAPH SERIES*, Research 21, 1978, entitled *PCP PHENCYCLIDINE ABUSE: AN APPRAISAL* and Research 64, 1986, entitled *PHENCYCLIDINE: AN UPDATE*.) The scientific names for PCP, phencyclidine hydrochloride, and Prozac, fluoxetine hydrochloride, rhyme, but in my observation they have **far more in common** than that. Never have I researched another drug so similar in action, effects and long-term withdrawal associated with Prozac than with those associated with phencyclidine (PCP, Angel Dust). Both drugs are powerful serotonin uptake blockers (Smith et al., 1977). Both were first in a whole new class of drugs. Both in the beginning were declared to have a large margin of safety in humans. In fact Kramer points out that "serotonin elevating drugs...are sometimes called 'serenics.'" Parke Davis, Co. promoted their drug in this way as well, marketing PCP as "Sernyl," signifying serenity. Yet Kramer goes on to say "The notion of serotonin-enhancing drugs as serenity-inducing makes the purported association between Prozac and violence all the more puzzling." Apparently he is not very familiar with phencyclidine and its notorious reputation for an association with violence. Perhaps it would help him to understand why this newer class of serotonergic drugs would also possess potential violent paradoxical reactions. To refer to a drug which has proven to be one of the most violence producing drugs ever on the market as "Sernyl," with the implication that it would produce serenity is beyond our comprehension now more than thirty years after its release. Thirty years from now how will we view the new serotonin reuptake inhibitors? To understand how long it takes for something to be done legally about these drugs, the Comprehensive Drug Abuse Prevention and Control Act of 1970 classified phencyclidine with the barbiturates and LSD in Section 202(c), Schedule III(b)(7) as...'having a depressant effect on the central nervous system"

(Munch 1974). PCP was released in 1957 and classed as a Schedule III drug (having no therapeutic use) thirteen years later in 1970. The case with LSD was that "Ninety percent of bad LSD trips are provoked by psychiatric propaganda which creates an atmosphere of fear rather than courage and trust. The bad trips and complications started happening before the psychiatrists knew about the complications to LSD...the bulk of lethal and non-lethal complications to LSD have not been reported in the medical or lay press. In a sampling of the psychiatrists in one city, fifty of them had been consulted about one or more LSD bad reactions and not one of these cases had been reported." *(THE BEYOND WITHIN, p. 253)*

Ronald K. Siegel explains that "PCP intoxication also can produce...perceptual distortions, and mental confusion can catapult the naive user into a state where s/he feels and fears loss of ego and identity, loss of contact with reality, and even permanent mental dysfunction. Consequently, panic ensues, and deviant behavior, including aggression, can occur." *(PCP PHENCYCLIDINE ABUSE: AN APPRAISAL, p. 284)* This type of intoxication is a dissociative state. Ex-Prozac patients consistently report these same fears as the reason for their fear of expressing to their doctors what is happening to them. PCP taken in low doses over a period of time completely changes the personality, chemically inducing schizophrenia, temporarily and sometimes indefinitely. The definition of the word hallucination comes from the Latin "hallucinari," meaning to prate, to dream, or to wander in mind. The accepted definition in psychiatry is: A false sensory perception in the absence of an actual external stimulus. *It may be induced by emotional and other factors such as drugs, alcohol and stress and may occur in any of the senses.* "Ninety-four percent of PCP users who have experienced hallucinations, experienced the type that included wandering in mind or attention (lapses of attention), mental confusion, clouding, difficulty in maintaining attention during complicated tasks, difficulty in maintaining thoughts during conversation, and preoccupation with subjective sensations...most of these users were distractable and when faced with frustration might become irritable, aggressive, or impulsive, often out of proportion to the reality of the situation." all these are indicative of schizophrenia. *(PCP PHENCYCLIDINE ABUSE: AN APPRAISAL p. 132)* Patient and patient family reports are indicating the same with those using Prozac for extended periods of time or in high doses.

Violence and a preoccupation with self-destruction are reported with both drugs. Dissociative states "as if in a dream" are reported with both. PCP creates a compulsion for alcohol and other drugs just as Prozac patients are reporting. PCP after chronic daily use causes severe bouts of depression upon discontinuation of the drug which last six months, a year or longer. Prozac patients, including those who took the drug for reasons other than depression and report that they had never before felt depression, are reporting the same type of long-term severe rebound depression upon discontinuation of Prozac. Withdrawal with PCP is long - lasting over a year with some who have used the drug for extended periods with severe depression persisting throughout the withdrawal period. Ex-Prozac patients are discovering the same type of withdrawal. And on and on goes the list of similarities in symptoms produced by both of these drugs thought in the beginning to be so safe and effective.

"In the 1950's D.W. Wooley first suggested that an abnormality of brain serotonin (5 hydroxytryptamine [5HT]) function might play a role in the pathogenesis of schizophrenia (Wooley and Campbell 1962; Wooley and Shaw 1954). This theory was based upon the similarity in chemical structure between 5HT and the hallucinogenic ergot alkaloids, and the observation that such compounds acted as antagonists of 5HT in peripheral smooth muscle compounds, lysergic acid diethylamide (LSD), and of others, such as psilocybin, N1, N4-dimethyltryptamine (DMT), 5-methoxy-N, N-dimethyltryptamine, bufotenine, and the B-carbolines, led to two major lines of investigation. "First, it was proposed that these compounds might be synthesized in significant amounts in the brains of schizophrenic patients as the result of abnormal metabolic activity..."Second, the actions of these compounds on brain serotonergic systems led to hypotheses that endogenous over- or under-production of 5HT [serotonin] might be related to the production of schizophrenic symptoms. The actions of LSD on brain 5HT have been most widely studied. In classic work of several investigators, it was shown that LSD suppressed the firing rate of serotonergic neurons in the raphe nucleus, causing increases in brain 5HT (serotonin)...Human bloodplatelets [blood levels] are the most widely adopted peripheral model of CNS [Central Nervous System] amine-containing neurons...A recurring finding has been *elevated* platelet concentrations in schizophrenic patients (for review, see Meltzer 1987). However, elevated platelet 5HT concentrations are not specific for schizophrenia; they are also found in mood disorders, organic brain disease (especially mental retardation), and childhood autism (Partington et al. 1973)..." (*SEROTONIN IN MAJOR PSYCHIATRIC DISORDERS*, p. 211, 212, 214)

Tonge and Leonard (1969) compared phencyclidine, Ditran, mescaline and LSD and their effect upon 5-HT serotonin and 5-HIAA serotonin. All four drugs increased brain 5-HT serotonin and decreased 5-HIAA over a three hour period. As we pointed out before inhibition of 5HT serotonin is known to result in a decrease of 5HIAA (serotonin turnover) while it increases extraneuronal content of the 5HT serotonin (Buus, et al. 1975; Nabeshima, et al. 1983).

Kenneth M. Johnson in 1978, thirty years after our official introduction to PCP, recommended that, "...Because of the suggestive nature of the foregoing studies with PCP and the proposed role of 5-HT in emotional and psychotic behavior, it is felt that a detailed biochemical study of the effects of PCP on serotonergic function is warranted..." *(PCP PHENCYCLIDINE ABUSE: AN APPRAISAL*, p. 46). This information on elevated serotonin levels and their connection to schizophrenia would imply that Prozac and the remaining SSRIs, along with any of the drugs which raise serotonin levels should all be classed as psychotomimetic drugs, over a period of use they are chemically inducing a psychosis mimicking schizophrenia. As early as 1986 Prozac's potential to induce psychosis emerged when an FDA Safety Reviewer uncovered that Lilly had withheld information of psychotic episodes in 52 patients during Prozac's clinical trials. It remains to be seen why no action was taken against Lilly for this withholding of pertinent safety information.

Another example of a psychotomimetic which chemically induces schizophrenia as we have just read is the drug of choice of the CIA, LSD. Both of these drugs, PCP and as we have just discussed in conjunction with LSD, can be used to chemically cause a complete change in personality. In fact, if you will remember, we already brought out the fact that LSD was originally marketed by Sandoz Pharmaceuticals as a drug which would chemically induce schizophrenia in *"normal subjects"* and would thereby help us to learn the cause of this condition. We have also discussed that these drugs too initially cause a rise in 5HT serotonin levels.

PCP taken in low doses over time generally will not cause the intensity of psychotic behavior we have come to associate with the drug, but will gradually cause Dr. Jeckyl to turn into Mr. Hyde. Most critical to note is that no known behavioral disturbance nor any evidence of psychiatric problems or mental disorders have preceded the psychotic reactions produced by the use of PCP. These included not only socially marginal individuals, but also those of substantial achievement without any indication of "premorbid psychopathology." In other words, these are the "normal subjects" Sandoz suggested be used as subjects to chemically induce schizophrenia in those who had never before experienced it. Over a period of time the use of PCP produced a sudden onset of paranoia, delusional thinking and auditory hallucinations, accompanied by unpredictable aggressive and violent behavior. This same sudden onset of symptoms is reported by patients using Prozac. Generally it too is produced over an extended period of use, but, just as with PCP, it can also happen soon after the introduction of the drug, depending upon the dosage of the drug and/or the patient's ability to metabolize Prozac.

A very frightening aspect of this PCP-induced psychosis besides that fact that it is generally overlooked as being drug-induced and is treated as if the patient is schizophrenic is that "about one fourth of the patients originally treated for phencyclidine psychoses return about a year later with schizophrenic ones in the absence of drug use...These later episodes have lacked the characteristic violence of the phencyclidine-induced ones..." (Luisada, 1976) We have already discussed the fact that cocaine has been found to do the same. We know that LSD causes flashbacks. What about Prozac and the other SSRIs? Can we expect the same from them? Considering the accumulation rate of Prozac and long-term flushing or washing out period, this could be considered a very likely possibility for some time. Patients and physicians should be aware of this, take precautions to keep the patient calm and avoiding stressful situations for some time to avoid the uncontrollable adrenalin rushes which could produce latent effects such as this. I am firmly convinced that patients can avoid latent effects if they will take precautions to avoid any or a major shock to their systems, whether the shock be emotional, chemical, mental, financial, spiritual, etc.

With PCP being used primarily as an anesthetic, it was placed in a controlled setting where reactions could be observed readily. It was also used in strong doses in order to create an anesthetic state, thus making any reactions more obvious or dramatic by their more rapid onset and increased intensity. In this way PCP's use was limited and observed reactions led to its removal from the market. Had PCP been used in low doses over an extended period of time as Prozac has, how long would it have stayed on the market? Would we have noticed what was happening or would we have been as confused about the effects of the drug as we have been with Prozac and the other SSRIs? The likelihood of this of this possibility is demonstrated by the fact that when used as a street drug in the lower doses PCP's dramatic dissociative effects are not so obvious. These effects emerge over time as the drug accumulates in the body. The most obvious to those around the PCP user is a gradual complete change in personality just as is being reported with the use of Prozac. PCP in low dose generally acts much like alcohol. In a mid-range dose it produces hallucinogenic properties. Then in high doses full psychosis is reached as we go into lower and lower levels of consciousness. As the drug accumulates over time within the body the effects felt from the use of the drug changes accordingly. Just as with Prozac, "... PCP has been shown to have a very large volume of distribution (i.e., very little of the drug is present in the blood stream), and to be primarily eliminated through metabolism (Cook et al. 1982a; Cook et al. 1982b; Woodworth et al., in press). Therefore, a more effective detoxification procedure is needed." *(PHENCYCLIDINE: AN UPDATE, p. 112)* [Note that the studies demonstrating the accumulative aspect of PCP were not published until twenty-five years *after* the drug was introduced. If Prozac's use were not so widespread, perhaps we could be more grateful that similar studies on it were published only seven years after its introduction.]

Prozac's actions appear to be slightly more like PCP than LSD when it comes to the production of anger or agitation. Recall the statements by Prozac users who have tried various illegal drugs earlier in life: "It was like half a hit of LSD, but it made me angry and aggressive too." "It was like a combination of speed and cocaine." Is this because of these drugs' similar effect upon cortisol levels? We have already noted that Prozac doubles cortisol levels with only a 30 mg. dose. The severe depression upon cessation of exposure to PCP would indicate that cortisol levels are strongly affected by this drug as well thereby producing the severe rebound depression. These intense bouts of depression last anywhere from six months to a year. This is considered to be the main reason those who use this drug find it so difficult to ever stop using it in spite of the suicidal and homicidal feelings it produces and the "bad trips" they experience. Those trying to stop the use of Prozac report this same reason for their defense of the drug and their fear of and inability to withdraw from the drug. Or could this anger and aggression be a result of the chemical induction of hypoglycemia by both drugs? Hypoglycemia is a common result of PCP use as well (McCarron, 1981).

The reported psychological effects from PCP are: increased anxiety, increased nervousness, social withdrawal and isolation, violent and aggressive behavior, paranoid delusions, auditory hallucinations, depression, suicidal and homicidal tendencies, personality changes, etc. *Thirty-three percent* of regular users reported a gradual change in mood, making them more irritable, angry, violent, depressed, lonely, isolated and antisocial. Some effects continued for several months to a year after discontinuation such as, short-term memory loss, slurred speech, disorientation, inability to recall certain words, etc. Patient reports from Prozac users demonstrate an identical pattern of adverse psychological effects. Most interesting to note with PCP intoxication is that as late as 1981 it was noted that even though PCP had been the subject of many reports, many problems in recognizing this type of intoxication in the medical field as well as the legal arena (McCarron, 1981).

"Whether chronic PCP use produces lasting changes in personality, biological functions, brain and nerve functions, reproductive functions, and in the health of the user's offspring remains unanswered." (PCP, The Dangerous Angel, 1985, p. 59) Over twenty years after the drug had been used in humans we still did not have the answers to these questions. Yet in early May, 1993 a national

news story on Prozac suggested that it appears to be safe for a pregnant woman to continue to use Prozac during the first trimester of her pregnancy because any apparent birth defects were no higher than with other drugs in that same class. An alcohol and drug abuse counselor let me know that she was absolutely irate at the misinformation in the article. Little critical information produced through the study referred to in this article had been stressed. What about the much higher rate of birth defects among Prozac mothers compared to those who are on no drugs? There was also no stress put on the fact that the miscarriage rate for those using Prozac was double the miscarriage rate for the other drugs. Miscarriage is generally due to a malformation or defect of the fetus or the poor physical condition or toxic condition of the mother. Just because the defect is being eliminated via a miscarriage before birth does not signify less risk with this drug. The truth is that we will not know for many years to come just how and what effect the drug has had upon children born to these mothers. We have no idea how the drug will alter the baby's brain function or any other body function until the child is old enough to detect those effects. Even aspirin is known to cause birth defects. Why would anyone consider taking a powerful mind-altering drug and not expect to see problems in offspring? What a terribly dangerous risk to take. Do not forget that Thalidomide was promoted as being "safe" for pregnant women...5000 deformed babies later we learned it was not true. How many babies with subtle defects, perhaps even complicated brain dysfunction as has been suspected with PCP, will it take before we learn our lesson with this drug? Cushing's syndrome which is the disease label for excess cortisol levels whether chemically induced by medications or a malfunction of the glandular system can produce such horrible deformities as dwarfism or masculinization of a female fetus or feminization of a male fetus. Because of Prozac's strong effect upon cortisol levels, these adverse effects of Cushing's should be considered possibilities. And any mother considering using Prozac during pregnancy should read the reports of birth defects already made to the FDA by doctors throughout the country. One that still stands out in my mind is a baby who died because the vital organs were outside rather than inside at birth. These are the stories that don't make front page news in the local newspaper - only in medical reports.

PCP can cause either CNS (Central Nervous System) stimulation or depression depending upon the dose (Balster and Chait 1978). It produces classic schizophrenic symptoms which fool even the professionals. Psychiatrists who are unaware of a patients' use of PCP will often not recognize the symptoms as drug reactions. This was often the case with LSD as well. Because of the out of character behavior it produces they will diagnose the patient as having an ongoing disease process, namely schizophrenia (Snyder 1980). Time should prove that this is exactly the dilemma in which we find ourselves in conjunction with Prozac. PCP is also a strong inhibitor of REM sleep through its potent affect upon serotonin (Martin et al. 1979, Ary and Komiskey 1980). The SSRIs are all strong REM inhibitors as well because of their action upon serotonin and the subsequent raising of cortisol levels.

PCP not only has some of the properties of a hallucinogen, but also possesses the properties of both a stimulant and a depressant. It is a virtual smorgasbord of drug reactions and is in a drug classification of its own. PCP, like Prozac, was also the first in a whole new class of drugs called the arylcyclohexylamines. Although many psychoactive drugs can be classified as either depressants, stimulants or hallucinogens, the arylcyclohexylamines defy any simple classification. They seem to possess mixed properties: hallucinatory, excitatory, sedative and cataleptoid-anesthetic. Patient reports surrounding the effects of Prozac would indicate that it too falls into all these types of classifications - hallucinatory, excitatory, sedative and anesthetic. The patient's reports of losing touch with reality, having memory lapses during the use of the drug, and describing it just as PCP users do - as though they are in a dream state are indicative of a dissociative state or hallucinogenic state. The dream state is a vivid hallucinogenic state.

We know that the amphetamine stimulants induce behavioral changes through serotonin (Lee, 1978; Nabeshima, 1983). Indications of a stimulant type effect reported by Prozac patients are often made using the exact same phrases as PCP users do to describe their experiences: feeling like superman or feeling increased physical strength, or feeling smarter or better than anyone else. When they first begin using Prozac or with an increase in their present dosage, they find they can think and perform better. As with all stimulants, this is not a lasting level of performance, as demonstrated by the need for larger and larger doses to attain the same effect. The patient finds he needs these higher doses over time to keep up that performance level just as someone on cocaine does. This need for continued use or an increase in dose leads them into dependence upon the drug. All of the preceding indications are descriptive of a stimulant profile.

The depressant effects appear as the patient finds that "what goes up must come down". We know that stimulants such as cocaine, or one more of us are familiar with on a milder scale, caffeine, produce a "high" followed by a "low." This in turn spurs the user on to use again in order to replace that most recent "low" with another "high". But when we bounce a ball we find that the higher the ball goes, the farther it falls. The extent to which it rises determines the extent to which it falls and so it is with the stimulant drugs - they produce an increase in depressive effects comparable to the increase in the highs they produce. Cocaine when used for the treatment of depression produces a depression far worse than the original depression when its use is discontinued. PCP produces indescribable depression upon withdrawal of the use of the drug. This depression is very intense and can last up to a year after a prolonged period of PCP use. Most of those who continue their use of the drug in spite of life threatening complications cite their inability to cope with the severity of the depression produced by the withdrawal as the reason for their continued use of PCP. They would rather face the "hell" they live through on the drug than to face the "hell" produced by withdrawal. When we consider the strong self-destructive tendencies produced by PCP, we may find also that the drug itself robs the user of his incentive or will power to save his life through discontinuing his use of the drug.

Prozac perfectly matches the profile in this depressant category also as patients describe their experience as a "roller coaster" in mood swings, constantly hitting highs and then lows. It also is producing terrible depression upon withdrawal (in fact some medical studies and the FDA's adverse reaction reports indicate that Prozac tends to produce more depression in the long run than it cures and the excess production of cortisol would indicate the same). The severe depression brought on by withdrawal compels the patient to begin their use of Prozac again. The most deceptive aspect of Prozac, which seems to set it apart (except for the benzodiazepines), is that of a *delayed* withdrawal. This is not always the case. It generally depends upon the term of use, occasionally not appearing for months after discontinuation of use of the drug. It is my opinion that this occurs because of the highly accumulative aspect of Prozac and the difficulty the body appears to have in flushing the drug out of the system. Added to that would be the high protein binding aspect of these newer drugs specifically designed to bind to brain tissue.

If physicians had been alerted to the stimulant properties of Prozac and the withdrawal aspect, they might have been watching for this severe long-term depression which appears upon discontinuation. This insight would have helped them to see that they patient is suffering what is known as "rebound depression" and should be assisted with their withdrawal rather than prescribing a restarting of the drug plus an *increase* in the dose. Or it would help them to see that the prescribing of anti-psychotic drugs or electric shock is not necessary as their patients are only suffering a long-term withdrawal rather than a progressive mental illness. Detoxification would be called for in this instance of a toxic psychotic reaction to a drug and\or severe withdrawal, not further drugging or use of invasive measures.

PCP too has a cumulative aspect. This is believed to be the reason that the

hallucinogenic type effects of the drug generally are not produced until after a prolonged period of use or in high dosages. At first the drug produces a euphoria, making the user feel that life is more complete and makes more sense. At first the mind could focus intensely on just one object and see the beauty there. A sense of oneness with society is reported. Mood states are intensified, with most users feeling happy or euphoric. Light was "felt." Music was "absorbed." Vision seemed distorted "like 2D." Feelings of "floating" are reported with actual visual hallucinations being a rarity. The large majority (80%) of regular users of PCP considered their first experience as pleasant and wanted to take the drug again. They reported it to be "fun," or "exhilarating." They reported feeling "happy" or "euphoric." It seemed to them to be a "perfect escape" or "a dream world."

The reports from Prozac users are identical. In the beginning it makes them feel good and gives them the desire to continue using it as their dependence upon the drug begins, then they report that the drug "turns" on them and becomes "a monkey on my back." Such is the deception surrounding the "peace" brought by the use of mind-altering drugs - it is not a lasting peace. This peacefulness is deceptive and only temporary as it is founded upon an individual's ability to withstand the full impact of the toxic effects and their metabolism. The chemicals wreak their havoc by causing abnormal stimulus to the brain and glandular system. They produce residual effects by accumulating within the brain and the body, generally the fatty tissues. In time the brain becomes accustomed to "expect" such abnormal stimulus by adjusting the various neurotransmitter systems to compensate for this stimulus. Then as so many report both with PCP and Prozac, "all hell breaks lose as the drug turns on you." Even though chronic PCP users have experienced this euphoric type sensation from the drug, they also experienced the severe depression. They state that they recognized the potential of the drug to bring one either to "the heights or depths of being." Prozac users simply call the drug "Prozac - Hell and Back."

CHAPTER 11

LILLY & POLITICS

Eli Lilly's continued silence concerning all the questions surrounding Prozac is beginning to ring loudly in the ears of the public. Why did they not disclose the information they already had on the link between their product and violence and suicide long before Harvard's Dr. Martin Tiecher had his test results published? Why have they not warned doctors, pharmacists or patients about their own study published a couple of years ago which shows that Prozac clearly multiplies by "10 fold or greater" many other drugs? Why are they even now ignoring all of these allegations of horrible emotional and physical side effects associated with Prozac while they continue to defend its safety?

They continue to stress that these problems are appearing only in a very small number of patients. Let's look at what they are calling a "small, insignificant number." Bonnie Leitsch, who is the past national director for the Prozac Survivor's Support Group, made this statement in early 1990, "Let's say this side effect [suicide] occurs in only one percent of the two million people now taking this drug...is it okay to flush those twenty thousand lives down the toilet to keep some people from feeling a little down?" How do we place a value on even one life lost, especially in such a violent fashion? Losing a loved one to a drug reaction which causes them to slip into a coma and die or heart failure, kidney failure, etc. would be difficult enough to deal with. But when the drug reaction produces insanity...an insanity that can produce in our loved one violence which takes their own life and/or the life of another, out of character behavior that is embarrassing to both patient and their family, coldness and insensitivity to loved ones even to the point of accusing them falsely of acts they have not taken against you, etc., how does a family recover?

If we look at current figures we find that, according to Eli Lilly, there are now 9 million prescriptions which have been filled for Prozac. Dr. Teicher's report indicates adverse reactions of suicidal and homicidal ideation in his study to be anywhere from 3% to 8%. This would mean that the number of patients we are talking about now would be *between 270,000 to 720,000* patients. But the study we looked at from Yale in this text which was released in March, 1991, indicates that one out of seven of their patients suffered intense suicidal preoccupation or intense feelings of violence. They state very clearly that from their observations this is *not a coincidence, but a reaction very directly related to Prozac.* If we use their one out of seven figure or approximately 15%, we are looking at an astounding figure of *1,350,000 patients, three quarters of a million patients experiencing the most serious of Prozac's adverse reactions - adverse reactions which affect not only the patient but all of society.* The study abruptly discontinued by Dr. Barbara Geller which peaked the interest of Ralph Nader's group gives us an astounding figure of *five out of eight* having these reactions to Prozac. That would be a figure which no one even wants to think of: *5,625,000 people being adversely affected by the most severe reactions to this drug - the homicidal and suicidal ideation.* (We should take into consideration that the last two studies involved adolescents who generally suffer a higher adverse reaction rate than adults.) Whatever the actual figures are for adverse reactions, it is obvious that the numbers are *incredibly high.* If medical journals reported up to an 8% figure in 1990 and in 1991 that figure jumped to almost double 15%, what might the medical studies released in 1992 reveal? *Remember that these are figures reported in **medical cases studies,** not from sources which Lilly would refer to as "media hype".*

The only public statement before publication of the first edition of this book other than a total denial of any possible problems with the drug was made August 28, 1990, in the *LOS ANGELES TIMES* by Rita Freedman, an analyst with Provident National Bank in Philadelphia. "I view the lawsuits as a non-event...", she said, adding that the issue of concern to Lilly is the possibility of additional lawsuits and more negative publicity about a drug that is very important to the company financially. The glaring ignorance of that position should be that if Prozac is producing hundreds or thousands of casualties from the severe emotional and physical side effects and all of the victims who survive file lawsuits, and the loved ones left behind file lawsuits, where are the profits Lilly would need to be concerned about then? Sounds logical until you realize that Lilly is bringing in approximately $100 million per month on Prozac alone. Each month of stalling the public's awareness of the dangers of the drug brings in an additional $100 million or more. With those profits a lot of lawsuits can be handled and a very large profit margin retained by the manufacturer.

It is also unfortunate that many victims and their families will remain unaware of the cause of the damages they have suffered. Many victims will also have their memories and judgement so badly impaired that they will not be able to determine that they have been damaged. Many of the adverse reactions masquerade as various physical and psychiatric ailments and doctors are telling patients, either out of ignorance or out of fear of a lawsuit, that there is no connection between their Prozac use and their ailment. Because of this many who would if they could file lawsuits are too critically ill to do so, or locked away in a mental hospital continuing to be drugged beyond their ability to judge, reason, recognize or even recall what has happened to them.

It is financially essential to any company to have ethical and moral business practices. You cannot make money from the pain and suffering of others without payment for those actions in the long run. Payment may not be immediate and may not come in a way one might expect, but universal laws of cause and effect will take their toll. They always have and always will.

As the first edition of this book was about to go to press Eli Lilly Pharmaceutical finally spoke to the public. Did they take the responsible position of addressing the issue of their product and the adverse reactions their customers are reporting? No, they attempted to divert the attention of the public from this unfolding Prozac produced pandora to the Church of Scientology, stating that they are the ones who have "stirred things up" on the Prozac issue, calling them a "cult of greed." In light of Lilly's over $100 million per month income this becomes the most obvious issue ever of the pot calling the kettle black. Besides being totally preposterous in light of all the incriminating medical reports and overwhelming onslaught of drug reaction reports made to the FDA, the fact remains that if there are problems with Prozac, does it matter who it is that is concerned enough to state that fact? Are they trying to make sure that we know who all is concerned enough to do everything in their power to raise public awareness of any problems with Prozac? If so, they had better lengthen their list because the Scientologists are only a small group of those who are concerned about the safety of Prozac. Lilly's attempt to have us focus on this group has been quite the diversion tactic. The actual list should include top medical researchers, consumer advocates, leading psychiatrists, the doctors making the reports of adverse reactions to the FDA, nurses, the general public, and ex-customers - the victims, which includes pharmaceutical executives, psychologists, psychiatrists, doctors, nurses, accountants, attorneys, housewives, students, people from every walk of life who have suffered incredible tragedy in their lives, but no Scientologists since they do not use the psychiatric drugs.

As someone who has worked for many years and continues to work with the heads of many businesses, both large and small, my opinion of a major company using this type of political ploy in the face of a flood of consumer complaints against their product is that it is completely inexcusable. When it involves a life and death situation and general well being of their customers, it is not only unethical, but immoral. The proper response from a company concerned about the consumer would be, "According to our customers, there seems to be a problem with this drug. Let's consider their input and take a closer look at these reports about our product." History has not shown Eli Lilly to have that type of ethical response in the past with their previous drugs which have been removed from the market. It took *outside pressure* to accomplish Oraflex's removal from the market in the mid-eighties, while Lilly continued to defend the efficacy and safety of their drug. The entire situation appears to be an exact "carbon copy" of the political maneuvering we now see happening with Prozac. It was removed from the market because of the high number of deaths it produced. That figure is far, far less than of the number of Prozac-related deaths that have been reported to the FDA. These stalling techniques, designed to milk the last dime out of the consumer have cost many lives with these previous products. The Prozac death count being reported to the FDA so far outweighs anything in the past it is difficult to comprehend. If you can "tell a book by it's cover," I'm afraid that Eli Lilly's past indicates a cover tainted with misrepresentation, to say the least.

We have just been given another reminder of this. Eli Lilly is currently being investigated by a federal grand jury in Maryland to see if they are complying with government regulations on drug manufacturing. After a four month inspection the FDA has found Lilly's submitted data to be inaccurate or incomplete "in nearly every system inspected." The FDA reported that even though they were told they had received complete information on a matter they found later that other records were withheld. It happened so often that the FDA could not determine if they had been given complete and accurate records. There were "objectionable" conditions in nearly every area inspected. The regional FDA director in Chicago, Burton Love, said many things were possible before this is over. There could be injunctions, seizures or recalls. Considering felony prosecution is also a possibility.

From 1978 to 1980 the FDA launched a campaign to slow down the widespread use of another of Lilly's psychoactive drugs, Darvon. It had been shown to be highly addictive and was often being used to commit suicide and addiction clinics were opening up to focus on Darvon addiction. The medical-educational campaign proved to be no match for Lilly's marketing efforts. Although Lilly was supposed to support the FDA in their efforts, an audit proved that they had continued to promote the drug to physicians. As a result sales hardly budged. Lilly's drop in profits at the expiration of Darvon's patent appeared to have solved the problem. Then Lilly began to market Darvocet-N. This was a combination of Darvon and another drug yet under patent, acetaminophen. Darvocet-N quickly rose to become the 10th most prescribed drug in the United States and Lilly's profits rather than the public is what remained protected.

Lilly also marketed DES, diethylstilbestrol, in the 50's, a synthetic estrogen prescribed to prevent miscarriage, which was found twenty years later to cause vaginal and cervical cancer or reproductive abnormalities in the patient's

312

female offspring. The chief of the University Department of Growth and Reproduction at Rigshospitalit in Copenhagen, Denmark, Neils Skakkeback, reports that in the male offspring similar problems have been found. The have suffered undescended testicles, poor quality semen leading to a higher possibility of infertility, testicular cancer and incomplete urinary channels. DES was also recently implicated in a study showing that the female offspring of those women using the drug have a seven times greater possibility of developing homosexual or bisexual responses (Ehrhardt et al., 1985). Lilly is currently involved in 250 lawsuits filed by the children and grandchildren of those who used this drug forty years ago. Even if a mother wants to avoid this drug she should know that it is used in cattle and other animals to boost weight for larger profits at the marketplace. So even if mothers are not directly using the drug, if they ingest meat and dairy products, there is still a very likely possibility that they are consuming DES indirectly in low doses. In fact the government has recently voiced concern over the various drugs passed on to the consumer in this way. There was a government-sponsored international conference held in Washington, D. C. on the subject, "Estrogens in the Environment." Many chemical pollutants are estrogenic and much concern over what that is doing to offspring has been voiced as of late.

At the moment Lilly is under fire for a new Hepatitis B drug. Studies have been halted because 5 out of the 15 individuals involved in the study died. One died after only the second dose. One of the remaining patients survived only because he was able to get a liver transplant. The fatality rate from hepatitis B is only 1.4%. The patients had a *far better chance* of living through the disease than they did of surviving the effects of Lilly's drug.

One of the warnings about Prozac is that it can bring on diabetes (hyperglycemia) and hypoglycemia, which often develops into diabetes later on. With this in mind, someone needs to ask what it might have to do with Eli Lilly being one of the two major suppliers of insulin products in this country today with two new types of insulin in the pipeline to be approved. An increase in diabetes would certainly increase Lilly's profits on diabetic related products. And they are major producers of antibiotics, so if their biggest moneymaker is causing severe adverse effects upon the immune system, it would certainly bring in revenues down the road.

During the inquest in the Joseph Wesbecker case the coroner testified that he asked doctors in Lilly's research department if they had any similar reports of violence resulting from the use of Prozac. Although they stated that they had no such reports (this was in November of 1989), Eli Lilly had already filed a

313

number of reports associating Prozac with hostility and violence with obvious intent to cause harm. One example: in July of 1989 a report documented that a female patient "was placed on 20 mg. of Prozac and showed signs of irritability and aggressive behavior. The dosage was increased to 40 mg. and the [patient] experienced an intense homicidal rage. She made plans to kill a man from her past." It goes on to say that when Prozac was discontinued the homicidal rage disappeared.

We have already mentioned unreported side effects, including psychosis and death associated with Prozac before Lilly obtained FDA approval to market Prozac. How many of us labor under the false notion that the FDA is our great protector from harmful substances? How many of us still labor under the false notion that the FDA tests drugs and then approves them, when in actuality, the pharmaceutical companies making the drugs and most definitely having a vested interest, are the ones who handle the testing. They then submit their results to the FDA for approval. If those drug companies are not completely thorough, open and honest in their reporting (and there appears to be no real incentives to encourage them to do so), then where is that protection we all feel so confident about? This corruption has gone on for many years. Morton Mintz's extremely well documented account in his book, *BY PRESCRIPTION ONLY,* documents the seriousness of the situation since the beginning of the century. Everyone should read it.

The law requires that drugs be tested before approval to make sure they are safe and have the desired therapeutic result. Yet the majority of this research is conducted by doctors at academic medical centers and paid for by pharmaceutical companies. If the researchers speak out as Martin Teicher attempted to do, they find their future position as a researcher threatened and their careers ruined since the pharmaceutical companies provide the majority of funding for these projects and therefore, can pull the strings. After FDA approval, based upon pharmaceutical company generated research, the drug remains on the market until the drug's adverse reaction profile is so out of line that it is pulled from the market and made a controlled substance. At this point it appears that the real research is begun on a substance. This is the point at which the government and other concerned organizations step in and begin to really look at a drug. Until that time *very little* is known about a drug other than "data" purchased with drug company funds. This leaves us all victims of whatever data can be bought or manipulated to shed a favorable light on a particular company's product. Drug companies have been stretching the truth about their products for decades.

314

According to Dr. Alan Hillman and his colleagues from the Univ. of Penn. in an article for the *NEW ENGLAND JOURNAL OF MEDICINE* about this testing process to determine safety, "They (the pharmaceuticals) fund projects with a high likelihood of producing favorable results....They exclude products that may compare favorably with the sponsor's own. Sometimes, only favorable clinical data are released to investigators....Negative studies may be terminated before they are ready for publication [in order to keep those unfavorable negative results from being made accessible to the general public]....Corporate personnel may seek to control the content and use of the final report, including the decision to publish." Of course it is generally understood by those who make so much money doing this research that if their data is not favorable the chances of an opportunity of doing additional research become less and less likely. So it is not surprising that Dr, Richard Davidson of the University of Florida reported that he found drug company- supported studies of new drugs were much more likely to favor their drugs than were studies supported by non-commercial entities.

Fred Gardner in the Northern California *ANDERSON VALLEY ADVERTISER* points out the lack of integrity of most periodicals in reporting who the sponsor of various studies are when they report the results of the study. "Concealing the sponsorship of a scientific study - when the sponsors have a direct interest in the results - violates the basic rules of science journalism as I learned them from Gerald Piel and Dennis Flanagan at Scientific American in the '60s. Our culture is getting more and more corrupt, the corporate flacks are getting more brazen, and rip-offs are occurring on a scale that seemed unthinkable not too long ago. As Carlos Puebla wrote about the last years of the Batista regime in Cuba: *'Robbery became the norm. They even lost regard for good form.'"*

On September 20, 1991, the FDA held a hearing to discuss a request that warnings be placed upon the labels of Prozac and other antidepressants, which was made by Ralph Nader's health research group, The Public Citizen. They felt that problems were serious enough that warning labels mentioning the possible side effects of "violence and suicide" should be put on the bottle to make consumers more aware of the rapidly mounting evidence that Prozac may chemically induce this reaction. Ten professionals sat on the FDA board. Although the FDA had felt that the financial interests held by these ten individuals would not sway their vote, so they had them sign a statement that they would not allow that to influence them. All five who admitted their interests at the beginning of the FDA hearing voted "against" the warning label.

Just one glaring example of those financial interests is the case of Dr. David Dunner who participated in the clinical trials on Prozac along with Dr. Claghorn who also sat on the panel. (Those who conduct clinical trials are paid by the pharmaceutical company to do so.) Dunner had 32 on-going grants from drug companies at the time of the hearing and had received over $1.3 million in research grants from Eli Lilly since 1982. Perhaps we need to question such blind faith in those who make life and death decisions which affect us on a daily basis. The blood and tears continue to flow while authorities with *admitted vested financial interests and blood on their hands,* continue to turn a deaf ear to the cries of this rapidly mounting number of victims.

Everyone heard on their evening news that the FDA ruled that there was "not sufficient evidence to warrant a warning label" for Prozac. The panel stated that a warning label might frighten patients from taking a drug which they may need. Their statement seemed an obvious slap in the face to the patient. It implicated that the FDA panel felt the patient nor his family were capable of investigating the available data and after being warned, make that judgement on their own.

The meeting had lasted for nine hours with no formal break. The time allotted for discussing their own personal tragedy surrounding the use of Prozac was limited to five minutes each for the first fifty people to respond. People gave *graphic accounts* of loved ones who had taken their lives after taking the drug, people shooting themselves in front of their children, mutilating their bodies, reports of lives lost or almost lost through horribly violent methods. They listened to pleas from so many to remove this drug from the market before more people are killed and more blood spilled.

One FDA panel member stated that she had been moved by these terribly tragic testimonials and that they should not be ignored. However, after a brief discussion the panel concluded that these personal tragedies were only "antidotal" reports and could not be considered in reaching a decision on the safety of these drugs. They "might order some relabeling" but wanted to discuss only double blind clinical/laboratory studies. The absurdity of this situation stands out when compared to the FDA decision just months before to pull a popular brand of popcorn off the shelves because a bad batch had made a handful of people sick. Out of 28,623 adverse reaction reports which include 1349 deaths there is obviously far more reason for concern about Prozac.

So while we wait for double blind studies, how many more lives will be affected? Just exactly how many drugs are we suppose to believe have ever been removed from the market because of double blind clinical studies? How ridiculous! Do they really believe that Lilly is going to order and pay enormous amounts of money for a double blind clinical study that might have the slightest possibility of devaluing their biggest money maker ever? *Drugs are generally removed because of antidotal studies, not because of double blind clinical studies!* All the babies born deformed by their mothers' use of Thalidomide became the "antidotal reports", *the living proof,* the cause for that terrible drug to be removed from the market. How dulled are our memories? We live in an antidotal world with many variables, not in a controlled clinical lab type of environment. Although it is important to learn the effects of these drugs in a controlled clinical setting, we also need to know what effects these drugs have upon us in *our* world, in real life situations. We have a great need to be aware of antidotal reports.

Dr. John Lombardo, chairman of the Department of Family Medicine at the Ohio State University and president of the American Medical Society for Sports Medicine addresses the issue of anecdotal data,"...Although it is important to base one's knowledge as a scientist on accurate data derived from well-designed experiments, one should never completely ignore the results of case reports and anecdotal evidence." *(ANABOLIC STEROIDS IN SPORT AND EXERCISE*, p. 91)

The FDA's statement in denying information to be placed on the label implies that the patient is not capable of judging for himself about the safety of a drug. To demonstrate why it is critical for that information to reach the patient we note a statement made by Craig Baskin, a group vice president of Duff & Phelps/MCM Investment Research Co., from the *AMERICAN MEDICAL NEWS*, June 24, 1991. He stated that the brand new anti-depressant, Zoloft, a self described more refined version of a serotonin uptake blocker, is cutting into Prozac's share of the market. Then he explained why Zoloft is a good investment, *"The advantage of Zoloft is that the patients haven't heard of it."* Now isn't that a comforting thought? Invest quickly before the patients learn what is happening in order to make your profits?! What great new adventures lie ahead with this drug and the next and the next? How long will we tolerate such blatant insults to the intelligence of today's consumer?! On the one hand we have those at the FDA who refuse to warn us of possible dangers and on the other hand we have those large companies who actually base their business income on the ignorance of the consumer or patient.

This "take the money and run before the consumer realizes what's hit him" attitude should wake us up to the fact that most of us are far too trusting of large pharmaceutical companies. Eli Lilly's history is not much different than all the rest. We should certainly realize by now that they are not charities nor angels of mercy nor benevolent non-profit foundations. All one has to do is look at the cost of drugs today. Prozac alone is bringing in over $100 MILLION per month for Lilly. These are the largest *for profit* companies in the business world! Their main focus is *PROFIT, PROFIT, PROFIT*. In February 1992 *CONSUMER REPORTS* tells us "the pharmaceutical industry has long been the nation's most profitable. The top 10 U.S. drug companies averaged 16 percent profit of sales in 1990, more than triple that of the average Fortune 500 company...Between 1980 and 1990, while general inflation was 58 percent, overall health-care costs rose 117 percent - and the cost of drugs rose 152 percent..." (p. 87)

If anyone really believes the focus of the pharmaceutical firms is in helping their fellow man achieve ultimate health, they had better look again. After reporting to their stockholders about the number of various lawsuits and legal investigations they were involved in at the end of 1992, Lilly reported, "While it is not possible to predict or determine the outcome of the legal actions pending against the Company, in the opinion of the Company such actions will not ultimately result in any liability that would have a material adverse effect on its consolidated financial position." Did they make the cold hard facts clear enough in that statement?

Society becomes the "laboratory" when a drug is not adequately tested before marketing. This makes the antidotal reports the FDA panel received testimony on in that hearing the results of *a very large laboratory study*. To give the reader a sense of what is happening in the real world (the world of "antidotal studies", Lilly's Prozac laboratory) I will mention just a few of my daily experiences over the last four years: Case #1: A petition which was circulating nationwide to ask Congress to investigate Prozac was left at a small new book store in a suburb of Salt Lake City, Utah, on a Friday afternoon. By Tuesday morning the owner called to report that the petition was already full and could be picked up. She expressed her amazement at how many of the 28 people who signed the petition in that three day period were grateful to have the opportunity because each had tried Prozac, had an adverse reaction to the drug, and discontinued using it. Case #2: One day I walked into the local post office and overheard two women discussing how walking every day was helping them to fight feelings of depression. I injected, "Anything you can do has got to be better than resorting to antidepressant drugs." Both sighed heavily in unison and said, "Boy, isn't that the truth!" The younger one added, "I had to run into the same telephone pole in front of my home three times before I figured out that it was the Prozac affecting me! I got off!" She then turned to her friend said, "And her son almost killed himself when he was on it! Now he is in jail for something crazy he did while on it. Why haven't they taken that off the market? Everyone you talk to has had problems with it!" Case #3: Just before Christmas 1993 I was having some gifts wrapped at a large department store. The girl wrapping the gifts had just begun to discuss the problems her sister was having on Prozac. She mentioned that the sister had been accusing her of all kinds of things. Unable to understand where these accusations were coming from, she was ignoring them. Someone a couple of people behind me stepped forward and anxiously asked, "Did you say something about helping people who have problems with Prozac? My sister is really in trouble on that drug! The person I know is gone." I told her that was almost always the first statement I hear from family members of those in trouble. She asked, "If we get her off Prozac will she think of her children again instead of nothing but having her hair or nails done? She used to be such a wonderful mother." Then I asked if her sister was still married. She replied that she had just filed for divorce adding, "The sister I knew would be crushed, completely heartbroken to see the way she has treated her husband in throwing him out of the house and keeping him from his children, but this person has not shed a tear."

How many more lives will be lost, how many families shattered, before Prozac takes its total toll on society? Will it be your life that will be lost as a Prozac consumer or will it be your life as an innocent bystander who is caught in the middle of this Prozac Pandora? Will it be your neighbor's family or a best friend's family or one of your own relatives whose family is shattered by a similar tragedy? These are questions we must all consider because whether we use the drug ourselves or not the possibility that its use may affect each of us personally is *very real*.

Although my instinctive gut response toward politics has been one bordering sheer repulsion, this research into Prozac has forced me to take a cold hard look at political connections to psychoactive drugs. When I uncovered the actual facts my nauseous repulsion toward politics became greatly magnified. Let us examine briefly a few of those facts. Psychiatry, the pharmaceutical giants and the CIA have been close friends from the days of the original CIA head Allen Dulles and Dr. Donald Ewen Cameron. Dr. Cameron served as head of the American Psychiatric Association, the Canadian Psychiatric Association and the World Association of Psychiatrists. These two men had similar goals - they were both obsessed with learning the process by which the human mind can be erased and reprogrammed - reprogrammed according to *their* specifications. After the Koreans were able to "brainwash" American soldiers during the Korean War there was a public outcry that seemed to so embarrass Dulles that he crossed every barrier of ethics, morality and decency, not to even mention limits of the law, in his search for the secret of mind control. He supplied Cameron with grants to carry out his inhumane torturous research. As I cannot personally stomach going into the details of this medical hypocrisy I will refer you to two extremely well documented accounts. I highly recommend them. The first is by BBC producer and investigative journalist, Gordon Thomas, entitled *JOURNEY INTO MADNESS, The True Story Of CIA Mind Control And Medical Abuse*. The second book *ACID DREAMS, The Complete Social History of LSD: The CIA, the Sixties, and Beyond* is by Martin Lee and Bruce Schlain. Two other books that also delve deeply into the politics are *THE MIND MANIPULATORS* by Alan Scheflin and Edward Opton and *THE BEYOND WITHIN* by Dr. Sidney Cohen.

These political connections between psychiatry, the pharmaceuticals and the CIA have continued over the years despite President John F. Kennedy's attempt just before his death to dissolve the CIA and his backing of legislation to make all psychoactive medications "controlled substances". Our past president George Bush sat on the board of Eli Lilly about the same time he headed the CIA. According to Eli Lilly's annual report of 1979 he resigned from their board of directors to seek the vice presidential nomination under Ronald Reagan. Keep in mind that a member of a board of directors generally holds a large amount of stock. Would such financial interest have influenced Bush's actions? Lilly's Prozac was approved by the FDA under Bush's administration. But that is not all...

Dan Quayle was another big player in Lilly's puppet administration. Quayle's close ties with Lilly go back to his home state of Indiana. To discover Mr. Quayle's connection we quote the footnote on page 151 of Dr. Breggin's *TOXIC PSYCHIATRY*: "If it turns out that Prozac received especially favorable treatment from the FDA, or that it had an extraordinary boost from certain media leaders, political influence may be at work. Eli Lilly, based in Indianapolis, was a large contributor to the senatorial campaigns of Dan Quayle. In addition, according to the October 1, 1988, *Washington Post*, 'Quayle's uncle, William C. Murphy, opened Lilly's government relations office in Washington in 1964 and his 1980 campaign manager, Mark D. Miles, went to work for the company in 1982 as director of communications' (p. A25). *Quayle was instrumental in passing legislation described by a Lilly spokesman as the most important drug measure before Congress at that time.*"

Then July 25, 1992 an announcement was made in *THE WASHINGTON POST* that Mr. Quayle would remain on the ticket as the Republican Vice Presidential candidate. The individual who made the announcement was "Mr. Prozac Promoter" himself, Mitchell Daniels, Eli Lilly's Vice President for Corporate Affairs. According to the September 11, 1992 issue of *THE SEATTLE TIMES*, "One of Quayle's closest political friends, Mitchell Daniels Jr., directs government relations while advising the Bush-Quayle campaign on media strategy on nights and weekends." He was co-host of a fundraiser which raised $600,000 for their campaign. It went on to point out that more than $185,000 has been donated to the campaign by top U.S. drug company executives with 13 out of 18 senior managers at Lilly on that list. The article taken from the *KNIGHT-RIDDER NEWSPAPERS* by Frank Greve and reprinted in the above mentioned issue of *THE SEATTLE TIMES* discusses in detail the questionable ethics of the White House Council on Competiveness, headed by Dan Quayle. The lead in reads, "A panel headed by Vice President Dan Quayle is giving the U. S. drug industry regulatory relief worth billions of dollars." The reactions have been clear cut, both from economist Peter Tamen, a pharmaceuticals specialist from MIT, "These are measures that drug companies love...They clearly show that the Competitiveness Council is on the side of drug companies," and Harvard business professor, Alfred Chandler Jr., who writes on competitiveness, "It's a total mystery to me why they'd be helping pharmaceuticals..." Just what part do all these connections play, if any, in Prozac still being on the market in spite of the fact that *the FDA has never in their history seen a situation like this before?*

The political ties become spine-chilling when this information is coupled with Dr. Frederick Goodwin's "Federal Violence Initiative." The public outcry to his statements and plan is what earned Dr. Goodwin his *pressured* resignation from the Alcohol, Drug Abuse, and Mental Health Administration after delivering his proposal February 11, 1992. Dr. Goodwin compared young inner city men to murderous, over-sexed Rhesus monkeys (Isikoff, 1992; Learyl, 1992; Rich, 1992). His proposal included plans to do testing on children as young as five years old to determine a potential pre-disposition to violence. The test would be an evaluation of 5HIAA serotonin levels with recommendation that 5HT serotonergic enhancing drugs would be in order to prevent these children from becoming violent offenders as they grow older. Of course we can see from the medical studies we have reviewed that given children these drugs would be the cause of exactly what we would want to prevent. After being pressured into resigning, Dr. Goodwin was *severely reprimanded* by being appointed to head the National Institute of Mental Health! What a nice "presidential style perk" it would be to have the nation's leading government psychiatrist propose that everyone needs a serotonergic drug like Prozac to be "non-violent" if you happen to have lots of stock in the company manufacturing the drug.

For additional information on the Federal Violence Initiative and the attempt to counteract this measure read Peter and Ginger Breggin's new book, *THE WAR AGAINST CHILDREN*, St. Martin's Press, 1994.

Dr. Martin Teicher deserves to be commended for the courage and integrity obviously required for him to come forward with his findings...the first in a long list of medical data which continues to replicate his and his colleagues discoveries. A true scientist will not bend under pressure and Dr. Teicher has proved himself to be classified as such. Last September 20, 1991, Dr. Teicher was invited to participate by making a presentation to the FDA panel investigating Prozac and other antidepressants. I was personally appalled and embarrassed by the manner in which the FDA panel did their best to ridicule and intimidate him and interrupt his presentation.

The experience quickly brought home for me a point a dear friend tried to make 20 years ago. At the time I found his statement quite puzzling and rather radical. My friend was Austria's most promising young physician at the time and had recently received honors from many other European countries. We met just after he had spent a week as the honored guest at Buckingham Palace. When I suggested that he might come to America one day to practice, he recoiled at the thought and said, "Never! I could not do my research and accomplish the great strides in medicine I intend to accomplish in my life! *Medicine in America is much too political!*" It was obvious that he was offended that I would think he had so little integrity or respect for his life's work. I now must apologize and say, "I understand now. Your words ring *loudly* and *clearly* in my ears my dear Peter! How right you were."

The following information is taken from the Freedom of Information Office, Center for Drug Evaluation and Research dated June 18, 1992 and contains only those reports filed on these drugs since 1985: (The big question is, "If all depressed people are at risk of suicide attempts", as Lilly puts it, why are there so few attempts made on the other drugs as compared to the ones on Prozac? As you can see the deaths linked to Prozac outnumber the others by an extraordinarily wide margin, even if the number of deaths associated with all the other drugs were combined. The total ADRs [Adverse Reaction Reports] for Prozac make the other drugs look like candy in comparison. Note also how high the number of reports that are in the anger type category.)

DEATHS: Prozac: 1313 / All other drugs combined: 861
TOTAL ADRs: Prozac: 23,067 / All other drugs combined: 15,274

Adverse Reactions	Prozac	Desyrel	Elavil	Tofanil	Ludiomil	Sinequan
Suicide Attempts	1,436	10	10	2	9	6
Rash (all types)	1,364	85	78	142	128	25
Overdose (all types)	895	98	167	100	136	188
Nausea (all types)	878	205	42	56	14	21
Insomnia	870	79	25	37	18	24
Pain	820	128	40	41	34	27
Agitation	815	84	26	34	18	27
Depression Psychotic	780	9	6	12	2	2
Depression	762	33	28	12	7	13
Nervousness	756	42	17	29	15	30
Headache	756	79	42	47	24	24
Anxiety	734	45	15	25	15	11
Hostility	643	13	10	6	5	5
Somnolence	619	109	60	86	92	220
Convulsion (all types)	579	83	67	71	318	58
React Aggrav	563	34	13	25	5	7
Tremor	499	58	53	70	29	11
Asthenia	474	68	18	41	17	23
Pruritus	434	33	15	30	22	7
Confusion	393	64	69	47	24	30
DEATHS	1,313	76	159	130	106	107
TOTAL ADR'S	**23,067**	**2,886**	**2,032**	**1,981**	**1,534**	**1,411**

Adverse Reactions	Pamelor	Ascendin	Wellbutrin	Nardil	Triavil	Amoxapine
Suicide Attempts	11	0	12	0	0	0
Rash (all types)	67	90	105	17	15	3
Overdose (all types)	60	186	76	47	31	8
Nausea (all types)	32	26	44	29	8	0
Insomnia	42	36	28	43	4	1
Pain	41	14	43	30	12	1
Agitation	18	36	44	15	7	0
Depression Psychotic	3	2	6	4	1	1
Depression	19	14	19	11	4	1
Nervousness	24	27	21	7	10	0
Headache	35	24	54	68	6	0
Anxiety	19	25	32	10	6	2
Hostility	14	3	19	6	1	0
Somnolence	24	29	22	35	14	1
Convulsion (all types)	38	182	239	41	9	7
React Aggrav	21	3	39	18	3	1
Tremor	30	26	48	26	14	0
Asthenia	15	16	17	27	7	0
Pruritus	17	11	51	15	1	1
Confusion	22	30	36	28	9	2
DEATHS	58	104	24	53	37	7
TOTAL ADR'S	**1,297**	**1,263**	**1,246**	**1,128**	**452**	**44**

Once again those total combined figures are:

DEATHS: Prozac: 1313 / All other drugs combined: 861
TOTAL ADRs: Prozac: 23,067 / All other drugs combined: 15,274

CHAPTER 12

CHEMICAL DEPRESSION

"The question is not 'Who is right?', but 'What is right?...Great progress can be made only by ideas which are very different from those generally accepted at the time. Unfortunately, it is not only literally true that the more someone sticks out his neck above the masses, the more likely he is to attract the eyes of snipers."

...Dr. Hans Selye

Chemicals interrupt sleep patterns and cause incredible stress. These chemicals are foreign substances to the body and foreign substances are toxins or poisons. We put chemicals in our soil, then we spray our plants with chemicals while they grow, then we spray them with chemicals again to ripen them, we water them with water loaded with chemicals, then we process them chemically and add chemicals to them to change them into "food", with all of the "essential nutrients", next we put chemicals on them to make them palatable once again and then we eat them and wonder how we acquired a "chemical imbalance." Then we take drugs (more chemicals) for all the symptoms produced by the massive amounts of chemicals we continuously ingest! How does one avoid a chemical imbalance of one kind or another in our chemically oriented society?

Have we become so technical and specialized that we can no longer think and reason with simple wisdom? Doesn't it naturally follow that if we are constantly introducing chemicals into our bodies that our chemical balance will suffer? How technical is it? How many specialized degrees does one need to understand such a simple deduction? We live in a society inundated with chemicals. Is it really any surprise to us or should it be that we now suffer diseases such as "multiple chemical sensitivity"? It is also believed that ADHD is produced by certain environmental toxins, such as lead and there is growing evidence that fluoride may be doing the same.

Pesticides put all of us at risk, but children in particular are at a greater risk. The amount of pesticides in food has been a problem for a long time, but a new study by the National Academy of Sciences concludes that pesticides may have an even greater impact on children. According to the study released in 1992, there is "potential concern" that some children may be ingesting unsafe amounts. The EPA joined with the Department of Agriculture in calling for a reduction in the use of pesticides on fruit and vegetables.

There is also concern that drugs may taint the nation's milk supply. The summer of 1992 investigators found that government inspectors do not test to see if most of the drugs given to cows wind up in milk. Ted Weiss, chairman of the House Government Operations subcommittee on human resources said that the FDA still cannot honestly assure the public that milk is safe. He pointed out that the FDA tests for only four out of 82 drugs that can be used in milk cows and that the most commonly used drugs have never been approved for use in dairy cows.

In our world today we tend to constantly strive to prove ourselves more intelligent than God or Nature by "improving" upon the foods we have been given, by processing them and changing them in any way we can. What exactly is processing? It is changing the chemical make-up by cooking, breaking down, adding chemicals, bleaching or colorizing to make the food more appealing to the eye, or to fatten the bank accounts of the manufacturers and distributors, etc., to the extent that, not only does the food no longer nurture our bodies, but it actually becomes a negative reaction in our systems depleting our bodies of necessary nutrients.

As an example, sugar is a wonderful food and vitally essential to our physical and mental health. It is an excellent fuel for our bodies when we get it directly from fruit, beets, sugar cane, maple sap, etc. But when we bleach and process all the good and natural nutrients out of it, what do we have? We have one of the most widely used chemical substances now known to man. In a refined state sugar must bind to nutrients already present in the body in order for it to be utilized. It, thereby depletes the body of essential nutrients causing a negative, rather than a positive effect upon us. Of course we would expect it or any other extensively processed food products to imbalance our body's chemical system.

Today the average per capita consumption of sugar is 130 pounds per year, yet two hundred years ago the average American ate less than one pound of sugar per year. This "excessive consumption of sugar has been conclusively linked to asthma, allergies, arthritis, cancer, heart disease, diabetes, hypoglycemia, Candida Albicans, tooth decay, obesity, headaches, gallstones, osteoporosis and inflammatory bowel disease, among others." (*ADDICTIONS, A NUTRITIONAL APPROACH TO RECOVERY,* p.22)

Dr. Abram Hoffer, a Canadian psychiatrist and author of *ORTHOMOLECULAR MEDICINE FOR PHYSICIANS* states, "Alcohol per se is almost a liquid replacement for the simple sugars. *Like the refined sugars it is devoid of all the elements of any food...It causes generalized malnutrition by forcing a dependence on other foods,* for nutrients are required to metabolize and neutralize the effects of alcohol...No one doubts alcoholics are more prone to anti-social and criminal behavior than are nonalcoholics...***The addiction to alcohol is very like the addiction to sugar.*** *" He then goes on to explain that hypersensitivity to the various elements in our diet (i.e. alcohol, sugar, food allergies, additives, and chemicals in our environment) can cause a decrease in judgment and an increase in impulsive behavior leading one to commit criminal acts.* .(If chemicals in the environment can effect us this way, what on earth do we think chemicals pumped directly into our brains will do?)

Many of us have heard that if sugar were to attempt now to pass the FDA approval process it would not be approved. The March 1993 issue of the *TOWNSEND LETTER FOR DOCTORS* gives us an idea as to why this is so. They give a list of ways in which sugar is known to be harmful. The reactions they list are: immune system suppression; mineral imbalance; hyperactivity; rise in triglycerides; reduces defenses against infection; reduces high density lipoproteins; chromium an copper deficiency; cancer of the breast, ovaries, intestines, prostate and rectum; increases fasting levels of glucose and insulin; interferes with absorption of calcium and magnesium; weakens eyesight; **raises serotonin;** causes hypoglycemia; produces stomach over-acidity; **increases adrenalin levels;** produces anxiety, irritability and difficulty concentrating; aging; alcoholism; tooth decay; obesity; contributes to duodenal and gastric ulcers; arthritis; asthma; Candida albicans (yeast infections); gallstones; heart disease; appendicitis; multiple sclerosis; hemorrhoids; varicose veins; elevates glucose and insulin responses in conjunction with the use of contraceptives; periodontal disease; osteoporosis; decrease in insulin sensitivity and glucose tolerance; decrease in growth hormone; increases cholesterol and systolic blood pressure; drowsiness and decreased activity; migraine headaches; food allergies; contributes to diabetes; toxemia during pregnancy; eczema, and it interferes with protein absorption. That is a very long list of health problems caused by such a popular product in our society. Most physicians do not have the time or feel that they may receive only a deaf ear if they attempt to warn or educate their patients about changing their diets. Considering how many other natural sweeteners exist which do not have these adverse effects, it seems it would be a valuable health insurance measure to switch.

A hypersensitivity to various substances is the inherited biological factor linking criminal behavior to a possible biological predisposition. Dr. Barbara Reed in her book *FOOD, TEENS AND BEHAVIOR* relates that there is a distinct relationship between biochemical roots and delinquency. She goes on to say that the typical teen junk food diet can lead to learning disabilities, delinquency and criminal behavior. Dr. Lendon Smith points out research indicating that seventy-five percent of prisoners were "hyperactive" as children. Much hyperactivity can be linked to hypoglycemia, which we will find has been connected to criminal behavior as well.

We have ignored the connection between our heads and our bodies for far too long. They cannot be separated; one affects the other. A blood stream full of chemicals will interfere with brain function and therefore, will as a consequence interfere with thought processes, judgement and behavior. Just as negative thoughts produce chemical reactions within us that in turn affect our bodies.

The research done by Dr. Glen Green, a Canadian researcher and Dr. El Kholy, an Egyptian researcher, shows that often the symptoms of pellagra, the vitamin B3 deficiency disease, are mistaken for schizophrenia (insanity). Dr. Kholy, in a seven year long study of incarcerated felons, found that eighteen percent of them had pellagra.

Pellagra causes obvious and sometimes dramatic mental and psychological symptoms. The psychological symptoms are depression, general anxiety, irritability, violence, periods of stupor or irrationality, etc. Physical symptoms include loss of appetite, diarrhea, vomiting, cracks in the skin, tongues become red and sore, etc. The head of the U.S. Public Health Service announced in 1908 that Pellagra was spreading dramatically. Between the years 1914 and 1929 it multiplied ten fold. Victims in the South were crowded into insane asylums before it was finally recognized that pellagra is caused by a vitamin deficiency. It is a deficiency in niacin, Vitamin B-3.

Tryptophan, the amino acid used by the brain to manufacture serotonin, is also converted to niacin in the body. Pyridoxine, Vitamin B-6, is involved in converting tryptophan to niacin. Because of this connection the symptoms of Vitamin B-6 deficiency are similar to those of Pellagra: depression, nausea, vomiting, irritability, confusion, weight loss, convulsion, anemia, dizziness, weakness, etc. Vitamin B-6 is essential for proper transmission of the nerve impulses we refer to as neurotransmitters. It is believed that this deficiency is a contributing factor in an alcoholic's experience with depression, sluggish thinking, hyperactivity or manic behavior.

Our excessive use of chemicals, refined sugar, stimulants, drug residue in animal products, the cumulative effects of chemicals in our water supply, massive amounts of protein consumption over several generations, etc. have all brought about serious health problems. One of those health problems is the effect of these chemicals upon the body's ability to balance blood sugar levels.

This is the result of "high living" and also the reason why diabetes was once known as the disease of the wealthy, since they were the only group who could afford these rich foods. Our increased wealth or abundance is now costing our health.

The medical terminology for this inability to control blood sugar is "hypoglycemia". It means that the pancreas becomes so accustomed to a constant barrage of stimuli that it just keeps right on working, even when there is no need to produce insulin. This extra insulin in the blood lowers the blood sugar level and the body cries out for something to raise that level back to normal. A rush of adrenalin will raise the sugar so most people react by reach for something that cause that rush and raise the blood sugar quickly (i.e., alcohol, coffee, nicotine, sugary snacks, etc.). This only further complicates the problem by causing the pancreas to become overstimulated once again. The combination of all these factors becomes a vicious cycle as the patient grows worse from his natural instinct to bring the blood sugar level back to normal. If the progress of the disease is not halted by the patient making strict changes in their dietary code, the pancreas does burn out and drastically slows down or quits and the patient has, at that point, developed hyperglycemia, diabetes.

It was surprising to me to find that there are doctors who now believe that there is little or no correlation between the amount of sugar one consumes and diabetes even though, as sugar consumption has increased in the United States, so has diabetes proportionally. It is also interesting to note that when sugar consumption dropped sharply during World War II, so did the rate of diabetes. Note though that the *TOWNSEND LETTER FOR DOCTORS* did include diabetes as a result of sugar consumption.

The first endocrine organ to come into contact with ingested foods or chemicals is the pancreas, so it should not be surprising that of all the endocrine glands, the pancreas is the most susceptible to damage by excess sugar. When we ingest sugar, our blood sugar level goes up. Insulin, a hormone secreted by the pancreas, is responsible for controlling the amount of sugar in the bloodstream. Malfunctioning of the pancreas can cause either excessively low or abnormally high levels of sugar in the blood.

Clusters of endocrine cells in the pancreas, called the islets of Langerhans, detecting an excess of sugar in the blood secrete insulin. They also stimulate the release of glycogen, a sugar stored in the liver and tissues. The combination of these two actions normalizes the blood sugar. When sugar is eaten excessively for a number of years, the pancreas can become overstimulated (the "falling into a groove" that Dr. Selye mentions) and secrete too much insulin. Or it can become incapable of stimulating the release of glycogen. This can make the blood sugar drop below normal, resulting in hypoglycemia. The instinctive reaction of eating more sugar to keep the sugar level normal, only causes further destruction through additional stimulation.

Researchers have also discovered that abnormally high (hyperglycemia) or abnormally low (hypoglycemia) blood sugar levels can occur in a person who has ingested a food or come in contact with a chemical to which he or she is sensitive. These substances are specific to each individual. Yet when the allergy-provoking substance is removed, the blood sugar level will return to normal.

Hypoglycemia can progress into hyperglycemia (diabetes) as the body reaches the exhaustive stage of distress. Just as with other overstimulated organs, the overworked pancreas eventually wears out and stops functioning correctly. The islets of Langerhans become exhausted and slow down or stop the secretion of insulin. The body has reached the point of exhaustion and can no longer attempt to compensate for the malfunctioning, as it did in hypoglycemia, and diabetes is the result.

Often, even if the islets continue to secrete insulin at a normal rate, the quality of the insulin may be insufficient. The essential ingredients of calcium and phosphorus needed to break down proteins into amino acids becomes imbalanced. These amino acids are the essential building blocks of hormones and neurotransmitters. Without these building blocks, insulin begins to diminish causing hyperglycemia or diabetes.

Now why, when we are discussing brain function and chemical imbalances, are we discussing the pancreas and blood sugar levels? Because the brain is fueled by blood sugar and without proper blood sugar levels, the brain cannot function properly. With the blood sugar levels depleted, the brain is actually starving to death. Brain cells are dying. This hypoglycemic reaction in the brain produces an effect similar to the effects of alcohol. There has been much written during the eighties to help us to understand that alcoholism is directly connected to low blood sugar - hypoglycemia. (Check the Recommended Reading section in the back for more information on this subject.)

As we have already discussed, when the blood sugar drops the individual instinctively reaches for something to bring the blood sugar up rapidly - generally alcohol or sugar. These are the worst substances to use because after initially raising blood sugar, levels then drop even lower than before. This causes the craving for more and more alcohol or sugar. This is often why a family history of alcoholism is moderately predictive of depression in near relatives. This glandular weakness of the pancreas is passed down to offspring and produces depression as a side effect. I always ask if there is any family history of alcoholism or diabetes. If there is, I want to know, and so should any physician, if the patient was ever evaluated for hypoglycemia before an antidepressant was prescribed. These patients tend to have a high rate of adverse psychiatric reactions.

The *TABER'S CYCLOPEDIC MEDICAL DICTIONARY* describes hypoglycemia as a condition in which the glucose in the blood is abnormally low, which is brought on by hyper-function of the pancreas. Then it goes on to list the symptoms: *"acute fatigue, restlessness, malaise (discomfort, uneasiness or indisposition), marked irritability and weakness.* In severe cases, *mental disturbances, delirium, coma, and possibly death."* As we look further into the symptoms we find *confusion, impaired memory, mood swings, irritability, depression, hyperactivity, inability to concentrate (attention deficit disorder?), negative attitude, hopelessness, anxiety, etc.* One list included symptoms in the order of frequency: *exhaustion, depression, insomnia, anxiety, irritability, headaches, vertigo, sweating, tremor (internal trembling), tachycardia (palpitation of heart), muscle pain and backache, anorexia, crying spells, phobias (unjustified fears), difficulty in concentration, numbness, chronic indigestion, mental confusion, cold hands or feet, blurred vision, muscular twitching or cramps, joint pain, anti-social behavior, restlessness, obesity, staggering, abdominal spasms, fainting or blackouts, convulsions, and suicidal tendencies.* Is any of this beginning to sound like what we so often label as "depression, anxiety, panic attack, etc."?

In 1988 Roy and Linnoila reported the results of a study on the correlation between violence and impulsivity and a hypoglycemic condition among legal offenders. They found a significant correlation between long term hypoglycemia and truancy, stealing, and crimes against property. They also tended to have a history of multiple offenses and a father who became violent if intoxicated (hypoglycemic tendencies are often passed down from parent to child). Insomnia and behavioral problems including poor impulse control were found to be consistent. Tempers flair easily with blood sugar imbalance which could tie in the adrenalin rush the body produces to raise sugar levels and an "akathisia type" reaction. Serotonin is believed to play a significant role in glucose metabolism and circadian rhythms (sleep patterns).

In Utah we consume high amounts of sugar. We are known as the ice cream capital of the nation. We also hold the record for Jello consumption. Besides the fact that these things are all high in sugar, jello is also known to have quite an impact in lowering serotonin levels. I believe this high rate of sugar use is the main reason why Utah also has one of the highest rates of diabetes in the nation. It should naturally follow that we would also have the highest rate of hypoglycemia, which is the beginning stages of pancreatic malfunction. We also have a rate of mind-altering drug use which is *three to four times the national average.* Just how often is hypoglycemia being mislabeled "depression" and treated as a psychiatric malady rather than a blood sugar problem which could be rectified by a good diet rather than a pill? *It is absolutely amazing to see how many patients had already been diagnosed as hypoglycemic before their doctors put them on Prozac. Rather than educate the patient, they hand them a pill which only blocks out their symptoms, while it magnifies the original problem and leads many into diabetes.*

Mental health is so closely tied to blood sugar balances that this is an area that very definitely should not be overlooked. This link has been obvious to psychiatry from the beginning. Why else would they have used glycemic shock, induced by injections of insulin to produce a coma, as a "therapeutic" treatment which was commonly used to treat schizophrenia?

Dr. James W. Long gives us this explanation of hypoglycemia and how brain function is affected by this condition in his book, *THE ESSENTIAL GUIDE TO PRESCRIPTION DRUGS 1992: "Since normal brain function is dependent upon an adequate supply of glucose, reducing the level of glucose in the blood below a critical point will cause serious impairment of brain activity.* The resulting symptoms are characteristic of the hypoglycemic state. Early indications are headache, a sensation resembling mild drunkenness and an inability to think clearly. These may be accompanied by hunger. As the level of blood glucose continues to fall, nervousness and confusion develop. Varying degrees of weakness, numbness, trembling, sweating and rapid heart action follow. If sugar is not provided at this point and the blood glucose level drops further, impaired speech, incoordination and unconsciousness, with or without convulsions, will follow. *Hypoglycemia in any stage requires prompt recognition and treatment. because of the potential for injury to the brain, the mechanisms and management of hypoglycemia should be understood by all who use drugs capable of producing it. "* (emphasis added)

Hypoglycemia is a potential listed side-effect of Prozac, the other SSRIs and many other drugs. DORLAND'S ILLUSTRATED MEDICAL DICTIONARY defines hypoglycemia as "an abnormally diminished content of glucose in the

332

blood, which may lead to tremulousness, cold sweat, piloerection, hypothermia, and headache, accompanied by confusion, hallucinations, bizarre behavior, and ultimately, convulsions and coma." From these descriptions of hypoglycemia it is easy to see how this disorder with its many psychiatric symptoms can be mistaken for a psychiatric disorder.

Hypoglycemia can be illusive or fickle as the pancreas either maintains or loses its ability to maintain blood sugar levels. Women during the stress brought upon their bodies by pregnancy can develop hypoglycemia which reverses itself after the pregnancy. Chemically induced hypoglycemia should also reverse as the chemical causing the stress upon the pancreatic function flushes out of the system. These stressors can cause damage that would necessitate longer healing time as the disorder persists. This illusive aspect of hypoglycemia makes it very difficult to obtain accurate test results in order to detect the disorder. Evaluation of symptoms is about the only method of detection. Altering the patients' diet to look for an alleviation of symptoms is far less intrusive than prescribing a mind-altering drug. As Dr. Long warns above, for many critical reasons, including potential damage to the brain, potential harm as a result of hallucinations and out of character behavior, it is extremely critical that physicians watch for this disorder, especially when giving the patient a drug capable of producing hypoglycemia.

There is a multitude of evidence from patient reports that Prozac is affecting the blood sugar balance and chemically inducing hypoglycemic reactions. According to patient reports, it can produce hypoglycemia in a patient who had no apparent blood sugar problems to begin with and diabetes in a patient who previously had hypoglycemia. Ex-patients report that it produced mood swings, confusion, blackouts, even deeper depression, hyperactivity, anxiety, exhaustion, compulsions for sugary foods, alcohol and stimulants, etc., etc., etc. Everyone of these symptoms can be directly linked to blood sugar problems. All are known to be hypoglycemic reactions.

Diabetics can drink alcohol and have it make them extremely drunk one day and the next time they have to drink excessively to even notice any effect. Prozac patients experience the same reaction with alcohol. These diabetics who drink can have long periods of time that are just "lost" for them [blackouts]; they remember nothing that has happened to them during these periods. Prozac patients are reporting identical experiences. We know that diabetes and hypoglycemia can be chemically or drug induced. But we need to know if the SSRIs are causing a temporary chemically induced diabetic state, even for a short period of time which is causing so many of these similar reactions. All these reactions are *far too similar* and the answer to this is extremely critical for the safety of the brain and for proper brain function as Dr. Long has just explained for us.

There are quite a few other purely biological illnesses which mimic depression. These include thyroid disorders, chronic viruses, etc. This is why a thorough physical examination is so critical before looking at the problem as potentially psychological. This can be time consuming and costly to a physician. Finding the cause of a patient who is "feeling down" is not always an easy thing to do. Searching for disorders such as hypoglycemia, low grade infections, thyroid problems, etc. can take a long time and often the patient is not willing to wait. Many want the answer quickly - too quickly at times.

Another habit that we have developed as a society is that of using "naturally" occurring substances which can overstimulate our body's own chemical reactions, such as caffeine, tobacco, alcohol, chocolate, etc. All these affect the pancreas as well. Also coffee, tea, and tobacco are all brain stimulants on a slightly milder scale than alcohol or other serious mind-altering drugs. Throughout time most of these substances have been used only for ritualistic purposes, but we have taken them out of the ritualistic setting and are now using them on a daily basis to *force ourselves to a level of peak performance.*

We know that cocaine and other illegal drugs can push one to perform beyond normal capacity, but we do not look upon this as an "acceptable" practice. If we are looking at degrees, we need to realize that the body becomes desensitized to milder stimulants and then requires stronger and larger amounts of stimulants in order to function normally. The milder stimulants do take their toll and can lead us to stronger ones over time. Once the stimulant or stimulants are withdrawn, the body will go through a withdrawal period - a cleansing, resting, recuperating and rejuvenating period - during which the price will be paid for forcing any body system beyond its capacity.

It would bring us far more satisfaction and peace of mind and body, and a much higher quality of performance to build our endurance level by caring for our real needs, nourishing our bodies rather than ignoring them, as we put on a "facade of perfection" by forcing our bodies to extremes.

Many patients who suffer Multiple Chemical Sensitivity report similar adverse reactions made by Prozac patients when it comes to concentration, learning disabilities, and memory problems. These are all indications of frequent exposure to toxic substances. According to the Office of Technology Assessment

1991, Walsh 1988, researchers believe that the hippocampus within the limbic system (the memory areas within the brain) is the main target for these toxins. Damage inflicted upon the hippocampus or upon the nerves leading to or from the area *may adversely affect the synthesis, storage, release, or inactivation of the neurotransmitters*. They explain that these toxins, with which we find our environment inundated, may disrupt the neurotransmitter balance leading to the release of a flood of excitory neurotransmitters which can damage neighboring cells. This is referred to as excitotoxicity. They state that this effect upon hippocampal function may have great and long-lasting impact upon behavior and cognitive function.

An area that needs to be addressed while we are discussing chemicals is the question surrounding the component of fluorine in the chemical structure of Prozac (fluoxetine hydrochloride) - C17/H18/F3/N/O/.HCl, Paxil and Luvox. What is fluorine? The definition in *Webster's New World Dictionary* (1989) is: "a corrosive, *poisonous,* pale greenish yellow gaseous chemical element, the most reactive non-metallic element, forming fluorides with almost all the know elements (symbol F)."

When fluorine is combined into a chemical structure such as fluoxetine hydrochloride (Prozac) it is assumed that it cannot then break loose from the structure to adversely affect the patient. Repeated reports from patients and physicians linking Prozac with severe abdominal pain and ulcerated esophagus and stomach linings and eating away of the roof of the mouth with liquid Prozac, is casting doubt upon this assumption. How can it be just a coincidence that as one reads through the many symptoms produced by a toxic reaction to fluoride, that these are identical to the symptoms being reported by Prozac patients? Both Prozac patients and individuals suffering from fluoride toxicity report these same reactions: forgetfulness, drowsiness, lack of coordination of thoughts, depression, behavior problems, complete personality changes, incoherence, neurosis, unusual excitement, lethargy, loss of appetite, weight loss, migraines, gastro-intestinal disturbances, nausea, bloody vomit, stomach or abdominal pain, teeth discoloration, joint pain and stiffness, muscle weakness and skin wrinkling from damage to the collagen structure, hives, rashes, kidney problems, ringing in the ears, allergies, thyroid problems, visual disturbances, edema, constipation or diarrhea, tremors, pulmonary irritations, heart failure, and most recently, cancer and other related immune system disorders, etc.

Fluoride has been a controversy for many years now. Dr. John Yiamouyiannis, in his book, *FLUORIDE - THE AGING FACTOR,* quotes Dr. John Forman, an allergist from Columbus, Ohio: "In our own practice, we have run down cases of hives, behavior problems, and several patients who others had labeled neurotics to be due to fluorine intoxication." The April 6, 1994 issue of the *VALLEY DAILY NEWS* in a Seattle suburb reported the case of the Wayne Mustonen family who had problems discovering the cause of their 5 year old daugther's nightly bouts with nausea and vomiting. Their concern heightened when their 3 year old daughter began the same pattern. They found their answer when they noticed it began for both children after brushing their teeth. "Fluoride in the toothpaste, not the brand itself, is likely to blame. In poison control centers it's a pretty common call," stated pharmacist and poison control specialist, Terri Bonck. (Keep in mind that nausea and vomiting should *never* be brushed off as insignificant. They are signs of liver impairment or toxicity and should be dealt with immediately before damage to this critical organ occurs.) The article as raised concern over another toothpaste ingredient, sodium laurel sulfate, which can also cause the user to become ill. Sodium laurel sulfate is the ingredient in so many shampoos as well. We know that chemicals go through the skin to affect us just as if we ingest them, yet we include them in everything from shampoo to lotion to deodorants. Even though aluminum has been suggested as the culprit in Alzheimer's, older Americans continuously ingest it in antacids and put it under their arms in their deodorants where it can pass readily through the skin and into the lymph system to be moved quickly to the brain. Why don't we think before we act?

The many reports of ex-Prozac patients who had developed allergies began to generate concern about what might be happening to the protein structures of the body. Once we begin to understand how fluoride affects proteins, we can begin to see what the possibilities may be with Prozac as well. In London, England Dr. John Emsley and his coresearchers in 1981 at King's College found that fluoride forms very strong hydrogen bonds which affect the size, shape and susceptibility to external conditions and enzymic activities of body proteins. Once the shape or conformation of the protein is distorted by the fluoride, the immune system can no longer recognize the distorted protein as its own and will destroy or reject it as a foreign protein. The immune system automatically rejects any protein that is foreign to it. An example we would all understand is what happens when an individual receives an organ transplant. In a transplant tissue types or protein makeup is compared to insure compatibility or in other words, to insure a closely matched protein structure. Then the patient is given an anti-rejection drug to trick the immune system into believing the transplanted tissue belongs to his body, thus interrupting the natural immune system rejection process. The immune system rejection response to its own altered proteins which have been produced by the hydrogen bonding of fluoride is observed in various ways, i.e., skin reactions, allergies, gastrointestinal disturbances, etc. These same hydrogen bonds are responsible for stabilizing the DNA structure and so the DNA is also affected by this process.

Fluoride is known to interfere with the immune system defenses by slowing the movement of white blood cells and interfering with their ability to attack and destroy foreign substances. Very small amounts of fluoride have been found to have a very significant effect upon our body's defenses. At Case Western Reserve University School of Medicine, a research dentist, Dr. J. Gabrovsek published a paper in 1980 voicing concern over cyclic AMP (a substance detected by blood or urine tests in fluoride toxicity which is known to drastically impair the rate of movement and the defence processes of white blood cells) levels and the effect of this upon the immune system. He stated: "Because of the inhibitory effects of NaF on phagocytosis and leukotaxis (the movement of white blood cells), which are basic defense mechanisms, I have doubts about the absolute safety of water fluoridation on a long-term basis." If he voiced that much concern over the amounts of fluoride in water, how much more concern should there be if fluoride toxicity is what is happening when a patient uses Prozac? Blood and urine need to be tested for AMP levels and fluoride levels in those who are using or have used Prozac. If this fluoride connection is tied in at all to the effects being reported by Prozac patients, the patients need to be made aware of this aspect as they would need to avoid fluoride in order to avoid it triggering latent reactions and more studies in this particular area are definitely in order.

After several generations of all these chemicals, we are really beginning to discover that we are having to account for it. What we now call "chemical depression" seems to be running rampant and it is a very serious problem in our society. But until we are ready to begin to repair the damage that has been done for generations, until we are ready to care for the body that is the house in which our brain resides, we will continue to suffer these serious problems of the mind. Plus we will turn to more and more of these deadly and dangerous mind-altering drugs which are rapidly proving themselves to be on the same level as those the "pusher" on the street corner has to offer.

Why is it that all nature obeys the basic laws of the universe, yet man seems to think because he has the "technical know how" he can break any or all of the laws and get away without suffering the consequences? Throughout time physical and moral pollution have gone hand in hand. As we pollute the earth, we inevitably pollute our bodies and therefore, our minds as well, thus affecting everything about us and our surroundings. There is a connection with everything. No one stands alone. We are all in this together. How bad do we allow things to get before we begin to accept responsibility for everything we touch in our lives and in our world?

CHAPTER 13

SOLUTIONS

"It is exciting to realize that each of us, every day, has the right and the opportunity to create the beginning of a new self and to challenge the old self that we no longer choose to accept."
        ...Shad Helmstetter, *THE SELF TALK SOLUTION*

"Taking drugs to escape from life is a cop out. One must learn to deal with the stresses and disappointments that are common to living. The problem will still be there when the trip, no matter how good, is over."
        ...Dr. Michael E.Trulson

From the story of Pandora's Box we read: "All at once, every evil and spiteful thing flew out, like a swarm of insects infesting the earth with pain and sorrow. Luckily though, Prometheus had locked hope in the box so that people were saved from total despair. Yet, thanks to Pandora, life on earth was never quite so joyful ever again." *PROZAC: PANACEA OR PANDORA?* was written to restore hope for those who have suffered paradoxical reactions to Prozac which have produced a scenario far too similar to what Pandora released from her box.

What is the solution? The National Prozac Survivor's Support Group has filed petitions with Congress gathered from across the country requesting a Congressional investigation and the removal of Prozac from the market. They are doing all in their power as individuals to alert others to the dangers they have personally encountered with this drug. The Citizen's Commission on Human Rights want Prozac taken off the market, charging that, "It makes sane people crazy and even those who seem to do 'well' on it begin to have problems over a period of time." Spokesman Michael O'Brien in an article of May 1990 in the *SAN FRANCISCO GUARDIAN* echoes the statement above, "It does alter the mind, but the thing is, it's a mind-altered state. A person on heroin thinks he's much better off, but that's not much of a recommendation for the drug. *The point is, what's the underlying problem? He's going to have to address it at some point.* This drug was promoted as having fewer side effects, but now we're finding out it's one of the worst. There is no evidence that the drug has got a value that offsets its harmfulness. It needs to be taken off the market."

Attorney Leonard Finz hopes the lawsuits will eventually force Lilly to remove Prozac from the market, "There are literally thousands of people out there who are having uncontrollable rages, and not understanding why. We're sitting on top of an explosive nightmare." And because he believes the FDA mainly reacts rather than acts, he wants a study to be done monitoring patients who are already taking Prozac. He would then discontinue the prescription of the drug while a six-month independent review of 1,000 patients could observe these patients for homicidal and suicidal reactions.

Dr. Peter Breggin suggests, "Since the antidepressants frequently make people feel worse, since they interfere with both psychotherapy and spontaneous improvement by blunting the emotions and confusing the mind, since most are easy tools for suicide, since they have many adverse physical side effects, since they can be difficult to withdraw from, and since there's little evidence for their effectiveness - it makes since never to use them....minor tranquilizers, barbiturates, opiates, alcohol, and perhaps antidepressants...effects are short-lived, with little or no evidence for sustained relief, and the hazards are considerable, including addiction, withdrawal reactions, rebound anxiety, mental dysfunction, and lethality. Even if these drugs were more effective or safer...Few psychiatrists would keep a pitcher of martinis at hand in the office to ease the anxiety of their patients; yet most are willing to reach into the drawer for a sample of 'alcohol in a pill', the minor tranquilizers. Both...accomplish the same thing - a brief escape from intense feelings by suppressing or sedating normal brain function....should doctors endorse this dangerous and self-defeating avenue as a form of medical treatment? As physicians or psychotherapists we should empower our patients to trust themselves and their capacity to triumph over frightening emotions...through self-understanding, improved self-control of their minds and actions, more courageous attitudes, and more successful principles of living..." (*TOXIC PSYCHIATRY*, p. 171, 265)

Dr. Malcolm Todd, past president of the AMA went right to the heart of the matter, "Thus far physicians have shown little objective interest in promoting health and preventive care. We actually have a **disease oriented cure system**, rather than a **health oriented care system** in this country today." It seems we have almost turned ourselves into walking, talking drug stores. Isn't it time to change our way of life and begin to take responsibility for our own health by caring for our bodies and minds? As Hippocrates said, "A wise man should consider that health is the greatest of gifts."

Pain, emotional as well as physical, is our own personal internal alarm system. When do we stop blocking out all physical, mental, spiritual and emotional pain with every kind of drug known to man and finally realize that *pain is one of our dearest friends? It is our alarm system, warning us that we have a problem that needs attention.* The proper reaction to pain should be to search out the cause and remove it from our life before it becomes a far more serious problem.

Instead, in our society, we tend to shut out all pain in any way we can. A true physician will search out the cause of pain in his patient and assist in repairing the problem, not in helping to cover it up, thereby causing it to fester and multiply.

It is as if we are saying, "Sure, I want to grow and become the person I know in my mind I really would like to be, but keep me from all those experiences that would help me become that person (i.e. pain, stress, turmoil, discomfort, etc.)." Learning to overcome these obstacles is what brings us the character growth and personal development we all long for in life. It appears we have begun to long for escape, or a "quick fix" (which we should know by now does not exist), rather than putting forth a little effort to gain optimum health as well as personal development.

After including the preceding comments about pain in the first edition entitled *THE PROZAC PANDORA,* I was elated to learn that Dr. Vogel echoes my belief that pain is an alarm, "...so does pain act as a warning of disruption in the harmonious workings of the body. Do you feel grateful for the warning...Will you try and find out what is causing the pain in order to treat it correctly? Oh no, for this is too time-consuming and we are not inclined to endure pain any longer than we have to. As soon as it arises we want to expel it. Of course, there are may proprietary drugs available for killing pain, which means you would have to be crazy if you continued to suffer longer than necessary! How short-sighted this attitude is! Consider how differently we react when it comes to repairing, say, our car or some other machine. What motor mechanic believes that the fault has been rectified if he simply plugs his ears so that he cannot hear the rattling? Will he not rather credit his trade by trying to get to the bottom of the problem and repair it before a wheel comes off or some other serious trouble develops? That is what we do with a machine, but the human body, which is much more delicate, we treat superficially, even though pain - that alarm bell - may be warning us that there might be something seriously wrong. In no way should pain ever be ignored or bypassed, which is what you are doing if you simply take a painkiller...nature is always ready to make amends for our mistakes; so if we are conscious of them and willing to learn from them we will avoid making the same ones again. How strange,...when an analgesic no longer gives the relief that it used to. Instead of admitting to ourselves that the analgesic effect did not mean that the cause of the pain had been cured and that we were acting contrary to nature, we foolishly take ever stronger drugs in order to suppress the pain at all costs." *(THE NATURE DOCTOR,* p. 23)

According to Dr. Hans Selye, "It is not to see something first, but to establish solid connections between the previously known and the hitherto unknown that constitutes the essence of scientific discovery. It is this process of tying together which can best promote true understanding and real progress." Let's explore the history of psychiatric treatments to see if we can tie together the past and present information and perhaps re-evaluate where we are at the moment.

Where have we come from, where are we now and where should we go from here? As early as 100 A.D. the Greek physician, Rufus of Ephesus, discovered that strong fever would cure many diseases, including mental symptoms, epilepsy and convulsions. In Africa people drank goat urine to bring on a fever to alleviate these symptoms. The American Indians employ sweat lodges as an essential part of their purification rites in religious ceremonies. The sauna and massage treatment has been an intrinsical part of Scandinavian culture for centuries. Modern medicine began to employ fever therapy in 1883. Dr. Julius Wagner von Jauregg, a Viennese psychiatrist, noticed that patients who contracted typhoid, which also produces a high fever, experienced a remission of their mental symptoms. Presuming the mechanism by which a cure was achieved was not through the body creating a fever in a which rid itself of the cause of the disease symptoms, but by shocking the body into an immune response. Dr. von Jauregg began to purposely infect the insane with malaria germs as a remedy. It worked and any type of therapy which would throw the body into shock became the accepted treatment. This shock to the system was customarily generated by either electricity (Electric Convulsive Therapy - Electric Shock) or toxic chemicals (drug therapy) - anything to cause a strong stress response by the body. Selye points out that those treatments we consider odd, such as blood-letting, injections with foreign substances or chemicals, etc., are not so different from our present therapies. They all have one thing in common: "they all cause wear and tear, making demands for adaptation; they all cause stress." And by causing stress they force the body into the adrenalin rush we want to avoid.

Obviously little or no thought was given to the possibility that during the high fever produced by the typhoid or malaria produced a flushing out an accumulation of poisons from the system, thereby alleviating disease symptoms. Recall Dr. Selye's explanation that *"Mere excessive accumulation suffices to block the machinery. It could induce the changes we consider characteristic of aging by the mere presence of ever larger amounts of inert waste products and the consequent inability to produce indispensable vital ingredients at the proper rate."* (*THE STRESS OF LIFE*, p. 431) When the organs of elimination are overloaded with toxins and cannot handle the increased volume, the skin, often referred to as the "third kidney" can assist in that elimination process through sweating those toxins out through the pores. As we discussed previously, it is now known that the body itself, even without any external adjunct, produces toxic chemicals within which cannot be flushed in any other way except through crying or *sweating*. Dr. William H. Frey, II, director of the Ramsey Dry Eye and Tear Research center in St. Paul, is one who believes that tears rid our bodies of the chemicals that build up during stress. Crying then will allow us to relax through this cleansing method.

While Dr. Selye reminded us about the fact that drug therapy is a chemical shock which causes wear and tear and stress to the body, Ronald K. Siegel reminds us of a critical point of information that most of us have either forgotten or have never even been made aware of before. He points out that the Greek term "pharmakoi" meant "human medicine" and was applied to *poisons and drugs.* *(PCP PHENCYCLIDINE ABUSE: AN APPRAISAL*, p. 273) The term "chemical shock" means to shock the body into an immune response via the ingestion or injection of toxic chemical substances or poisons.

After all we now know about stress - how each stressor takes such an enormous toll on our health while the effects accumulate - why would we want to create stress as a "remedy" for any disease? We now know that stress is the cause of disease. Whether the stress is brought on by physical, chemical, emotional, mental or spiritual stressors, the result is the same - disease. The excess adrenalin produced by the stress response forces the body to work beyond its present ability, depleting energy supplies, weakening the immune system, lowering coping capabilities. In the mind, the excess adrenalin lowers the level of consciousness. Remember that mania, depression, dancer, etc. can all be induced by a series of consistent stressors, even mild stressors. If we want to keep the body from developing a pattern of over reacting to stress or becoming keyed up at inappropriate times, we should be avoiding consistently stressful situations, not intentionally causing the body to go into a stress response from various chemicals, electricity, disease germs, goat urine, additional artificial adrenaline - any stimulant or toxic substance.

It should be very obvious at this point that we should avoid stress as much as possible. We are surrounded by stress in our lives. In this day and age we stumble across enough stress without looking for it. Although complete avoidance of stress is unrealistic, we can learn to keep its damaging side effect of "distress" at a minimum. There are many simple common sense (unfortunately "common" sense is not too common any more) solutions: spend less time trying to "keep up with the Jones" and more time with loved ones; perhaps a career change would alleviate stress; nature is incredibly soothing and healing - try gardening, a trip to the mountains, lying in the grass, listening to running water is so soothing, even petting a dog or cat has been demonstrated to be very healing; play soft classical music throughout the night to calm a nervous or fussy baby who refuses to sleep - this will help both you and the baby to catch up on much needed sleep (with more sleep the baby should grow and develop better and be healthier as well); learn to take naps as the experts in the chapter on sleep disorders suggested and go to bed earlier; learn how to release traumas from the past so that you will have the tools to deal with similar traumas without overreacting *(FEELINGS BURIED ALIVE NEVER DIE* is an excellent source); cut stimulants or chemical stressors out of your daily diet; find some simple old home remedies to use rather than popping a pill (an additional chemical stressor) for every little thing that comes up in life, relying on pills only very briefly when you know of no alternative; learn more about your own strengths so that you can utilize those strengths in overcoming difficulties; gain wisdom and knowledge in many areas so that you feel more capable of handling a large variety of situations in life; do not be self centered - learn to serve and care for others - since they say that blood is thicker than water, if you have trouble caring about others, do a little genealogy and you will quickly discover how closely related all of us are; etc. The time is long past due for us to begin to treat ourselves with kindness, concern, caring, nurturing, etc.

We need to ask if our use of drugs has gone on for enough generations now that in order to create an effect we must use heavy duty, super strength drugs, which are so toxic that we can hardly tolerate or survive them. Have we pushed the situation about as far or further now than we can safely do so? How long can our systems and our children's systems and their children's systems be able to tolerate this chemical shock? We have pushed it to the point now that our immune systems are shot with hundreds of thousands sick and dying from immune deficiency diseases. Our minds are going quickly. Sanity almost appears to be an illusion in our society. What will it take for nature to teach us a few simple lessons? "Surely even orthodox medicine must begin to conclude form experience that 'wonder' drugs do not get to the root of the disease and that nature can neither be circumvented nor overpowered with impunity. The wild animal is often wiser than civilized man when it comes to knowing what nature requires for healing and recuperation. In future, therefore, refuse to be guided by misguided views and dulled instincts. [Common sense is not so common any longer.] If we follow nature's lead, it can only be for our good. If, on the contrary, we ignore its direction, we are the ones who will suffer." *(THE NATURE DOCTOR,* p. 22)

Perhaps the time has arrived in America for us to follow the example set by the majority of the world, the far older, more experienced and presumably, because of their experience, wiser cultures. Modern medicine is the "new kid on the block" and is fast proving just how many hazards it poses. Why have we had such an aversion to investigating alternative methods? Do they not fit into our capitalistic mode of thought because of the inability to produce huge bank accounts for large pharmaceutical companies? Many profits are lost as people learn simple ways of caring for themselves, thereby eradicating and avoiding disease. We do finally appear to be awakening now to what others have seen for centuries. Many are beginning to use various alternative healing methods with much success. The *NEW ENGLAND JOURNAL OF MEDICINE* announced that last year 34% of Americans turned to various alternative treatments. The absolutely staggering cost of standard medical treatment for the remaining 66% of the population was $939 billion. The cost of alternative treatment was 33 times less, at only $14 billion. This cost factor alone is overwhelmingly persuasive.

Other cultures have for many more years than we have even dreamed of practicing modern medicine, turned to diet, herbs, fasting, yoga, exercising, bio-feedback, oxygen therapy, lymphatic massage; aromatherapy, acupuncture, acupressure, deep breathing exercises , sauna baths, various types of water therapy, magnetic therapy treatments, meditation, chelation, etc. In many cultures these practices are often included as a part of their religion. These healing methods may sound strange or odd to us, but when we kill and maim as many people as we do with our modern drug therapies, perhaps it is time for us to give these long proven methods the consideration they deserve. We need to recognize our weaknesses as a society in order to grow. One of the greatest weaknesses we have developed has been that as the result of graft and politics we are becoming an arrogant and closed minded culture. Without an open mind we become stunted, damned if you will, in our learning, growth and progression. With an open and searching mind, one remains young at heart and excited about life and knowledge, and healthier in both mind and body. We should be willing to explore all avenues and options to bettering our lives.

Rest is perhaps the most essential element in physical, emotional and mental health. Have you noticed that you have more control over your life when you feel rested and at peace? We know that stress, the product of excess adrenalin and the opposite of a restful state, has been proven time and time again to be the worst enemy we face when it comes to health. When you are working to make changes in your life, virtually any progress you are striving to make, can be accomplished as long as you are well rested. You feel strong, determined, in complete control and able to cope with life as long as you approach it in a rested state. Loss of control comes when we are tired, frustrated, upset, exhausted, frazzled, etc. We achieve rest in many ways, the most obvious being sleep. Sleep gives our bodies and our minds ability to replenish and rebuild. Prozac, as well as many other drugs, robs us of this most essential ingredient. The increase in adrenalin flow prevents sleep. When you are keyed up for a crisis by this excess adrenalin you are ready to fight or flee, not sleep. The excess adrenalin must be used up. This is why so many Prozac users stay up all night cleaning house, working in the office, etc. The patient is constantly being pushed beyond his natural abilities by this stimulant effect of Prozac. When he does attempt to rest he cannot sleep (insomnia is one of the most prevalent of the side effects). While he is awake he is often in a state of mania, hypomania or akathisia - being driven to move incessantly and being constantly bombarded by a barrage of thoughts and words popping in and out of the brain. The appearance of mania or hypomania can be mistaken by the patient and even by those around the patient as greater efficiency and performance. These patients assume that with all this movement they must be accomplishing more. Yet many are on the verge of losing their jobs because their performance is so poor. Because of the constant raising of cortisol levels, this stimulant effect carries over even after discontinuation of the drug. Until the drug is completely flushed from the brain and the body can normalize the adrenergic and noradrenergic systems. Sleep will continue to be disrupted even if it does not seem apparent through any other means of detection other than brain waves. Unable to attain the rest which he needs to overcome his health problems, the patient reaches a state of total exhaustion with little or no ability to cope or carry on with life. Doctor and patient assume he must need more of the drug to cope so the dose is increased providing a more stimulating effect and the cycle begins again on a higher and more dangerous level, making the subsequent drop extend to a new all time low.

Other avenues to a restful state are also blocked through the effects of Prozac.
Meditation and prayer become impossible because of the constant barrage of single words and thoughts which inhibit concentration. In addition to this, the patients report an inability to **feel** spiritual feelings or to receive answers to prayer while using Prozac. This is most likely caused by the chemical interference produced by Prozac in the frontal lobes of the brain. Dr. Breggin explains for us, that this is the location in the brain where those feelings are accessed. "The frontal lobes are the seat of higher human functions, such as love, concern for others, empathy, self-insight, creativity, initiative, autonomy, rationality, abstract reasoning, judgement, future planning, foresight, willpower, determination, and concentration. The frontal lobes allow is to be fully 'human' in the full sense of that word; they are required for a civilized, effective, mature life." *(TOXIC PSYCHIATRY,* p. 53)

It would appear that Prozac leaves the patient little means of achieving this most precious commodity of peace or rest. How does he attain the ability to cope and bring about desired changes in his life? This is a sad state of affairs in light of the fact that since most depression is brought on because the patient initially experienced an inability to cope or make changes in his life. Prozac, because of its stimulant effect, and its anesthetic effect may mask all this for a short time, but eventually the price for such abuse will have to be paid.

Looking at other cultures throughout the world one is struck by the emotion and feelings freely displayed by all. Emotions are not buried. Perhaps we are now beginning to learn as a nation that burying emotions, rather than expressing them or dealing with them, can be hazardous to our health. After an experience with Prozac, where feelings are chemically blocked, the patient begins to really grasp the great importance of feelings and the expression of those feelings. Whether the feelings are pleasant or unpleasant, these patients begin to see that the ability to access any of those feelings is *a very essential element* for good mental health. Many ex-Prozac patients speak of the guilt they now feel because they could feel no love, even for newborn babies, while on the drug. Many report cutting themselves just to see if they could still feel. Others speak of ingesting more and more stimulants to see if that would bring back "any feeling of any kind" just so they could feel something, anything again. Programs designed to assist those dealing with grief stress that the body generates toxic chemicals during the grieving process which cannot be eliminated any other way but through the shedding of tears or sweating. Crying is an essential release mechanism emotionally and physically. It should seem obvious by now that treating these conditions with additional foreign chemicals, mind-altering drugs, in an attempt to balance a chemical imbalance is self defeating and absurd. This process only creates more serious imbalances while it robs the brain and glandular system of their ability to maintain or restore balance. The best thing about sweating out these toxic chemicals through sauna treatment, etc., is that by going out through the skin you in large part bypass the kidneys and liver. This alliviates the excess stress they are under produced by the toxic condition.

Much has been said throughout this text about permanent brain damage resulting from the use of these drugs. On this issue I want it clearly understood that I personally am convinced, through my own personal experience with serious life-threatening illness, that our bodies and minds are extremely resilient and have the ability to recover most miraculously in far more instances than we presently believe, if they are given the opportunity to do so. This process may take far longer than we would expect or wish, requiring much patience by us and those around us, nevertheless hope remains. I also believe it is a far less difficult task to recover from a physical illness when the patient regains the control over his mind and thoughts. With the problems brought about through paradoxical reactions from these mind-altering drugs the patient finds he does not possess as much mental control to focus on getting well.

Dr. Frances Pottenger did some very interesting research over several generations of cats on the nutritional deficits created by denatured food. His research focused not only on the immediate effects, but the effects in offspring and then their offspring as well. "One of the experiment's more startling discoveries is that once a female cat is subjected to a deficient diet for a period of 12 to 18 months, her reproductive efficiency is so reduced that she is never again able to give birth to normal kittens. Even after three or four years of eating an optimum diet, her kittens still show signs of deficiency in skeletal and dental development. *When her kittens are maintained on an optimum diet, a gradual reversal and regeneration takes place.*" So even though the mother seems unable to produce healthy offspring, she is at least able to produce a kitten, which, after applying the proper laws of nature, will be able to reverse the inherited adverse effects and regenerate their bodies. This should give us all grant hope or faith in our ability to overcome not only the damage we have caused to ourselves through wrong choices, but also any inherited weaknesses.

After winning his own battle with death, Norman Cousins in his book *ANATOMY OF AN ILLNESS AS PERCEIVED BY THE PATIENT*, expresses this same thought, "I have learned never to underestimate the capacity of the human mind and body to regenerate - even when the prospects seem most wretched. The life-force may be the least understood force on earth. William James said that human beings tend to live too far within self-imposed limits. It is possible that these limits will recede when we respect more fully the natural drive of the human mind and body toward perfectibility and regeneration." Norman Cousins has done a great deal to help us learn more about the chemical reactions which are produced by our emotions. Scientists have now discovered that emotions themselves trigger a chemical reaction within the body and the brain. Those emotions we consider good emotions actually set off a positive reaction in the system which generates health and life-giving properties. Those emotions we consider bad emotions give off a negative reaction in the system, fostering a foundation for disease and death. Prozac blocks out too many - necessary, life-generating emotions. It tends to dull the higher feelings while enhancing the animalistic feelings. We all know that life isn't always easy to go through or always a lot of fun. Even if we had been promised a rose garden, we need to realize that rose gardens have thorns. When Prozac affects the mood centers to block out what we would classify as "bad" feelings, it also blocks out the "good" feelings. Aren't feelings there to let us know we do exist and to increase our awareness of ourselves and our surroundings? Is it worth cutting those unpleasant feelings out of our life if we at the same time cut out feelings of love, concern, empathy, hope - all the good feelings? Without feelings are we really alive? Are we human? And if we can no longer feel, is life "real" for us and worth living? How terribly depressing it must be to feel nothing.

Most will agree that we are here in this world to experience life and learn and grow from those experiences. Why would we block out life's experiences with Prozac, alcohol, or any other mind-altering or mood-altering substance? It is through overcoming those experiences or in learning to adapt to what life hands us that we grow and gain the wisdom we need to live life to its fullest and to assist others - our children, our mates, our friends, and fellowman with our acquired wisdom in overcoming their problems in life. Being robbed of those experiences, good or bad, is robbing us of the growth we want to achieve in life. These are the things which bring us joy and satisfaction and happiness and keep us from feelings of helplessness, worthlessness and depression.

We need to realize also that we cannot treat the body and think that it will not affect the mind, nor can we treat the mind and have no effect upon the body. In a living being the two are inseparably connected. Life ceases to exist when a separation occurs. Treating the mind and ignoring the body appears to produce the same result. Certainly one cannot function without the other. We have become too specialized in our treatments and methods of practicing medicine. We need to look at the whole body and not just the various separate parts in order to make proper diagnosis and in the treatment of disease. Hippocrates told us, "I will give no deadly drugs to anyone" and "Our natures are the physicians of our diseases". And Thomas A. Edison gave us the answer in a nutshell when he said, *"The doctor of the future will give no medicine, but will interest the patient in the care of the human frame, in diet and in the cause and prevention of disease."*

John Finnegan in his book, *ADDICTIONS, A NUTRITIONAL APPROACH TO RECOVERY*, echoes what I have been saying from the onset of this book. "One wonders how many times history need repeat itself. Freud declared that cocaine brought peace, happiness, and boundless creative energy, only to find himself and one of his best friends addicted to the drug. During the 1960's, thousands of people seeking enlightenment from hallucinogens damaged their nervous systems, freaked out, jumped off buildings or became psychotic. The newest addition to the hallucinogenic line-up is Ecstasy, which has yet another following that believes love, peace and happiness can be found in a chemical. Coming down from Ecstasy can lead to serious depression and insanity...Any substance that greatly increases the stimulation of the nervous system will at the very least deplete the neurotransmitters and create a corresponding depression. At worst, the drug can cause a malfunction in the delicate biochemical pathways and create a drug-induced psychosis. It is *a law of physics that applies to all levels of life - every action creates an opposite reaction...What is needed are foods, nutrients and herbs that nourish, strengthen, and build up the nervous system. And, above all, to see that love and peace are created by how we live, what we live for, and what we seek and see inside ourselves. "* (P. 27)

Herbs have certainly stood the "test of time" in other countries around the world and for many have added to a very long physically and mentally active life, reaching well into later years. This has been foreign to us in our culture. Yet, many ex-Prozac patients are finding that in order for them to escape their Prozac-induced nightmares without severe withdrawal, there are herbs to assist them. They are using gota kola, ginkgo, cayenne, Matol, barley green, pycnogenol, etc. and reporting that these are also helping them in restoring their ability to concentrate and helping to restore memory. Make sure that your source for information on these alternatives is a well informed one. Caution should be taken with anything you are using. The general rule of thumb with all herbs is that they should be gradually tapered onto and off again just as with medication. Those who have been on Prozac for long periods or had reactions to it find they have to start with very small doses of these and go up very slowly to avoid latent reactions. (We should note here that there has been a problem with using super blue green algae. Patients have reported effects identical to the symptoms those on Prozac are reporting. It has been discovered that some of the algae has been grown in fluoridated water and have high concentrations of fluoride. This could be the connection.) Yet care should be taken that we not exchange a chemical stressor for an herbal stressor. Just as an example, guarana has a lot of caffeine in it and should be avoided.

Ginkgo is an herb which is convincing the medical community to finally take a serious look at herbal healing properties. It has undergone intense medical scrutiny. Ginkgo has been the subject of over 300 scientific studies. It is successfully addressing many of the conditions which affect the elderly. Tens of millions of elderly Europeans have been successfully treated with ginkgo for conditions of the eyes, ears, heart and peripheral circulation. But results with conditions affecting the brain such as memory loss (especially in Alzheimer's patients), cognitive function and even cerebral disorders have been phenomenal.

The brain is especially sensitive to oxygen deprivation. One of the most exciting aspects of ginkgo is its ability to stimulate circulation and oxygen flow to the brain, thereby enhancing cognitive function and memory. Human studies have shown this increase in blood flow in patients with cerebrovascular disease. With ginkgo treatment the increase in cerebro-circulation is evident both in the disease-damaged areas of the brain, as well as the healthy areas. Other circulation enhancers, natural or synthetic, are not known to have this aspect. It increases oxygen transport at the blood-brain barrier, yet inhibits the permeability of toxins into the brain and nervous system. In a French double-blind study involving 166 patients with cerebral disorders researchers found that *those who had been the most severely affected benefited the most*. Patients specifically improved in communication, mental alertness, mobility, orientation, short-term memory and a wide variety of other factors. A new study out of London's Whittington Hospital confirmed marked improvement of cognitive function.

Studies conducted on rats, young and aged, showed that ginkgo actually increased the number of the type of brain receptors thought to be responsible for memory. According to French researcher K. Drieu, the major effect of ginkgo appears to be due to its ability to restore cell membrane integrity. It is intriguing to note how many of the complaints of adverse reactions stemming from Prozac use are addressed in these studies indicating the various applications of this herb - depression, short-term memory loss, cognitive function, indications of chemically induced brain disorders, muscle cramping, ringing in the ears, vision impairment, pain in limbs, etc. Because of its stimulant properties upon the circulatory system ginkgo has also proven useful in numbness, cramping, sensitivity to cold, deteriorating vision, ringing in the ears, etc.

Ginkgo is only an example of many herbal options. There are many which are just as effective. Find what works for you. Be aware that caution should be used in whatever mode of therapy we choose. (I emphasize this because after being on Prozac far too many patients become impulsive and do not show wisdom in making decisions about proceeding cautiously during the withdrawal period.) Some patients report that after having an adverse reaction to Prozac, using ginkgo makes them feel as if they are on Prozac again with the same disturbing side effects. These reports generally come from those who have been off Prozac for some time before using ginkgo. Those who begin to use it as they are tapering off Prozac seem to do much better and feel it has been very helpful in assisting them with their withdrawal. They also report that if they use too much it causes headaches and they know to cut back the amount. The adverse reactions being produced after a period of Prozac abstinence could be due to ginkgo's ability to increase oxygen transport at the blood-brain barrier, thus facilitating a much too rapid flushing of Prozac from the brain, where we know it has accumulated in large quantities. Flushing the drug too rapidly would be like being on high doses of Prozac. You must keep in mind that it took time for you to accumulate that much drug residue and you need to give yourself at least that same amount of time in order to remove it safely at the same pace. Always proceed slowly, cautiously and with wisdom with any method you use. While the drug is still in your system, you are still being affected by it as if you were still on it, but you will notice your ability to control your own actions and ability to think begin to gradually return.

Aromatherapy is the use of natural oils from botanicals, rather than chemical agents, in order to produce an effect upon the limbic system. Several patients have reported that they have used aromatherapy to take themselves off Prozac and overcome their depression. Although I remained curious to the many reports of altered sense of smell produced by Prozac, for quite some time I remained skeptical about the reports of successful results coming from the use of aromatherapy. My ignorance of aromatherapy prevented me from understanding how this might be possible. But while studying multiple chemical sensitivity, the understanding surrounding the potential benefits of this type of treatment began to dawn on me. According to Dr. Claudia S. Miller, M.D., M.S. in "Possible Models for Multiple Chemical Sensitivity: Conceptual Issues and Role of the Limbic System" presented to the Conference on Multiple Chemical Sensitivity; Association of Occupational and Environmental Clinics; Washington D.C.; September 20-21, 1991, *there are three physical routes through both the nose and mouth whereby substances can directly and immediately affect, stimulate, or even cross over into the brain.* Of course when we consider the increasing problems drug enforcement officials have with inhalants, and look at chemical warfare agents such as mustard gas, etc., we see very clearly how powerfully the brain can be affected in this manner. Mood, smells, short-term and long-term memory are all linked together and stored in the limbic system. Stimuli produced by various odors in the limbic system (olfactory brain) release many various neurotransmitters. The cells of the olfactory membrane are brain cells. It is through the olfactory membrane that the central nervous system has direct contact with the environment - its only exposure to the environment. The well known British aromatherapist, Robert Tisserand, reports that chemically produced oils, rather than natural oils, have been used experimentally in paramilitary use. He states that these chemicals produce very unpleasant emotions and in one instance he personally observed people ran from the building in a panic after being exposed to these odors. Scientists the world over are now exploring the sense of smell and the possibilities of various aromas in therapeutic treatments as well.

Aromatherapy has been practiced throughout recorded history. Fragrant oils were used in the Israelite temples and in many other cultures they were offered to the gods as gifts. The use of aromatic essences in healing became a lost art for many years until the French chemist Dr. Rene-Maurice Gattefosse revived this science around the turn of the century and he became known as the father modern aromatherapy. He declared, "...doctors and chemists will be surprised at the wide range of odoriferous substances which may be used medicinally...the antiseptic and antimicrobial properties of which use is currently made, the essential oils are also antitoxic and antiviral...In the future their role will be even greater." Between 1920 and 1930 Italian scientists conducted studies on the psychological effects of essential oils. A study published in 1922 by Dr. Renato Cayola and Dr. Giovanni Garri reported both calming and stimulating effects upon the nervous system with the use of various oils, along with their bacteria destroying capabilities. Pablo Rovesti from the University of Milan treated patients for depression with a combination of jasmine, sandalwood, orange blossom, verbena, and lemon oils. For anxiety or hysteria he suggested bergamot, neroli, cypress, orange leaf, lime, rose, violet leaves, and marjoram. Patchouli was used for many years in sanitariums to prevent psychotic reactions. Bergamot is a standard recommendation for manic depression. A combination of lemon, juniper berry, and cypress are used on the feet, over the kidneys and under the arms to assist in pulling foreign chemicals out of the body. The oils are applied to the skin after being mixed with a carrier oil such as grapeseed oil or almond oil. Or they are pumped through a diffusor, similar to an air freshener, into a room where the patient can inhale them and recuperate in the comfort of their own home. French physician Dr. Jean Valnet became interested in Gattefosse's work and began using oils for disinfecting and healing during World War II. In 1964 he wrote a book entitled *AROMATHERAPIE, TRAITEMENT DES MALADIES PAR LES ESSENCES DES PLANTES*. In 1982 his book, an excellent resource and highly recommended, was translated and published as *THE PRACTICE OF AROMATHERAPY*. In it he too makes an impassioned plea "for curtailing our use of dangerous chemical therapies and antibiotics, offering ***demonstrable proof*** of the vital power of plant medicines to prevent and heal disease and strengthen the immune system." It is an excellent book for professionals. A few of Valnet's students took the art to England where today they have professional aromatherapists and it is taught in several schools. I have been absolutely fascinated by the information I have gleaned in the field of aromatherapy, and look forward to learning much more. Two other books I have found very informative and quite simple to use for the layman are: *AROMATHERAPY, The Complete Guide to Plant and Flower Essences for Health and Beauty,* by Daniele Ryman and *THE COMPLETE BOOK OF ESSENTIAL OILS AND AROMATHERAPY* by Valerie Worwood.

In exploring alternatives it is also interesting to note that there have been several medical studies done on the efficacy of prayer in healing. MEDICAL TIMES, Vol. 97, No. 5, pp.201-203, May 1969, detailed a triple-blind study entitled, "The Efficacy of Prayer: A Triple-blind Study", by Plant J. Collipp M.D. Patients, parents, physicians and those praying for the patients were all unaware of the study being conducted. It involved ten children who were dying of leukemia. Ten families were asked to pray for the ten children. After fifteen months of prayer, results showed that out of the ten children seven were still alive and out of the eight in the control group not being prayed for only two were alive. Overall the group which was prayed for fared far better and the study concluded: "Among the plethora of modern drugs, and the increasing ingenuity of our surgeons, it seems inappropriate that our medical literature contains so few studies on our oldest and, who knows, perhaps most successful form of therapy [i.e., prayer].

March 3, 1986, cardiologist Randy Byrd, reported in the MEDICAL NEWS his study on 393 coronary care unit patients at San Francisco General Hospital. The group was divided in half and patients and physicians were unaware of the study. Those offering prayers were given the names, diagnosis and condition of the patients and asked to pray each day for "beneficial healing and quick recovery". Those praying included Jews, Catholics, Protestants. Each patient had 5 to 7 people offering prayer in his behalf. Distance was not considered important.

The results showed that those being prayed for did far better and had fewer complications. Only three required antibiotics, compared to 16 of those not prayed for. Six suffered pulmonary edema, compared to three times that amount in the unprayed for group. None of those prayed for required incubation (insertion of a breathing tube into the trachea) as compared to 12 of the unprayed for group. So from these studies it would be obvious that before we do anything else, perhaps we should all remember to say our prayers. In fact on The Larry King Show, July 11, 1992, his guest, a Dr. Jeffery, stated that prayer is proving to be so effective that it is his opinion that the doctor of the future will actually be required to pray for his patients. (Check references for several other studies involving the efficacy of prayer.)

Each of us has "heros" in life who we look up to and emulate. If we all could realize that we have chosen our own particular heros because we see something of ourselves within them, then we would begin to see our true worth, our real identities and our inner potential. We would begin to see that we are literally a combination of all those heros in embryo and that as we go through life's experiences we will begin to see their strengths beginning to emanate from us.

As we work to overcome life's obstacles we begin to understand that through this process we begin to recognize that the battles we all face are "gifts" helping us to grow and develop the same strengths we admired in those "heros". Armed with that knowledge we will be able to find within us the resources we need to face anything in life. We all have many inner strengths of which we seem to be unaware until we face a situation in life which forces us to draw upon those hidden strengths. This is a critical growth process that is often blocked out as an individual reaches for a drug rather than accepting the experience he is faced with by life and learning from the experience. Through reaching for a drug to escape, our inner strengths remain hidden from us.

Gandhi has always been one of my "heros". Gandhi with his frequent fasts appeared frail when judged by our standards of a "healthy" appearance. Yet contrary to our present belief system about abstaining from food, his fasting produced the physical stamina and endurance far beyond someone only a third his age. Paul Bragg, one of America's leading health enthusiasts, had the wonderful opportunity of spending a period of time getting to know Gandhi. He says in his classic book on fasting (long one of my most treasured possessions) *THE MIRACLE OF FASTING*, p.194, "Gandhi was *inexhaustible*. I have been an athlete all my life and a high mountain climber...but I have never seen a human who had the physical staying power and limitless energy as Gandhi...His internal strength was so powerful that weak people felt strong after seeing him and hearing his words. He gave of his unlimited strength to the discouraged and the sick. He brought light where there was darkness...This physically small man was a spiritual giant. He led the millions of people on the sub-continent of India to independence from the mighty British Empire without striking a single physical blow. And yet, with all his power and influence, he was completely without arrogance."

The "Mahatma" taught his people to fast and purify their bodies and minds, promising as a result that *joy would be their lot in life regardless of their circumstances.* He said, "The light of the world will illuminate within you when you fast and purify yourself. Fasting will bring spiritual rebirth to those of you who cleanse and purify your bodies." He felt fasting was an excellent method of both passing toxins from the body and allowing the organs an opportunity to rest from their labors and regenerate themselves. (As we learn in *FIT FOR LIFE,* digestion uses up more energy than any other activity - even running.) He might also have pointed out that fasting is the *least expensive* healing method known to man, definitely within everyone's budget and accessible to all.

Christ often encouraged a fast. His conviction of the great importance of the "law of the fast" was demonstrated by the forty day and forty night fast He accomplished in preparation for His greatest task of all - the mission of taking upon Himself the sins of the world and then having the courage to die for us in order to overcome the bonds of death. His long fast was a beautiful example of dedication and a witness to Himself and to us of his own internal strength. In our crazy world, who couldn't use a little extra internal strength or a witness of our own strength to help us believe in ourselves? We would do well to follow the examples of both Christ and Gandhi in this matter. For many years now I have personally benefited greatly from periodic fasts. Nothing clears the mind as quickly and efficiently as a fast. In fact Arnold Ehret, another of my heros because his ideas assisted me in saving my own life years ago, points out "There is nothing easier to heal than insanity by fasting...After a fast comes a clearer mind. Unity of ideas comes to take the place of differences." *(MUCUSLESS DIET HEALING SYSTEM*, p. 41) Unfortunately he was writing before the mind-altering drugs became so widely used. Clearing the mind is much more difficult after the encumbrance of chemical build-up in the brain is greater. Fasting assists in alleviating anxiety and pain, builds energy levels because energy is not depleted as a result of digestion, adds to a completely relaxed state and helps you to sleep like a baby. *The internal peace that comes from fasting regularly is beyond description!* The peace and tranquility we all search for must be built within ourselves before we are able to demonstrate it outwardly to bring peace within our families, our communities, nations, and the world.

The type of fast I have found most beneficial for myself and others living in this age of so much accumulated chemicals in our bodies and minds and our weaken immune systems is the lemon - pure maple syrup - purified water fast. (Gandhi generally used lemon and honey in water.) This lemon drink comes from Stanley Burroughs book *HEALING FOR THE AGE OF ENLIGHTENMENT.* One cup of fresh squeezed lemon juice and one cup of pure maple syrup (not the sugar water with maple flavoring - it will not work at all) are poured into a gallon bottle which is then filled with purified water. You may want a little more or little less maple to sweeten to your taste. For optimum benefit at least one gallon is consumed daily. Although it is most beneficial to do a complete abstinence from food and just drink the lemon drink, it is not always possible for those who are very weak or debilitated or toxic from an extended use of drugs or exposure to chemicals. They find that it is generally safer and more beneficial for the first few years of fasting to eat one or perhaps two light meals per day while drinking the gallon of lemon each day. If doing a straight lemon drink fast, it is often necessary to use a mild herbal laxative for the first couple of days if you are not accustomed to fasting regularly. If some of the lemon pulp is left in the drink and not strained out it will assist in moving the bowels. Keeping the elimination process moving is critical as you want all toxins to move out of the body, not recirculate through the intestinal wall.

The ingredient of pure maple syrup as a sweetener balances blood sugar unlike any other ingredient, facilitating one's ability to fast and not experience overpowering hunger pains. Most importantly in attempting to recover from the adrenalin rushes which patients continue to report after Prozac use by balancing the blood sugar the adrenalin rush the body utilizes to normalize blood sugar balance is eliminated. Diabetics can generally do a straight lemon drink fast of ten days with no problem. It is a very gentle fast. But an extensive fast including just the lemon drink should not be done even by healthy individuals for a ten day period more than three or four times a year. Many find it easier for them to do a day or two each week. Everyone has their own preference. A fast should *never* be ended with a heavy meal or cooked foods. The first few meals should be very light, ie., fresh vegetable juices, salads, etc. Paul Bragg's *MIRACLE OF FASTING* is an excellent guide book for someone to learn about fasting.

Lemon is an excellent cleanser and healer especially for the liver and the body as a whole. "Lemon essential oil is called 'polyvalent' (cure all) by French phytotherapists, who classify it as tonic, stimulant, stomachic, carminative, diuretic, antiseptic, bactericidal, and antiviral. It was still being used as an antiseptic and disinfectant in hospitals up to the First World War...Lemons also help the symptoms of premenstrual tension and insomnia. Every day for the seven days leading up to a period, drink a hot, freshly squeezed lemon drink last thing at night and first thing in the morning. For menstrual period pain, massage an oil made from 4 teaspoons almond oil and 8 drops lemon oil on the stomach, clockwise." I too have had many women tell me that all their PMS symptoms have disappeared with the use of the lemon drink just as an adjunct to their daily diet the week before their period.

The most critical recuperative measure is in regulating the excess adrenalin flow after Prozac use. The majority of adverse after effects such as insomnia, anxiety or panic attacks, mania, exhaustion, depression, etc. most likely stem from this over reaction to stressors brought on by the body being accustomed to being forced by the drug to pump the excess adrenalin. Many answers are still needed in this area. One well known method of calming adrenalin flow is to take three deep breaths through the nose, hold and let out slowly through the mouth when you first feel it building. Determine what causes adrenalin rushes or stress responses for you and avoid them if possible, at least until you regain control over your the overreactions to stressors, or while recuperating.

Emotionally do everything possible to avoid upsets or arguments. This is not easy when you cannot control the adrenalin which fuels the anger. If you do become upset you can walk or work off the excess adrenalin immediately in order to use it up in a constructive way. Most ex-SSRI patients who have had adverse reactions report that they need to avoid gory or violent movies. These make them feel that they may be losing control. These are the types of things which stir up stress responses as well so that may explain this reaction. It probably would be beneficial to turn off the news as well. Competition sports is another adrenalin pumping activity. You and your loved ones know yourself best, you will know what to avoid.

Physically, do not allow yourself to become over tired. The body views exhaustion as a crisis situation and will begin to pump adrenalin to bring you out of that exhausted state if you continue to give it the signal to keep pushing. We need to learn to rest when we are tired. Learn to take naps and go to bed earlier. All body systems will be at an exhaustion point after a prolonged period of being chemically revved up. Because of this you will find yourself needing far more rest than ever before. If you want to correct the problem now in order to avoid more serious problems in the future, you will be patient with yourself and take the time needed for rest and recuperation. Exercise is critical. Walking or bicycling is best. Start out slowly. Exercise can also help to normalize disrupted sleep patterns if the exercise is engaged in during the middle of the time period you want to be awake. A hypoglycemic diet is considered a standard procedure among those having the greatest success in rehabilitation from damage brought on by chemicals. The diet consists mainly of grains and vegetables with very little or no meat and no refined sugar, alcohol or stimulants. It is critical to keep the blood sugar balanced in order to avoid the body's normal reaction of a rush of adrenalin to normalize it for you. It can throw you into a spin resulting in the highs and subsequent lows you are working to avoid.

As all the body steroids, both adrenal and sex hormones come from cholesterol, and we are searching for a way to lower the hormone level, a diet low in cholesterol should be advantageous. Meats generally are not only high in cholesterol, but are full of artificial steroids. The tissues are also saturated with the animal's own body steroids generated by the stress response to its own death. The consumer then ingests the excess steroids with his steak, hamburger, etc. Dr. Vogel recommends using wisdom in our diets also, "Surely nutritional therapy has yielded convincing proof of the importance of proper diet in treating most ailments and a doctor should not overlook the potential benefits, especially when it can contribute so much to his patient's welfare...I am firmly convinced that there is no illness in which a proper diet does not play a part, whether it concerns the laying of a good foundation from which to counteract the patient's sensitivity or the provision of healing factors...Only unadulterated. Unrefined foods should be eaten, just as the Creator provided them in nature. In preparing them we should be guided by the same principle: food should be left in its natural state as far as possible. Cooked animal protein, such as meat, is detrimental according to my experience. For best results, adopt a predominantly vegetarian diet and include plenty of raw foods. Curds or cottage cheese, as animal derived protein, are good for you." *(THE NATURE DOCTOR,* p. 269)

Dr. Vogel is correct in pointing to the statistics. Those who maintain a vegetarian diet have proven to live longer, healthier lives than their carnivorous counterparts. A recent and very thorough, German study of 1,904 vegetarians over an 11-year span showed that death from any cause among vegetarians is one half that of the general population. The included in the study were both "strict" vegetarians who ate no meat of any kind and "moderate" vegetarians who occasionally ate meat, poultry and fish. *(Vegetarian Times,* June 1993, p. 14) Many excellent books have come out on diet over the last decade or so. A couple of the best are *DIET FOR A NEW AMERICA* by John Robbins and *FIT FOR LIFE* by Harvey and Marilyn Diamond.

Vitamins and minerals are depleted by drugs and must be replaced. Excess adrenalin flow found in Cushing's disease is associated with a drop in potassium. The most successful and popular drug withdrawal and rehabilitation programs for both illegal and legal substances always include a vitamin and mineral supplementation and exercise program (generally walking). They recommend using the most natural vitamin supplement possible. (See list of sources at end of chapter.) The reason for this is most likely that with the natural vitamins there are no artificial substances which would interact and possibly cause an interaction with the drug residue in the patient's system. Vitamin C is always listed as the most critical ingredient these programs use. Unfortunately I have found that most ex-Prozac patients cannot handle vitamin C except for the acerola C because of stomach problems. Three books I would recommend in assisting with this are: *ADDICTIONS, A NUTRITIONAL APPROACH TO RECOVERY*, by John Finnegan, *HIDDEN ADDICTION AND HOW TO GET FREE,* by Phelps and Nourse and *UNDER THE INFLUENCE* by James Milam. I am sure there are many others but these are ones I have reviewed.

Various herbs and oils are known to have anticonvulsant, antispasmodic and calmative properties. Sage is known to be an antispasmodic and calmative which balances the nerves and parasympathetic system. Lavender and bergamot are both antispasmodics and calmatives. While living in Germany I learned to love chamomile tea. I just liked the taste. I didn't know it was good for me. Chamomile as an herb or aromatic oil is known to be an anticonvulsant with very soothing and calming properties. Because of these particular properties we should be able to assume that chamomile would be very advantageous in normalizing adrenalin flow and assisting in withdrawal. Study the alternatives available to you. Learn about your choices in life. Take charge of your own life and health. Truth and knowledge do set us free from many things, including the terrible bondage of disease.

Just as this edition of *PROZAC: PANACEA OR PANDORA?* was about to go to press I read the best selling book *EMBRACED BY THE LIGHT* by Betty Jean Eadie. Anyone suffering depression or pain or loss of a loved one should most definitely read this book. I want to quote here a portion of the book which encapsulates what I have been saying in this chapter. After experiencing a near death experience Betty described what she learned from reviewing her life, "It all seemed so simple...It sank into the deepest part of my soul, changing my outlook on trials and opposition forever: 'You needed the negative as well as the positive experiences on earth. Before you can feel joy, you must know sorrow.' All of my experiences now took on new meaning. I realized that no real mistakes had been made in my life. Each experience was a tool for me to grow by. Every unhappy experience had allowed me to obtain greater understanding about myself, until I learned to avoid those experiences. I also saw myself growing in ability to help others...*Some experiences were sad and some were joyful, but all were calculated to bring me to higher levels of knowledge.*"

SOURCES FOR NATURAL VITAMINS:

BE Professional Products
13375 South 2200 West
Riverton, Utah 84065
801-254-4148
(acerola vitamin C source also)

Ethical Nutrients-Metagenics
23180 Del Lago
Laguna Hills, CA 92653
1-800-692-9400

Great Health
2663 Saturn St.
Brea, CA 92621
714-996-8600

Omega Nutrition (flax)
309-8495 Ontario St.
Vancouver, B.C.
Canada V5X 3E8
604-322-8862

San Francisco Herb and Natural
Food Company
1010 46 Street
Emeryville, CA 94608
800-523-5192 (CA)
800-227-2830 (U.S.)

Standard Process
Box 38
Campbell, CA 95009-0038
800-662-9134

Sunrider International
3111 Lomita Blvd.
Torrance, CA 90509-2840
800-448-8786
213-534-4786

Threshold Distributors (flax)
P.O. Box 533
Soquel, CA 95073
800-438-1700

Yerba Prima
P.O. Box 2569
Oakland, CA 94614
415-632-7477

ESSENTIAL OIL SOURCES:

Oils may be obtained through any local health store. Aura Casia or Now are both good products or my own personal source for therapeutic grade oils is:

Elsa Kartchner
5475 Sweetwood Circle
Murray, Utah 84123
801-268-9111

CHAPTER 14

A RELIGIOUS ISSUE?

One of the first individuals to become aware of the Prozac-violence and suicide connection and bring it to public attention was Dennis Clark, a spokesman for the Citizen's Commission on Human Rights (CCHR). Dennis is a brilliant researcher and a compassionate human being. CCHR was originally organized by the Church of Scientology. In April, 1991, Eli Lilly began to make accusations that the Church of Scientology was "the entity" behind all this backlash or bad press Prozac was beginning to experience. In May, 1991, *TIME* picked up Lilly's story. Then in defense of their stand against Prozac, during the first two weeks of June, 1991, the Church of Scientology ran full page ads every day in *USA TODAY* exposing the political ties between *TIME* and Eli Lilly. They also published Lilly's past history of harmful drugs. The battle was on and the attention of the public, as well as professionals, was diverted from the real issue of serious adverse Prozac reactions. The political mud slinging became all anyone heard about, rather than the scientific evidence. And anyone who said anything negative about Prozac instantly became labeled a "Scientologist."

I had heard nothing of the Citizen's Commission on Human Rights, nor knew anything about The Church of Scientology's ongoing battle with psychiatry until long after research for the first edition of this book began. My concern about Prozac came first of all through the warnings and information Lilly included with each prescription (which, if translated into layman's terms, should be enough to raise anyone's eyebrows). Secondly concern was raised by observing serious reactions to the drug in friends and family who were using it and their persistent inquiries made to me about the drug. Then in early February, 1991, I voiced my concern about Prozac and the serious problems surrounding it to one of the leaders of my own church, a retired chemist. At the mere mention of the word Prozac he surprised me. He immediately became very serious and began shaking his head and repeating over and over and over again, *"very, very, very dangerous drug."* Occasionally he would stop to inject the reasons for his feelings and the concern held by his colleagues in leadership positions in the church. Although at that time I too had a deep concern about Prozac and its safety, I didn't even begin to see how very true his words would prove to be after three years of research.

The Prozac issue is not necessarily a religious issue, it most definitely is a moral and ethical issue, as well as a serious public health issue, yet, when patients report losing spiritual feelings or any ability to feel love or guilt which affects one's moral behavior and values, perhaps religions need to be more concerned about this drug and its analogues. Religious groups are finally beginning to ask many questions. The BBC felt it was enough of an issue to do a documentary which should be airing soon on the ethics of Christians using a drug like Prozac. Most religious denominations teach self control, a mastering of one's appetites and passions, etc. As we use a drug which has enough power to alter our behavior, we give up our control. Control is maintained through our thoughts. Drugs which are mind-altering alter our thoughts and therefore, alter our behavior. We give up our agency to act on our own to a substance. As one survivor put it, "I felt some else's brain was in my body." Another discussed the loss of spirituality and ability to love, "I lost all natural ability to love. It became a spiritual dullness. You cease to know right from wrong. And because there is no wrong, you're right 100% and to hell with anyone else."

Remember what Dr. Kramer says in his book, *LISTENING TO PROZAC*. I quote, "In the *THANATOS SYNDROME*, the last novel by the Southern writer Walker Percy, a maverick doctor finds that plotters have introduced an insidious chemical, Heavy Sodium, into the water supply. On Heavy Sodium, shy and anxious women - the first example is 'a housebound Emily Dickinson' - become erotic, bold, competitive, slim, un-self-conscious, and insensitive to the point of perfunctoriness. They shake off 'old terrors, worries, rages, a shedding of guilt like last year's snakeskin.'

"Percy was writing before Prozac was marketed, but *Heavy Sodium is like Prozac in so many respects that we must credit him with creating the art that life imitates.* To Percy, the drug's effects are all to the bad. One Heavy Sodium, people are 'not hurting, they are not worrying the same old bone, but there is something missing, not merely the old terrors but a sense in each of her - her what? her self?' Heavy Sodium *reduces a person to his or her ignoble, animal being*, a point Percy emphasizes by having the book's villains, overdosed on Heavy Sodium, take on the posture and behaviors of apes. *By reducing human self-consciousness, the drug robs individuals of their souls.* What links men and women to God is precisely their guilt, anxiety, and loneliness.

"Percy's novel of ideas, written from a Catholic viewpoint, presages much of the controversy that followed the medical community's discovery of Prozac. Like Percy, medical ethicists asked: Is it a good thing?" p. 250

How many have repeated to me over and over again during the last three years, "This drug tore my soul right out!" They look at the cover of Dr. Kramer's book with a person lifting their head off to reveal a blank face and they say, "That is exactly what Prozac does. It rips your head off and there is nothing left!" It is inconceivable to me that Dr. Kramer emphasizes the similarity between Prozac and Heavy Sodium, admits their effects of reducing one to an "animal being" and "robbing one of his soul" and then goes on to explain that if we can get rid of painful emotions such as guilt, we won't have those emotions to hold us back in life. We can go forward aggressively and boldly living our lives. There will be no need to waste time worrying about who we might hurt, nor be embarrassed about our actions, nor worry whether or not we really have enough money in the bank to write out that check, nor be concerned about whether or not whatever it is we are using or consuming actually belongs to us, etc. We can just go on through life without any obstacles, obstacles such as guilt or embarrassment.

These feelings should serve as our internal check and balance system. It should be clear what could happen with those feelings being erased. Why would we pollute the seat of our spirit, our mind, with these toxins which rob us of all those feelings we hold most dear? Is it worth losing so much for a short period of numbness or being insensitive to emotional or physical pain? In blocking the bad feelings, we also block the good feelings. Elder Boyd K. Packer, one of the twelve apostles of the Church of Jesus Christ of Latter-Day Saints spoke in the October 1989 worldwide General Conference. He spoke of drugs which numb or dull the senses, legal as well as illegal drugs. He said, "The Holy Ghost communicates with the spirit through the mind more than through the physical senses. This guidance comes as thoughts, as feelings, through impressions and promptings...The scriptures teach us that we may *"feel"* the words of spiritual communication more than hear them,...even though an angel spoke to some, they 'were past *feeling*, that [they] could not *feel* his words' (Book of Mormon, 1 Nephi 17:45)" He then concludes that the use of these drugs *"draw curtains which close off the light of spiritual communication."* Patients who have used the SSRIs consistently report no longer being able to pray or feel the Holy Spirit. They generally report losing those higher feelings.

I personally am proud to say that I am a very staunch and active member of the Church of Jesus Christ of Latter-Day Saints (Mormon). This has been the case throughout my teenage years and adult life. I even devoted two and a half years to serve as a missionary for the church. Guy McConnell, the National Director of the Prozac Survivor's Support Group (PSSG), is Baptist. Bonnie Leitsch, the Assistant National Director, is a staunch member of her faith, the Assembly of God, and all the other directors of PSSG in the various states have their own religious preferences, i.e., Catholic, Presbyterian, Methodist, Jewish, etc., etc., some are atheists and none are Scientologists.

The Prozac Survivor's Support Group, as a whole, feels that too much emphasis has been placed upon this battle between the Church of Scientology and Eli Lilly. They want the real issues about Prozac brought into focus before others have to suffer as they and their families have suffered. The problems surrounding Prozac are so obvious and far-reaching that *everyone* is becoming aware of how it is affecting their lives. Scientology is not the issue here although Lilly would like us to believe that in order to avoid someone taking a hard look at their "golden goose." How far are they going to go? Is Lilly going to declare war on all religious denominations as one by one they step forward and speak out? They have done everything they can to divert the attention from the real issues surrounding Prozac by resorting to name calling and mud slinging. It is well past time to directly address all the problems connected with their drug - those they admit to and those they continue to publicly ignore and deny in spite of the onslaught of negative medical reports and overwhelming number of adverse reaction reports.

CHAPTER 15

THE BIRTH OF *PROZAC: PANACEA OR PANDORA?*

Four years ago when I began to notice several friends and neighbors who were beginning to experience problems in their lives and beginning to act very much unlike the persons I had known, I did not even begin to suspect it might be reactions to their "medication". I was completely unaware, as so many others are unaware, that doctors prescribe drugs that alter a patient's thoughts and behavior. I watched these people for almost a year develop behaviors so completely out of character for them that I could not understand how they could be so different from the persons I had always known them to be.

One friend, who was aware of my knowledge of medicine and health, began to ask me in depth questions about his medication. His persistence and very obvious concern peaked my interest enough that that I finally stopped by the local pharmacy and picked up a package insert on Prozac. At first reading I immediately became very concerned that this may be the cause that three out of four of these individuals, all Mormon with a very strict health code, were now drinking or abusing drugs. This was definately out of character behavior for every one of them. The package insert made it very clear to me that the adverse effects upon the pancreas could produce this effect and that the major concern about this drug should be its adverse effects upon both the liver and the pancreas. If Prozac had the effect upon the pancreas that the package insert explained it did, it should at the very least, be chemically inducing hypoglycemia, thereby causing alcoholism or a craving for other drugs, caffeine, sweets, etc.

I watched one neighbor just two blocks away who had been a close friend. She was thin, active, always doing things with her four children - so "vibrant and alive" had always been my impression of her. I had admired her and thought how I wished I could be a little more like her in many ways. Three years after I first met her, her husband filed for a divorce. After sixteen years of marriage, this naturally devastated her. I have been through a divorce. It is far from pleasant, but it is certainly not reason enough to give someone a powerful mind-altering drug. Her doctor prescribed Prozac. As I began to see the changes in her I assumed they must be a reaction to the stress of the divorce. She and I stopped spending much time together. I soon discovered that this was the case with her other friends as well, she was cutting off or no longer associating with many of them. About this time she also concluded that she must be an alcoholic as she began drinking and felt she could not stop. The next step was hospitalization because of a nervous breakdown. (Mixing Prozac and alcohol should be enough to do that for anyone.) As she began to experience additional reactions, more drugs were added to the Prozac prescription. Seizures developed next and antiepileptic drugs were added. Now four years later, few who knew her before even recognize her. She is no longer on Prozac. After three years of use, it has now been replaced with very strong anti-psychotic drugs and antiepileptic drugs. Her ex-husband now has custody of the children because of her condition. She sits in her house alone in a stupor with a blank look on her face and her lower lip protruding. The divorce is no longer a concern to her. The brain damage and mental retardation brought on by the toxic effects of the drugs are painfully apparent. She is overweight now, mostly edema and abdominal bloating, and dresses in very odd looking clothing. Her once long strawberry blonde hair is now cropped short and plain. She appears old and worn out and sleeps off and on while visiting with you. Such have been the results of her long-term Prozac use coupled with other powerful mind altering drugs and electric shock (now we know how Prozac multiplies the effects of the other drugs by at least ten times to cause such toxicity). I say as all the other families who have a loved one on Prozac say over and over again, "My friend is dead. The person I knew is gone, just completely gone." Her four children lost their mother four years ago when she was prescribed Prozac. The fun loving, vibrant human being we knew left. If she were aware enough to even begin to realize what tragedies her children have met as they have grown up without their mother, she would be absolutely devastated. Her children meant so much to her. Now their lives too have been tragically altered by the negative impact of going through their teenage years without their mother's influence.

Living in Utah where the use of Prozac is apparently the highest in the nation, I have had far too much experience to draw upon. Most people here know many on the drug. Most people know many who have been on the drug for quite some time. Although I had some concerns that day after first reading a Prozac package insert, I had no clue to what I had stumbled onto or where my investigation would lead me as I searched for answers for my friends. Dr. Michael DeCaria, a local and very well respected psychopharmacologist, became impressed with my insight into Prozac and the initial concerns I expressed about the drug. When he learned of my writing experience he encouraged me to begin writing an article for a local magazine. He expressed that he felt society had suffered a great loss that I who possessed so much natural ability had not persued my medical career. I was overwhelmed by his compliments and encouragement and took his advice. I began to write and I finished my degrees concentrating on forensic and biological psychology and drug abuse counceling.

When the news spread that I was writing an article on Prozac, the Western Institute of Neuropsychiatry in Salt Lake City invited me to speak, requesting that I present the "con" side of a pro and con Prozac lecture. After much prompting I finally agreed and thus began my education on the politics of medicine in this country today. Although I was told that each side would have half an hour to present and then the audience would be allowed to ask questions, I was to find that I would be given five minutes and the other side thirty minutes. Three psychiatrists, two of which needed their lips surgically separated from Eli Lilly's bureaucratic derriere, discussed the "wonders" of Prozac. As they turned the meeting over to the audience to ask questions, one man identified himself as an attorney, and asked, "What do I do with all these people who are afraid to tell you - their doctors, what they are experiencing on this drug? They fear that if they do so you will just commit them to a psychiatric hospital."

One at a time many of the audience came forward after the meeting to express to me how disappointed they were that I had not been allowed to speak. They had wanted to hear what I had to say. It became quite clear to me that I had been used as token symbol - proof that both sides of the Prozac issue had been addressed. The experience made me begin to really question why physicians would go to such lengths to defend a drug. In May of 1991 at the request of many of the audience from that meeting, I held a public meeting to present the material I had previously gathered on the con side of Prozac. At the end of my presentation the group of individuals attending, many who had suffered adverse reactions, concluded that something needed to be done to alert citizens in our area of any possible problems arising from Prozac. They proposed that we form our own local branch of the national Prozac Survivor's Support Group. In spite of my vigorous protests they unanimously voted me in as director. Although I spent much of the evening coming up with reasons as to why I could not fill the position, all reservations I had about acting as a support for those on Prozac were completely removed for me the following morning by a 20-year-old young man who jumped to his death right outside my downtown office window. As he was dying he told the officer he had been using Prozac. After that I *absolutely had to know* if Prozac was causing such terrible reactions in the lives of so many people.

My magazine article quickly took on the length and form of a booklet and the first edition entitled *THE PROZAC PANDORA* was published in the fall of 1991. It came out just before I testified to the FDA about the seriousness of the problems in Utah with the use of Prozac. Since that time I have continued researching and writing to finish this second edition for publication. I became committed enough to mortgage my home to fund my project. For almost four years now I have devoted full time to the study of Prozac and the other mind-altering drugs, documenting cases and assisting the victims of adverse drug reactions. I have interviewed in depth nearly 1000 patients and/or families of Prozac patients - generally an average of one hour per patient. How many doctors have the opportunity to take such time for specific in depth study? They are far too busy with an overload of patients to even keep up with the general information on drugs, much less learn about specific drugs.

Let me share with you a little about me which may give you some insight as to why I would embark on such an endeavor as this. I grew up in the very small southeastern Arizona community of Safford. To a child's imagination life was exciting and stimulating growing up in the famous Indian territory of those great Indian chiefs, Cochise and Geronimo. Even at an early age I examined intensely why people made the choices they make and why they do the things they do. I felt much injustice had been done to my neighbors the American Indians. In all of our childhood Cowboy and Indian battles I fought for who I, in my childhood wisdom, deemed "the oppressed" as I cheered on the Indian nation and led them down those dusty Arizona trails to victory in all our battles. My mother shared some of the family genealogy with us children by letting us know that on her side we were one eighth Cherokee through my great, grandmother Phoebe Ellen Choate. This added a whole new dimension to our vivid imaginations. In my five-year-old mind I was convinced that I was an Indian princess and the *only* way I would ever marry would be on a white horse. I would then ride off into the sunset just as the Indians on television were married.

My Uncle Claude's authentic stagecoach in the backyard made these Cowboy and Indian battles seem even more real to me and all of my neighborhood friends, who could in the twinkle of an eye transform themselves into real life cowboys and Indians. We would ride that stagecoach and his old saddle draped across a saw horse for hours on end. The old West really came alive in that backyard. My observation at a very early age was that the Indians were the ones who actually "won" the real life cowboy and Indian battles (I never understood why we use the term "win", since no one ever really "wins" in a war, everyone loses.). It seemed to me that they were the real victors in that war because they introduced the white man to tobacco, a drug which has destroyed far more white men over the years than any of the battles the Indians fought to defend their land. Yet I could not overlook the white man's introduction to the Indian of "spirits" or "fire water", which has been the means of breaking the spirit of many a noble Indian warrior and their descendants since then. This observation in childhood served as my first insight into mind-altering substances and the havoc they cause in personal lives and in our society in general.

I must admit that from early in life I have always been unorthodox. Although there seemed to be much pressure brought to bear for conformity in our society, being a carbon copy of everyone else seemed boring and unproductive to me. I have always felt that we all have our own unique individual qualities and should magnify them to the fullest extent in order to contribute our part in life. Although very serious and introspective in my outlook on life, even in childhood, I have always loved to laugh. Perhaps my grandmother, Rita Higgins Blake, a truly elegant lady and my dearest friend in my youth, played a large part in developing my spunkiness. I learned to have great respect and love for her. She had learned to be a true survivor through painful adjustments in life as she fought to adapt to the loss of her beloved husband, Andy, early in life. (Ironically the day this book went to press I learned that my grandfather's death had been the long-term result of being sprayed with mustard gas during World War I. Thanks to chemical warfare I never had the opportunity of meeting my grandfather.) Part of that survival instinct she possessed also stemmed from the fact that she came from a strong pioneer background. Her parents had crossed the plains with Brigham Young and then went on to settle in Arizona.

As I mention in my dedication, the influence of my great, great grandfather, Charles A. Thomas has played an important part in my life. Charles and his wife, Edith adopted my great grandmother, Sarah Fletcher, when she was yet a small child in Missouri. They were on their way West from New York to Tombstone, Arizona to embark upon a whole new world. Charles was a man of integrity who honored people for their individual qualities regardless of their station in life. In his day there was little difference between the right side of the law and the wrong side of the law. Keeping as much peace as possible was the most important factor. Once while serving as mayor of Tombstone he put his own life on the line as he stood between his sheriff, Wyatt Earp, and his friend, Johnny Ringo, to prevent the loss of either life. As I stand between giant multimillion dollar pharmaceutical companies and their unsuspecting victims to stop the loss of any more lives, I have an idea of how my great, great grandfather felt that day on that dusty Tombstone street. This time the battle is not fought with guns, but with words. In his day it was acceptable to tar and feather someone, but now the practice is to taunt and fault the opposition. In this way the real issues can be clouded by the diversion.

When I first uncovered the research which demonstrates the similarity in action between Prozac and the other SSRIs in comparison to the psychedelic drugs I approached a well respected scientist with the information. I knew of his interest because he had been approached two years before by two doctors who were looking for a leading expert in the field of psychoactive drugs to help their brother. Their brother was an attorney who had experienced terrible long-term reactions while on Prozac for only five months. Help had been impossible to find. Every new doctor wanted to try another drug to stop his reactions and the reactions continued to become more and more severe with each new drug. After working with this patient for over a year, this doctor could offer no hope either. He tried everything he could think of, but he was baffled. He remained convinced that the patient was suffering what drug experts would call post drug syndrome. The symptoms were electric surges throughout the body which would leave him breathless and wondering if after the attack he could begin breathing again or retain the ability of his heart to continue beating, constant ringing in the ears, plus a large majority of the other side effects we have discussed. The doctor felt sure that what the patient was suffering was the result of damage to the cholinergic nervous system, like he had seen in conjunction with illicit drug use. This is something that we are being told does not happen with Prozac use.

He was still looking for answers when I shared with him my new found research. Obviously shocked, he responded, "That means that LSD has the same effect upon serotonin as the Serotonin Reuptake Inhibitors! No wonder!" He asked for a copy of the research material. I then requested that he go public with this very critical information. He sighed deeply and replied, "Lilly will crush whoever comes forward with this information." It was clear that he felt the action may put an end to his career and that I was on my own - thanks once again to the politics in medicine in America. I have already begun to see what can be done to discredit those willing to stand for a cause and speak out against injustices. I have learned how much power and influence is exerted by an infinite advertising budget. I have learned that when you have friends in high places you can manipulate the media, but no one could stand by and witness the tragedies I have seen with my own eyes and hear what I have heard with my own ears and not cry out in warning. Somehow I understand how my great, great grandfather felt standing alone between two loaded guns on that Tombstone street over a hundred years ago. My great grandfather put everything on the line to save those two lives and I intend to continue to follow his example throughout my life.

APPENDIX A

SIDE EFFECTS DEFINED

The reader is encouraged to acquire a package insert which Lilly distributes with Prozac. It is becoming increasingly difficult to get one from a doctor or pharmacist as many now even refuse to hand them out, but it should be available through Lilly Pharmaceutical. It is recommended that you go through it thoroughly with a medical dictionary in order to fully understand all terms.

Below are medical definitions of a few of the Prozac side effects listed by the pharmaceutical company which may be less familiar to the reader than the others. (Most of these are also listed side effects of the other SSRIs.) According to the report filed with the FDA by Ralph Nader's consumer protection group, "fluoxetine is most frequently associated with anxiety, insomnia, hypomania, nervousness, nausea, akathisia (a syndrome characterized by motor restlessness and marked anxiety), anorexia, and diarrhea." The following definitions are taken from Taber's Cyclopedic Medical Dictionary, Edition Fifteen, compiled by Clayton L. Thomas, M.D., M.P.H.

Agitation: Excessive restlessness, increased mental and physical activity, especially the latter.

Akathisia: Inability to sit down because the thought of doing so causes severe anxiety. Patient has a feeling of restlessness and an urgent need of movement and complains of a feeling of muscular quivering.

Author's note: This side-effect is considered *most dangerous*. It has been described in studies as the drug induced feeling which seems to be the trigger for the impulsive suicidal attempts associated with Prozac. It has also been found in many clinical studies to be the cause behind extremely bizarre and very violent behavior in patients using other mind-altering psychiatric drugs. Akathisia is described as "a drug induced psychosis or drug induced insanity".

Ataxia: Defective muscular coordination, especially that manifested when voluntary muscular movements are attempted.

Asthenia: Lack or loss of strength; debility (generally brought on by stress - common among combat soldiers)

Ataxia: Defective muscular coordination, especially that manifested when voluntary muscular movements are attempted.

Depersonalization: The belief that one's own reality is temporarily lost or altered. The patient feels estranged or unreal and may have the sensation that the extremities have changed size. Feeling of being automated or as if in a dream may be present.

Hypesthesia: Lessened sensibility to touch.

Hypoglycemia: Deficiency of sugar in blood. A condition in which the glucose in the blood is abnormally low. Brought on by hyper-function of the pancreas. [The pancreas over reacts producing too much insulin which drops the blood sugar level below normal.]

Hypomania: Mild mania and excitement with moderate change in behavior.

Hysteria: Histrionic (hysterical) personalities are conspicuously egocentric...esteem and admiration of other is important to them...emotional immaturity...lively manner lends itself to easily established superficial relationships, but these persons are rarely deeply involved emotionally... Their relationships are affected by a seemingly insatiable need for affection and protection; ie, they tend to be dependent. Promiscuous entanglements with many partners are possible because of the histrionic person's lack of real involvement with any of them. The crises that arise from these relationships are managed with manipulative behavior that may include suicidal threats and shrewd exploitation of emotional susceptibilities in other people. Insight fails to develop in histrionic persons because they can easily repress or forget unpleasant or discreditable experiences; responsibility for misfortunes and failures usually is ascribed to others. Dissociation... drastic modification of one's sense of personal identity. These modifications can include fugues, hysterical conversion reactions, short-term denial of responsibility for one's acts or feelings, trance states, chance-taking, and pharmacologic intoxication to numb unhappiness.

Mania: A form of psychosis characterized by exalted feelings, delusions of grandeur, elevation of mood, psychomotor overactivity, and overproduction of ideas. Additionally, U.S. News and World Report, March 5, 1990, p. 53, describes mania: "Mania shares this departure from reality. Possessed of limitless energy, thoughts racing, manic-depressive patients in the elated phase of the illness may stay up all night, insist they are in touch with creatures from outer space, become uncharacteristically promiscuous or run up thousands of dollars in credit-card bills."

Neuralgia: Severe sharp pain along the course of a nerve.

Neuropathy: Any disease of the nerves.

Paranoid personality: characterized by projection of their own hostilities and conflicts onto others. These persons are markedly sensitive to interpersonal relationships and tend to find hostile and malevolent intentions behind trivial, innocent, or even kindly acts by others. Often their suspicious attitudes lead to aggressive feelings or behavior or bring about rejection by others, which seems to justify their original feelings; however, they are unable to see their own roles in this cycle. Their behavior may be designed to prove their adequacy, while their sense of superiority becomes exaggerated and is accompanied by belittlement of others...They may be litigious, especially when they feel a sense of righteous indignation...**Some of these are transitory paranoid states due to toxic conditions**, a paranoid type of schizophrenia, and paranoid states due to alcoholism [or intoxication from drug interaction].

Psychosis: A term formerly applied to any mental disorder, but now generally restricted to those disturbances of such magnitude that there is personality disintegration and loss of contact with reality.

Tremor: 1. A quivering, esp. continuous quivering of a convulsive nature. 2. An involuntary movement of a part or parts of the body resulting from alternate contractions of opposing muscles.

From TABER'S CYCLOPEDIC MEDICAL DICTIONARY

Iatrogenic disorder - Any adverse mental or physical condition induced in a patient by effects of treatment by a physician or surgeon. Term implies that such effects could have been avoided by proper and judicious care on the part of the physician.

Pharmaco- Combining form meaning drug, medicine, poison.

APPENDIX B

REFERENCES - ADVERSE REACTIONS

The following are some medical review articles on adverse effects associated with fluoxetine [Prozac] and where the title is not completely explicate, a short summary of the contents which the reader may find interesting.

Achamallah NS; Decker DH. Mania induced by fluoxetine in an adolescent patient [letter] *AM J PSYCHIATRY* 1991 Oct:148(10):1404

Ahmad S. Fluoxetine and glaucoma [letter] *DICP* 1991 Apr:25(4):436

Ananth J; Elmishaugh A. Hair loss associated with fluoxetine treatment [letter] *CAN J PSYCHIATRY* 1991 Oct;36(8):621

Austin LS; Arana GW; Melvin JA. Toxicity resulting from lithium augmentation of antidepressant [fluoxetine & haloperidol (Haldol)] treatment in elderly patients. *J CLIN PSYCHIATRY* 1990 Aug:51(8):344-5

Baldwin D; Fineberg N; Montgomery S. Fluoxetine, fluvoxaminie and extra-pyramidal tract disorders. *INT CLIN PSYCHOPHARMACOL* 1991 Spring;6(1):51-8 (Basal Ganglia Diseases and mental disorders/chemically induced.)

Bell IR; Cole JO. Fluoxetine induces elevation of desipramine level and exacerbation of geriatric nonpsychotic depression [letter] *J CLIN PSYCHOPHARMACOL* 1988 Dec:8(6):447-8

Black DW; Wojcieszek J. Depersonalization syndrome induced by fluoxetine [letter] *PSYCHOSOMATICS* 1991 Fall;32(4):468-9

Bodkin JA; Teicher MH. Fluoxetine may antagonize the anxiolytic action of buspirone [letter] *J CLIN PSYCHOPHARMACOL* 1989 Apr:9(2):150

Browning WN. Exacerbation of symptoms of multiple sclerosis in a patient taking fluoxetine [letter] *AM J PSYCHIATRY* 1990 Aug:147(8):1089

Budman CL; Bruun RD. Persistent dyskinesia in a patient receiving fluoxetine [letter] *AM J PSYCHIATRY* 1991 Oct:148(10):1403 [Chemically induced basal ganglia diseases, drug-induced dyskinesia with Prozac.]

Buff DD; Brenner R; Kirtane SS; Gilboa R. Dysrhythmia associated with fluoxetine treatment in an elderly patient with cardiac disease. *J CLIN PSYCHIATRY* 1991 Apr:52(4):174-6

Chouinard G; Steiner W. A case of mania induced by high-dose fluoxetine treatment [letter] *AM J PSYCHIATRY* 1986 May;143(5):686

Ciraulo DA; Shader RI. Fluoxetine drug-drug interactions: I. Antidepressants and antipsychotics. *J CLIN PSYCHOPHARMACOL* 1990 Feb:10(1):48-50 ("As clinical experience with fluoxetine grows, so do reports of drug interactions. The most common adverse interaction appears to be inhibition of drug metabolism. Other antidepressants are so affected, and toxicity may result if proper dosage adjustments are not made...Fluoxetine has been greeted with an enthusiasm that claims some advantages. We should be mindful that any unique therapeutic benefits may be accompanied by a unique adverse effects profile and a special propensity for drug-drug interactions."

Ciraulo DA; Shader RI. Fluoxetine drug-drug interactions. II. *J CLIN PSYCHOPHARMACOL* 1990 Jun:10(3):213-7

Cohen BJ; Mahelsky M; Adler L. More cases of SIADH with fluoxetine [letter] *AM J PSYCHIATRY* 1990 Jul:147(7):948-9

Cole JO; Bodkin JA. Antidepressant drug side effects. *J CLIN PSYCHIATRY* 1990 Jan;51 Suppl:21-6. ("Frequently encountered adverse effects are emphasized, but some of the more serious rare ones are also considered. Where possible, guidelines for management of these effects are provided, although there are not invariably ways of avoiding them...It is an unfortunate fact that the research literature does not treat these issues thoroughly, despite their great clinical importance.")

Cunningham M; Cunningham K; Lydiard RB. Eye tics and subjective hearing impairment during fluoxetine therapy [letter] *AM J PSYCHIATRY* 1990 Jul:147(7):947-8

DeMaso DR; Hunter TA. Combing fluoxetine with desipramine [adverse effects] [letter] *J AM ACAD CHILD ADOLESC PSYCHIATRY* 1990 Jan:29(1):151

Dorval GS; Meinzer AE. Appearance of obsessive-compulsive symptoms in depressed patients treated with fluoxetine [letter] *AM J PSYCHIATRY* 1991 Sep:148(9):1262-3 (Obsessive-compulsive disorder was chemically induced with Prozac treatment.)

Downs JM; Downs AD; Rosenthal TL; Deal N; Akiskal HS. Increased plasma tricyclic antidepressant concentrations in two patients concurrently treated with fluoxetine [see comments]. (Comment in: *J CLIN PSYCHIATRY* 1990 Mar:51(3):126) *J CLIN PSYCHOPHARMACOL* 1989 Feb:9(1):63-5

Ellison JM; Milofsky JE; Ely E. Fluoxetine-induced bradycardia and syncope in two patients [see comments] *J CLIN PSYCHIATRY* 1990 Sep:51(9):385-6

Fallon BA; Liebowitz MR. Fluoxetine and extrapyramidal symptoms in CNS lupus [letter] *J CLIN PSYCHOPHARMACOL* 1991 Apr:11(2):147-8 [Chemically induced basal ganglia diseases, dyskinesia, systemic Lupus. Neurologic examination revealed organic mental disorders.]

Feder R. Bradycardia and syncope induced by fluoxetine [letter: comment] (Comment on: *J CLIN PSYCHIATRY* 1990 Sep:51(9):385-6) *J CLIN PSYCHIATRY* 1991 Mar:52(3):139

Feder R. Fluoxetine-induced mania [letter] *J CLIN PSYCHIATRY* 1990 Dec:51(12):524-5

Fluoxetine and extrapyramidal side effects [letter; comment] (Comment on: *AM J PSYCHIATRY* 1989 Mar:146(3):399-400) In: *AM J PSYCHIATRY* 1989 Oct:146(10):1352-3

Gardner SF; Rutherford WF; Munger MA; Panacek EA. Drug-induced supraventricular tachycardia: a case report of fluoxetine. *ANN EMERG MED* 1991 Feb:20(2):194-7

Gernaat HB ; Van de Woude J ; Touw DJ. Fluoxetine and parkinsonism in patients taking carbamazepine [letter] *AM J PSYCHIATRY* 1991 Nov:148(11):1604-5

Ghaziuddin M; Tsai L; Ghaziuddin N. Fluoxetine in autism with depression [letter] (Comment on: *J AM ACAD CHILD ADOLESC PSYCHIATRY* 1990 Nov:29(6):985) In: *J AM ACAD CHILD ADOLESC PSYCHIATRY* 1991 May;30(3):508-9

Goldbloom DS; Kennedy SH. Adverse interaction of fluoxetine and cyproheptadine in two patients with bulimia nervosa. *J CLIN PSYCHIATRY* 1991 Jun:52(6):261-2 (Chemically induced psychosexual dysfunction)

Gommans JH; Edwards RA. Fluoxetine and hyponatremia [letter] *N Z MED J* 1990 Mar 14;103(885):106

Gupta S; Major LF. Hair loss associated with fluoxetine [letter] *BR J PSYCHIATRY* 1991 Nov; 159:737-8

Guthrie S; Grunhaus L. Fluoxetine-induced stuttering [letter-comment] (Comment in: *J CLIN PSYCHIATRY* 1990 Jul:51(7):310-1) *J CLIN PSYCHIATRY* 1990 Feb:51(2):85

Hadley A; Cason MP. Mania resulting from lithium-fluoxetine combination [letter] *AM J PSYCHIATRY* 1989 Dec;146(12):1637-8 [Substance-induced psychoses, manic disorder chemically induced.]

Hahn SM; Griffin JH. Comment: fluoxetine adverse effects and drug interactions [letter] *DICP* 1991 Nov;25(11):1273-4

Halman M; Goldbloom DS. Fluoxetine and neuroleptic malignant syndrome. *BIOL PSYCHIATRY* 1990 Sep 15:28(6):518-21

Hansen TE; Dieter K; Keepers GA. Interaction of fluoxetine and pentazocine [letter] *AM J PSYCHIATRY* 1990 Jul:147(7):949-50

Herman JB; Brotman AW; Pollack MH; Falk WE; Biederman J; Rosenbaum JF. Fluoxetine-induced sexual dysfunction. *J CLIN PSYCHIATRY* 1990 Jan:51(1):25-7

Hersh CB ; Sokol MS : Pfeffer CR. Transient psychosis with fluoxetine [letter] *J AM ACAD CHILD ADOLESC PSYCHIATRY* 1991 Sep:30(5):851-2 (Substance induced psychosis by Prozac.)

Hoehn-Saric R; Lipsey JR; McLeod DR. Apathy and indifference in patients on fluoxamine and fluoxetine. *J CLIN PSYCHOPHARMACOL* 1990 Oct:10(5):343-5 (Chemically induced impulsive behavior and fatigue.)

Hoehn-Saric R; Harris GJ; Pearlson GD; Cox CS; Machlin SR; Camargo EE. A fluoxetine-induced frontal lobe syndrome in an obsessive compulsive patient. *J CLIN PSYCHIATRY* 1991 Mar:52(3):131-3

Hon D; Preskorn SH. Mania during fluoxetine treatment for recurrent depression [letter] *AM J PSYCHIATRY* 1989 Dec:146(121638-9

Humphries JE; Wheby MS; VandenBerg SR. Fluoxetine and the bleeding time. *ARCH PATHOL LAB MED* 1990 Jul:114(7):727-8

Hwang AS; Magraw RM. Syndrome of inappropriate secretion of antidiuretic hormone due to fluoxetine [letter] *AM J PSYCHIATRY* 1989 Mar:146(3):399

Jafri AB; Greenberg WM. Fluoxetine side effects [letter] *J AM ACAD CHILD ADOLESC PSYCHIATRY* 1991 Sep:30(5):852(Patient with depression has mania chemically induced by Prozac.)

Jenike MA. Severe hair loss associated with fluoxetine use [letter] *AM J PSYCHIATRY* 1991 Mar:148(3):392

Jerome L. Hypomania with fluoxetine [letter] *J AM ACAD CHILD ADOLESC PSYCHIATRY* 1991 Sep:30(5):850-1 (Manic disorders are chemically induced with Prozac.)

Kahn DG. Increased plasmanortriptyline concentration in a patient co-treated with fluoxetine [letter] *J CLIN PSYCHIATRY* 1990 Jan:51(1):36

Koizumi H. Fluoxetine and suicidal ideation [letter] *J AM ACAD CHILD ADOLESC PSYCHIATRY* 1991 Jul:30(4):695

Lebegue B. Mania precipitated by fluoxetine [letter] *AM J PSYCHIATRY* 1987 Dec:144(12):1620

Lensgraf SJ; Favazza AR. Antidepressant-induced mania [letter] *AM J PSYCHIATRY* 1990 Nov:147(11):1569 (Adverse effects of mania, organic mental disorders chemically induced.)

Levinson ML; Lipsy RJ; Fuller DK. Adverse effects and drug interactions associated with fluoxetine therapy. *DICP* 1991 Jun:25(6):657-61 ("Although fluoxetine has been promoted as a safe antidepressant, a recent literature search revealed a number of case reports of adverse effects and drug interactions attributed to its use. This review familiarizes healthcare professionals with some of the currently known interactions and adverse effects and suggests ways of avoiding such events in clinical practice." ADVERSE EFFECTS/SUICIDE)

Lipinski JF Jr; Mallya G; Zimmerman P; Pope HG Jr. Fluoxetine-induced akathisia: clinical and theoretical implications [see comments] (Comment in: *J CLIN PSYCHIATRY* 1990 May:51(5):210-2; Comment in: *J CLIN PSYCHIATRY* 1990 May:51(5):212) *J CLIN PSYCHIATRY* 1989 Sep;50(9):339-42

Lock JD; Gwirtsman HE; Targ EF. Possible adverse drug interactions between fluoxetine and other psychotropics [letter] *J CLIN PSYCHOPHARMACOL* 1990 Oct:10(5):383-4

Lyiard RB; George MS. Fluoxetine and anorgasmia [obsessive-compulsive disorder][letter] *AM J PSYCHIATRY* 1989 Jun;146(6):804-5

Mandalos GE; Szarek BL. Dose-related paranoid reaction associated with fluoxetine. *J NERV MENT DIS* 1990 Jan:178(1):57-8

Mann JJ; Kapur S. The emergence of suicidal ideation and behavior during antidepressant pharmacotherapy. *ARCH GEN PSYCHIATRY* 1991 Nov:48(11):1027-33

March JS; Moon RL; Johnston H. Fluoxetine-TCA interaction [letter] *J AM ACAD CHILD ADOLESC PSYCHIATRY* 1990 Nov:29(6):985-6

Marik PE; van Heerden W; Steenkamp V. Fluoxetine-induced syndrome of inappropriate antidiuretic hormone excretion [letter] *S AFR MED J* 1990 Dec 15:78(12):760-1

Mars F; Dumas de la Roque G; Goissen P. Acute hepatitis during treatment with fluoxetine [letter] *GASTROENTEROL CLIN BIOL* 1991;15(3):270-1

Masand P; Gupta S; Dewan M. Suicidal ideation related to fluoxetine treatment [letter] *N ENGL J MED* 1991 Feb 7:324(6):420

Matthew P; Quinn D; Marcoux GS; Falkenberg K. Fluoxetine and neuroleptic synergistic effects [letter] *J AM ACAD CHILD ADOLESC PSYCHIATRY* 1991 Jan:30(1):154-5

McGrath BJ; Stoukides CA. Fluoxetine and suicidal ideation. *DICP* 1991 Jun:25(6):607-9

Metz A; Shader RI. Adverse interactions encountered when using trazodone (Deseryl) to treat insomnia associated with fluoxetine. *INT CLIN PSYCHOPHARMACOL* 1990 Jul:5(3):191-4

Metz A. Interaction between fluoxetine and buspirone [letter] *CAN J PSYCHIATRY* 1990 Nov:35(8):722-3

Miller LG; Bowman RC; Mann D; Tripathy A. A case of fluoxetine-induced serum sickness *AM J PSYCHIATRY* 1989 Dec:146(12):1616-7

Mirow S. Cognitive dysfunction associated with fluoxetine [letter] *AM J PSYCHIATRY* 1991 Jul:148(7):948-9.

Modell JG. Repeated observations of yawning, clitoral engorgement, and orgasm associated with fluoxetine administration [letter] [see comments] (Comment in: *J CLIN PSYCHOPHARMACOL* 1989 Oct:9(5):384) *J CLIN PSYCHOPHARMACOL* 1989 Feb:9(1):63-5

Montgomery SA; Gabriel R; James D; Hawley C; Burkitt P. The specificity of the zimelidine reaction. *INT CLIN PSYCHOPHARMACOL* 1989 Jan;4(1):19-23

Montgomery SA; Gabriel R; James D; Hawley C; Burkitt P. Hypersensitivity to zimelidine without cross reactivity to fluoxetine. *INT CLIN PSYCHOPHARMACOL* 1989 Jan;4 Suppl 1:27-9

Nakra BR; Szwabo P; Grossberg GT. Mania induced by fluoxetine [letter] *AM J PSYCHIATRY* 1989 Nov;146(11):1515-6

Neill JR. Penile anesthesia associated with fluoxetine use [letter] *AM J PSYCHIATRY* 1991 Nov:148(11):1603 (Impotence and penile diseases are chemically induced.)

378

Nguyen T; Middleton RK. Fluoxetine in bulemia. School of Pharmacy, University of California, San Francisco 94143.

Odenheimer GL. Management of patients with Alzheimer's disease. *PHARMACOTHERAPY* 1991:11(3):237-41

Olfson M; Wilner MT. A family case history of fluoxetine-induced skin reactions. *J NERV MENT DIS* 1991 Aug:179(8):504-5

Ooi TK. The serotonin syndrome [letter] *ANESTHESIA* 1991 Jun:46(6):507-8.

Pearson HJ. Interaction of fluoxetine with carbamazepine (Tegritol) [letter; comment] (Comment on: *J CLIN PSYCHIATRY* 1989 Jun:50(6):226-7) *J CLIN PSYCHIATRY* 1990 Mar:51(3):126

Preskorn SH; Beber JH; Faul JC; Hirschfeld RM. Serious adverse effects of combining fluoxetine and tricyclic antidepressants [letter] *AM J PSYCHIATRY* 1990 Apr:147(4):532 (Adverse effects of Prozac and tricyclic chemically induced delirium and epilepsy.)

Reccoppa L; Welch WA; Ware MR. Acute dystonia and fluoxetine [letter] *CLIN PSYCHIATRY* 1990 Nov:51(11):487

Reed SM; Glick JW. Fluoxetine and reactivation of the herpes simplex virus [letter] *AM J PSYCHIATRY* 1991 Jul:148(7):949-50

Rosenthal E; Bodokh I; Chichmanian RM; Pesce A; Vinti H; Reboulot B; Cassuto JP. Lyell's syndrome in 2 HIV infected patients... *PRESSE MED* 1991 Sep 28:20(30):1459

Sacristan JA; Iglesias C; Arellano F; Lequerica J. Absence seizures induced by lithium; possible interaction with fluoxetine [letter], *AM J PSYCHIATRY* 1991 Jan:148(1):146-7

Settle EC Jr; Settle GP. A case of mania associated with fluoxetine. *AM J PSYCHIATRY* 1984 Feb:141(2):280-1 [A depressed woman with no history of mania experienced an episode during treatment with Prozac. "This side effect appears to be a universal property of effective antidepressants, including this new, purely serotonergic agent."]

Sholomskas AJ. Mania in a panic disorder patient treated with fluoxetine [letter] *AM J PSYCHIATRY* 1990 Aug:147(8):1090-1

Skowron DM; Gutierrez MA; Epstein S. Precaution with titrating nortriptyline *after* the use of fluoxetine [letter] *DICP* 1990 Oct:24(10):1008

Spier SA; Frontera MA. Unexpected deaths in depressed medical inpatients treated with fluoxetine. *J CLIN PSYCHIATRY* 1991 Sep:52(9):377-82 (Complications, arrhythmia, mortality, sudden death, brought on through the adverse effect of toxicity in elderly patient and mortality caused through complications of lung diseases in middle aged patient.)

Staab JP; Yerkes SA; Cheney EM; Clayton AH. Transient SIADH associated with fluoxetine [letter] *AM J PSYCHIATRY* 1990 Nov:147(11):1569-70

Stein MH. Tardive dyskinesia in a patient taking haloperidol and fluoxetine [letter] *AM J PSYCHIATRY* 1991 May;148(5):683

Steiner W; Fontaine R. Toxic reaction following the combined administration of fluoxetine and L-tryptophan: five case reports. *BIOL PSYCHIATRY* 1986 Sep:21(11):1067-71

Steiner W. Fluoxetine-induced mania in a patient with obsessive-compulsive disorder [letter] *AM J PSYCHIATRY* 1991 Oct:148:(10):1403-4

Sternbach H. The serotonin syndrome. *AM J PSYCHIATRY* 1991 Jun:148(6):705-13 ("The serotonin syndrome is most commonly the result of the interaction between serotonergic agents and monoamine oxidase inhibitors. The most frequent clinical features are changes in mental status, restlessness, myoclonus, hyperreflexia, diaphoresis, shivering, and tremor…The incidence of the syndrome is not known…Discontinuation of the suspected agent..typically resolves [it], but confusion can last for days, and death has been reported. The serotonin syndrome is a toxic condition requiring heightened clinical awareness for prevention, recognition, and prompt treatment. Further work is needed to establish the diagnostic criteria, incidence, and predisposing factors…"

Stoll AL; Cole JO; Lukas SE. A case of mania as a result of fluoxetine-marijuana interaction [letter] *J CLIN PSYCHIATRY* 1991 Jun:52(6):280-1

Stoukides JA; Stoukides CA. Extrapyramidal symptoms upon discontinuation of fluoxetine [letter] *AM J PSYCHIATRY* 1991 Sep:148(9):1263 (Chemically induced basal ganglia diseases, dystonia, substance withdrawal syndrome, torticollis produced in conjunction with Prozac.)

Suchowersky O; deVries J. Possible interactions between deprenyl and Prozac [letter] *CAN J NEUROL SCI* 1990 Aug:17(3):352-3 (Complications produce Parkinson's Disease.)

Tanquary J; Masand P. Paradoxical reaction to buspirone augmentation of fluoxetine [letter] *J CLIN PSYCHOPHARMACOL* 1990 Oct:10(5):377

Tate JL. Extrapyramidal symptoms in a patient taking haloperidol and fluoxetine [letter] [see comments] (Comment in: *AM J PSYCHIATRY* 1989 Oct:146(10):1352-3)*AM J PSYCHIATRY* 1989 Mar:146(3):399-400

Turner SM; Jacob RG; Beidel DC; Griffin S. A second case of mania associated with fluoxetine [letter] *AM J PSYCHIATRY* 1985 Feb:142(2):274-5

Vincent A; Douville M; Baruch P. Serum sickness induced by fluoxetine [letter] *AM J PSYCHIATRY* 1991 Nov:148(11):1602-3

Vishwanath BM; Navalgund AA; Cusano W; Navalgund KA. Fluoxetine as a cause of SIADH [Letter] *AM J PSYCHIATRY* 1991 Apr:148(4):542-3

Ware MR; Stewart RB. Seizures associated with fluoxetine therapy [letter] *DICP* 1989 May:23(5):428

Weber JJ. Seizure activity associated with fluoxetine therapy. *CLIN PHARM* 1989 Apr:8(4):296-8

Yaryura-Tobias JA; Kirschen H; Ninan P; Mosberg HJ. Fluoxetine and bleeding in obsessive-compulsive disorder [letter] *AM J PSYCHIATRY* 1991 Jul:148(7):949

Absence seizures induced by lithium; possible interaction with fluoxetine [letter] (Epilepsy, absence/chemically induced with fluoxetine-lithium combination.)

Acquired abnormalities of platelet function [letter;comment] (Comment on: *N ENGL J MED* 1991 Jan 3;324(1):27-39) In: *N ENGL J MED* 1991 Jun 6;324(23):1670-2 [Chemically induced blood platelet disorders-platelet aggregation, skin temperature - adverse effects of Prozac.]

Additional cases of suicidal ideation associated with fluoxetine [letter; comment] (Comment on: *AM J PSYCHIATRY* 1990 Feb:147(2):207-10] *AM J PSYCHIATRY* 1990 Nov:147(11):1570-1

If the reader would like more case reports to investigate relating to the adverse effects which are chemically induced by Prozac [fluoxetine], please refer to the over 28,000 case reports of adverse reactions in the files of the United States Food and Drug Administration Office, Washington, D.C.

REFERENCES AND RECOMMENDED READING

Truth helps us unravel the mysteries of life and makes the problems posed by life easier to overcome. Truths can be found in all the great writings we have available to us. We should learn of one another and have an "unquenchable thirst" for all truth. We have so many wonderfully informative books available to us that it is difficult to single out only a few. I encourage you to read as much as possible from the sources where I have gleaned this information.

Aghajanian GK, Foote WE, Sheard MH: Action of psychotogenic drugs on midbrain raphe neurons. *J PHARMACOL EXP THER* 171:178-187, 1970.

Aghajanian GK, Foote WE, Sheard MH: Lysergic acid diethylamide: sensitive neuronal units in the midbrain raphe. *Science* 161:706-708, 1968.

Akindele MO, Evans JI, Oswald I. Monoamine oxidase inhibitors, sleep and mood. *EEG CLIN NEUROPHYSIOL* 1970;29:47-56.

Alcena, V., & Alexopoulos, G.S. (1985). Ulcerative colitis in association with chronic paranoid schizophrenia: A review of steroid-induced psychiatric disorders. *JOURNAL OF CLINICAL GASTROENTEROLOGY*, 7(5), 400-404.

Alpert, E., & Seigerman, C. (1986). Steroid withdrawal psychosis in a patient with closed head injury. *ARCHIVES OF PHYSICAL MEDICINE AND REHABILITATION*, 67, 766-769.

Anderson GM, Minderaa RB, van Bentem PPG, et al: Platelet imipramine binding in autistic subjects. *PSYCHIATRY RES* 11:133-141, 1984.

Anderson GM, Minderaa RB, Cho SC, et al: The issue of hyperserotonemia and platelet serotonin exposure: a preliminary study. *J AUTISM DEV DISORD* 19:349-351, 1989.

Anderson GM, Freedman DX, Cohen DJ, et al: Whole blood serotonin in autistic and normal subjects. *J CHILD PSYCHOL PSYCHIATRY* 28:885-900, 1987.

Angelieri F. Partial epilepsies and nocturnal sleep. In: Levin P, Koella WP (eds.) *SLEEP 1974.* Basel: Karger, 1975:196-203.

Angst J. Recurrent brief depression. A new concept of mild depression. In: Abstracts of the XVIth CINP congress, Munich. *PSYCHOPHARMACOLOGY* 1988; 96: (suppl): 123.

Annitto, W.J., & Layman, W.A. (1980). Anabolic steroids and acute schizophrenic episode. *JOURNAL OF CLINICAL PSYCHIATRY*, 41(4), 143-144.

Appleton, Nancy. *LICK THE SUGAR HABIT*, New York; Avery, 1988.

Archer, J. (1991). The influence of testosterone on human aggression. *BRITISH JOURNAL OF PSYCHOLOGY*, 82, 1-28.

Arne'-Bes MC, Calvet U, Thilbege M, Arbus L. Effects of sleep deprivation in an EEG study of epileptics. In: Sterman MB, Shouse MN. Passouant P (eds.) *SLEEP AND EPILEPSY.* New York: Academic Press, 1982:339-346.

Asberg M, Thoren P, Traskman L: 5HIAA in the cerebrospinal fluid - a biochemical suicide predictor? *ARCH GEN PSYCHIATRY* 33:1193-1197, 1976.

Asberg M, Bertilsson L, Tuck JR, et al. Indoleaminic metabolites in the cerebrospinal fluid of depressed patients before and during treatment with nortriptyline. *CLIN PHARMACOL THER* 14:277-286, 1973.

Askenasy JJ, Weitzman ED, Yahr MD. Rapid eyemovements - Expression of a general muscular phasic event of the REM state. *SLEEP RES* 1983;12:172.

Atsumi Y, Kohima T, Matsu'ura M et al. Polygraphic study of altered consciousness - Effect of biperiden on EEG and EOG. *ANN REP RES PSYCHOTROP DRUGS* 1977;9:171-178 (in Japanese).

Baldessarini, R. J. & Marsh, E. (1990), Fluoxetine and side effects (letter). *ARCH. GEN. PSYCHIATRY,* 47:191-192.

Ballenger J, Goodwin F, Major L, et al: Alcohol and central serotonin metabolism in man. *ARCH GEN PSYCHIATRY,* 36:224-227, 1979.

Balster, Robert L. Clinical Implications of Behavioral Pharmacology Research on Phencyclidine, in: Clouet, Doris H., Ph.D. ed. *PHENCYCLIDINE: AN UPDATE,* National Institute of Drug Abuse Research Monograph Series 64, 1986.

Banki CM, Arato M. Amine metabolites and neuro endocrine responses related to depressions and suicide. *J AFFECT DIS* 1983; 5: 223-232.

Barbaras G, Ferrari M, Schemp P et al. Childhood migraine and somnambulism. *NEUROLOGY* 1983;33:948-949.

Bargmann, Eve, M.D., Wolfe, Sidney M., M.D., Levin, Joan, and The Public Citizen Health Research Group, *STOPPING VALIUM and Ativan, Centrax, Dalmane, Librium, Paxipam, Restoril, Serax, Tranxene, Xanax,* 1982.

Barker SA, Monti JA, Christian ST. N,N-Dimethyltryptamine: an endogenous hallucinogen. *Int Rev Neurobiol* 22:83-110, 1981.

Barker, S. (1987). Oxymetholone and aggression. *BRITISH JOURNAL OF PSYCHIATRY,* 151, 564.

Bechinger D, Kriebel J, Schlager M. EEG following sleep deprivation. An important tool for diagnosis of epileptic seizures. *Z NEUROL* 1973; 205:193-206.

Benson, Herbert, *YOUR MAXIMUM MIND,* (New York: Times Book, 1987), pp. 6-7, 9, 46.) Note: Dr. Benson is Associate Professor of Medicine at the Harvard Medical School and Chief of the Section on Behavioral Medicine at the New England Deaconess Hospital.)

Bental E, Lavie P, Scharf B. Severe hypermotility during sleep in treatment of cataplexy with clomipramine. *ISR J MED SCI* 1979;15:607-609.

Bergstrom RF, Peyton AL, Lemberger L. Quantification and mechanism of the fluoxetine and tricyclic antidepressant interaction, *CLINCIAL PHARMACOLOGY AND THERAPEUTICS,* Vol. 51, 3:239-248, 1992.

Bertilsson L, Tuck JR, Siwers B. Biochemical effects of zimelidine in man. *EUR J CLIN PHARMACOL* 18:483-487, 1980.

Bertilsson L, Asberg M, Thoren P. Differential effect of chlorimipramine and nortriptyline on cerebrospinal fluid metabolites of serotonin and noradrenaline in depression. *EUR J CLIN PHARMACOL* 7:365-368, 1974.

Besset A. Effect of antidepressants and sleep. *ADV BIOSCI* 1978;21:141-148.

Bjerkenstedt L, Edman G, Flyckt L, et al. Clinical and biochemical effects of citalopram, a selective 5HT reuptake inhibitor - a dose-response study in depressed patients. *PSYCHOPHARMACOLOGY* (Berlin) 87:253-259, 1985a.

Blandina P, Goldfarb J, Craddock-Royal B, et al. Release of endogenous dopamine by stimulation of 5-hydroxytryptamine receptors in rat striatum. *J PHARMACOL EXP THER* 1989;251:803-809.

Blaustein, Mordecai P., Bartschat, Dieter K., Sorensen, Roger G. Phencyclidine (PCP)

Selectively Blocks Certain Presynaptic Potassium Channels in: Clouet, Doris H., Ph.D. ed. *PHENCYCLIDINE: AN UPDATE*, National Institute of Drug Abuse Research Monograph Series 64, 1986.

Blier, P. et al. (1988), Electrophysiological assessment of the effects of anti-depressant treatments on the efficacy of 5-Ht neurotransmission. *CLIN. NEURO-PHARMACOLOGY*, 11(Suppl. 2):S1-S10.

Blier, P., de Montigny, C., Chaput, Y. (1987), Modifications of the serotonin system by antidepressant treatments: implications for the therapeutic response in major depression. *J CLIN PSYCHOPHARMACAL.* 7:24S-35S.

Blier, P. et al. (1990), A role for the serotonin system in the mechanism of action of antidepressant treatments: preclinical evidence. *J. CLIN. PSYCHIATRY*, 51:14-20.

Boarder MR. The mode of action of indoleamine and other hallucinogens, in *ESSAYS IN NEUROCHEMISTRY AND NEUROPHARMACOLOGY*, Vol 2. Edited by Youdim MBH, Lovenberg W, Sharman DF, et al. New York, John Wiley, 1977, pp 21-48.

Borman, M.C., & Schmallenberg, J.C. (1951). Suicide following cortisone treatment. *JOURNAL OF THE AMERICAN MEDICAL ASSOCIATION*, 146, 337-338.

Bost RO, Kemp PM. A Possible Association Between Fluoxetine Use and Suicide, *JOURNAL OF ANALYTICAL TOXICOLOGY*. Vol. 16, March/April, 1992.

Bouchard RH, Pourcher E, Vincent P. Fluoxetine and extrapyramidal side effects. *AM J PSYCHIATRY* 1989;146:1352-1353.

Bowden CL, Koslow SH, Hanin I, et al. Effects of amitriptyline and imipramine on brain amine neurotransmitter metabolites in cerebrospinal fluid. *CLIN PHARMACOL THER* 37:316-324, 1985.

Bowersox SS, Drucker-Colin R. Seizure modification by sleep deprivation: A possible protein synthesis mechanism. In: Sterman MB,

Shouse MN. Passouant P (eds.) *SLEEP AND EPILEPSY*. New York: Academic Press, 1982:91-104.

Brandes L, et al. Stimulation of Malignant Growth in Rodents by Antidepressant Drugs at Clinically Relevant Doses, *CANCER RES.* July 1992.

Brawley P, Duffield JC. The pharmacology of hallucinogens. *PHARMACOL REV* 24:31-66, 1972.

Brecher, Harold and Arline. *FORTY SOMETHING FOREVER, A Consumer's Guide to Chelation Therapy and Other Heart Savers*, Health Savers Press, 1992.

Brennan D, MacManus M, Howe J, et al: "Neuroleptic malignant syndrome" without neuroleptics (letter). *BR J PSYCHIATRY* 1988; 152:578-579.

Brink, Susan, "Singing the Prozac blues", *U.S. NEWS & WORLD REPORT*, November 8, 1993

Brod TM. Fluoxetine and extrapyramidal side effects. *AM J PSYCHIATRY* 1989;146:1352-1353.

Brody, S. (1952). Psychiatric observations in patients treated with cortisone and ACTH. *PSYCHOSOMATIC MEDICINE*, 14, 94-103.

Brosen K, Skjelbo E: Fluoxetine and norfluoxetine are potent inhibitors of P450IID6 - The source of sparteine/debrisoquin oxidation polymorphism. *BR J CLIN PHARMACOL* 36:136-137, 1991.

Brower, K.J., Blow, F.C., Bereford, T.P., & Fuelling, C. (1989). Anabolic androgenic steroids and suicide. *JOURNAL OF CLINICAL PSYCHIATRY*, 50(1), 31-33.

Brower, K.J., Blow, F.C., Eliopulos, G.A., & Beresford, T.P. (1989). Anabolic androgenic steroids and suicide. *AMERICAN JOURNAL OF PSYCHIATRY*, 146(8), 1075.

Brower, K.J., Blow, F.C., Young, J.P., & Hill, E.M. (1991). Symptoms and correlates of anabolic-androgenic steroid dependence.

BRITISH JOURNAL OF ADDICTION, 86,759-768.

Brower, K.J., Eliopulos, G.A., Blow, F.C., Catlin, D.H., & Bereford, T.P. (1990). Evidence for physical and psychological dependence on anabolic-androgenicsteroids in eight weight lifters. AMERICANJOURNALOF PSYCHIATRY, 147(4), 510-512.

Brower, K.J. (1989). Rehabilitation for anabolic-androgenic steroid dependence. CLINICAL SPORTS MEDICINE, 1, 171-181.

Brown, G..L., Ebert, M.H.,Goyer, P,F., Jimerson, D.C., Klein, W.J., Bunney,W.E.,& Goodwin , F.K. (1982). Aggression, suicide, and serotonin: Relationships of CSF amine metabolites. AM. J. PSYCHIATRY, 139,741-746.

Brown, G.L., Linnoila, M. & Goodwin, F. K. (1990), Clinical assessment of human aggression and impulsivity in relation-ship to biochemical measures. In: VIOLENCE AND SUICIDALITY: PERSPECTIVESIN CLINICAL AND PSYCHO-BIOLOGICALRESEARCH, eds. H. M. van Pragg, R. Plutchik & A. Apter. New York: Brunner & Mazel, pp. 184-217.

Brown, G.L., Goodwin, F.K., Ballenger, J.C., Goyer, P.F., & Major, L.F. (1979). Aggression in humans correlates with cerebrospinal fluid amine metabolites. PSYCHIATRYRESEARCH, 1, 131-139.

Browne,Ronald G. Discriminative Stimulus Properties of PCP Mimetics in: Clouet, Doris H., Ph.D. ed. PHENCYCLIDINE: AN UPDATE, National Institute of Drug Abuse Research MonographSeries 64, 1986.

Browning WN. Exacerbation of symptoms of multiple sclerosis in a patient taking fluoxetine. AMER J PSYCHIATRY 147; 1089 (1990).

Burns R.S.; Lerner S.E. The effects of PCP in man: A review. In: Domino, E.F. ed. PCP (PHENCYCLIDINE): HISTORICAL AND CURRENT PERSPECTIVES. Michigan: NPP Books, 1981. pp. 449-469.

Burns, R.S.; Lerner, S.E.; Corrado, R.; James,

S.H.; Schnoll, S.H. Phencyclidine--states of acute intoxication and fatalities. WEST J MED 123(5):345-349,1975.

Burns and Lerner, Guest Editors, CLINICAL TOXICOLOGY, Aug. 1976.

Burroughs, Stanley, HEALING FOR THE AGE OF ENLIGHTENMENT, 1976.

Buterbaugh, Gary G. & Michelson, Hillary B. AnticonvulsantProperties of Phencyclidineand Ketamine in: Clouet, Doris H., Ph.D. ed. PHENCYCLIDINE: AN UPDATE, National Institute of Drug Abuse Research Monograph Series 64, 1986.

Buus, Lassen, J., R. F. Squires, J. A. Christensen and L. Molander. Neurochemical and pharmacological studies on a new 5-HT-uptake inhibitor, FG 4963, with potential antidepressant properties. PSYCHOPHARMACOLOGIA 42:21-26, 1975.

Byyny, R.L. (1976). Withdrawal from glucocorticoid therapy. NEW ENGLAND JOURNAL OF MEDICINE, 295(1), 30-32.

Cadilhac J. Tricyclics and REM sleep. In: Guilleminault C, Dement WC, Passouant P, eds. NARCOLEPSY, New York: Spectrum, 1976:605-624.

Cadilhac J. Complex partial seizures and REM sleep. In Sterman MB, Shouse MN, Passouant P (eds.) SLEEP AND EPILEPSY. New York: Academic Press, 1982:315-324.

Callahan A., Fava M, Rosenbaum J. Drug Interactions in Psychopharmacology, PSYCHIATRIC CLINICS OF NORTH AMERICA, Vol. 16, Num. 3, Sept. 1993, p. 647-671.

Caporael, LR. Ergotism: The Satan loosed in Salem?, SCIENCE, (1976), 192, 21-26.

Carlton PL. Potentiation of the behavioural effects of amphetamines by imipramine. PSYCHOPHARMACOLOGIA 1961;2:364-376.

Cassano GB, Asiskal HS (eds). SEROTONIN-

RELATEDPSYCHIATRICSYNDROMES. Royal Society of Medicine Services, London & New York, 1991.

Cepeda C, Pacheco MT, Cruz ML, Almanza X, Velasco M. Phasic paradoxical sleep precipitates focal motor and limbic seizures. NEUROSCI LETT 1984; 47:179-184.

Charney, D.S., Woods, S.W., Krystal, J.H., & Henninger, G.R. (1990). Serotonin function and human anxiety disorders. ANNALS OF THE NEW YORK ACADEMY OF SCIENCES, 600, 558-573.

Charney DS, Kales A, Soldatos CR et al. Solmnambulistic-like episodes secondary to combined lithium-neuroleptic treatment. BR J PSYCHIATRY 1979; 135:418-424.

Chase MH, Morales FR. Subthreshold excitatory activity and motoneurone discharge during REM periods of active sleep. SCIENCE 1983; 221:1195-1198.

Chase MH. The motor functions of the reticular formation are multifaceted and state-determined. In: Hobson JA, Brazier MAB (eds). THE RETICULAR FORMATION REVISITED. New York: Raven Press, 1980:449-472.

Chen CN. The use of clomipramiine as an REM sleep suppressant in narcolepsy. POSTGRAD MED J 1980;56:86-89.

Choi PYL, Parrott AC, & Cowan D. (1989). Adverse behavioral effects of anabolic steroids in athletes: A brief review. CLINICAL SPORTS MEDICINE, 1, 183-187.

Ciraulo DA, Shader RI. Fluoxetine drug-drug interactions, II: antidepressants and antipsychotics J CLIN PSYCHOPHARMACOL, 1990;10:210-217.

Ciraulo DA, Shader RI. Fluoxetine drug-drug interactions, I: antidepressants and antipsychotics J CLIN PSYCHOPHARMACOL, 1990;147:207-210.

Clark, L.D., Bauer, W., & Cobb, S. (1952). Preliminary observationson mental disturbances occurring in patients under therapy with cortisone and ACTH. NEW ENGLAND JOURNAL OF MEDICINE, 246, 205-216.

CLINICAL TOXICOLOGY in August of 1976 was devoted to it (Burns and Lerner, Guest Editors, 1976)." p.22

Clouet, Doris H., Ph.D. ed. PHENCYCLIDINE: AN UPDATE, National Institute of Drug Abuse Research Monograph Series 64, 1986.

Coccaro, Emil F, Murphy, Dennis L. eds. SEROTONIN IN MAJOR PSYCHIATRIC DISORDERS, American Psychiatric Press, Inc., Washington, DC, London, England, 1990.

Coccaro, E. F., (1989), Central serotonin and impulsive aggression. BR J PSYCHIATRY, 155:(Suppl. 8)52-62.

Cohen HB, Duncan II RF, Dement WC. (1967) SCI. 156:1646.

Cohen JC, Hickman R (1987) Insulin resistance and diminished glucose tolerance in powerlifters ingesting anabolic steroids. JOURNAL OF CLINICAL ENDOCRINOLOGY AND METABOLISM, 64, 960-963.

Collipp, Plant J., The Efficacy of Prayer: A Triple Blind Study, Department of Pediatrics, Meadowbrook Hospital, Meadow, New York, MEDICAL TIMES, May, 1969, Vol. 97, No. 5, pp. 201-203.

Conacher, G.N., & Workman, D.G. (1989). Violent crime possibly associated with anabolic steroid use. AMERICAN JOURNAL OF PSYCHIATRY, 146(5), 679.

Connell PH. Amphetamine psychosis. MAUDSLEY MONOGRAPH. London: Oxford University Press, 1958.

CONSUMER REPORTS, High Anxiety [Xanex], January 1993, p. 19

CONSUMER REPORTS, Miracle Drugs or Media Drugs, March 1992.

CONSUMER REPORTS, Pushing Drugs to

Doctors, February 1992, p. 87-94

Cook, C.E.; Brine, D.R.; Jeffcoat, A.R.; Hill, J.M.; Wall, M.E.; Perez-Reyes, M.; and Di Guiseppi, S.R. Phencyclidine disposition after intravenous and oral doses. *CLIN PHARMACOL THER* 31(5):625-634, 1982a.

Cook, C.E.; Brine, D.R.; Quin, G.D.; Perez-Reyes, M.; and Di Guiseppi, S.R. Phencyclidine and phenylcycloexane disposition after smoking phencyclidine. *CLIN PHARMACOL THER* 31(5):635-641, 1982b.

Cousins, Norman. *ANATOMY OF AN ILLNESS AS PERCEIVED BY THE PATIENT,* 1979, W. W. Norton & Company, New York.

Crawford N, Sutton M, Horsfield GI: Platelets in the carcinoid syndrome: a chemical and ultrastructural investigation. *BR J HAEMATOL* 13:181-188, 1967.

Crowner, Douyon, Convit, Gaztanaga, Volavka, Bakall; Psychopharmacology Bulletin, Vol. 26, No. 1, 1990.
Dasgupta, K., Additional cases of suicidal ideation associated with fluoxetine [letter]. *AM J PSYCHIATRY,* 1990:147:1570

d'Orban, P.T. (1989). Steroid-induced psychosis. *LANCET,* 2, 694.

D'Souza T, Shraberg D. Intracranial hemorrhage associated with amphetamine use. *NEUROLOGY* 1981;31:922-923.

Dabbs, J.M., Frady, R.L., Carr, T.S., Hopper, C.H., & Sgoutas, D.S. (1988). Saliva testosterone and criminal violence among women. *PERSONALITY AND INDIVIDUAL DIFFERENCES,* 9(2), 269-275.

Dabbs JM & Morris R. Testosterone, social class, and antisocial behavior in a sample of 4,462 men. *PSYCHOLOGICAL SCIENCE,* 1, 209-211, 1990.

Dabbs, J.M., Frady, R.L., Carr, T.S., & Besch, N.F. (1987). Saliva testosterone and criminal violence in young adult prison inmates. *PSYCHOSOMATIC MEDICINE,* 49(2), 174-182.

Dahl M, Dam M. Sleep and epilepsy. *ANN CLIN RES* 1985;17:235-242.

Damluji, N.F.& Ferguson, J.M. (1988), Paradoxical worsening of depressive symptomatology caused by antidepressants. *J. CLIN. PSYCHOPHARMACOL.,* 8:347-349.

Dasggupta K. Additional cases of suicidal ideation associated with fluoxetine. *AMER J PSYCHIATRY* 147;1570(1990).

Daskalov DS. Influence of the stages of nocturnal sleep on the activity of a temporal epileptogenic focus. *SOV NEUROL PSYCHIATR* 1975;8:37-45.

Davane CL: Pharmacokinetics of the selective serotonin reuptake inhibitors. *J CLIN PSYCHIATRY* 53(suppl):13-20, 1992.

Davidson, J.M., Camargo, C.A., & Smith, E.R. (1979). Effects of androgen on sexual behavior in hypogonadal men. *JOURNAL OF CLINICAL ENDOCRINOLOGY AND METABOLISM,* 48(6), 955-958.

Declerck AC, Wauquier A, Sijben-Kiggen R, Martens W. A normative study of sleep in different forms of epilepsy. In: Sterman MB, Shouse MN. Passouant P (eds.) *SLEEP AND EPILEPSY.* New York: Academic Press, 1982:329-337.

DeLisi LE, Neckers LM, Weinberger DR, et al: Increased whole blood serotonin concentrations in chronic schizophrenic patients. *ARCH GEN PSYCHIATRY* 38:647-650, 1981.

Depue, R.A., & Spoont, M.R. (1986). Conceptualiziinga serotonin trait: A behavioral dimension of restraint. *ANNALS OF THE NEW YORK ACADEMY OF SCIENCES,* 487,47-62.

DESERET NEWS, "Prozac may not add to risk of bearing defective babies", May 5, 1993.

Dewan MJ, Masand P. Letters to the Editor; Prozac and Suicide, *THE JOURNAL OF FAMILY PRACTICE,* Vol. 33, No. 3 (September, 1991), p. 312.

Dimeff, R., & Malone, D. (1991). Psychiatric disorders in weightlifters using anabolic steroids. *MEDICINE AND SCIENCE IN SPORTS AND EXERCISE*, 23(2) (Suppl.), S18.

Dixon, R.B., & Christy, N.P. (1980). On the various forms of corticosteroid withdrawal syndrome. *AMERICAN JOURNAL OF MEDICINE, 68, 224-230.*

Doctor: Steroid rage led to killing. (1988, June 2). *SUN-SENTINEL* (Ft. Lauderdale, FL).

Doghramji K, Connell TA, Gaddy JR. Loss of REM sleep atonia: Three case reports. *SLEEP RES* 1987;16:327.

Domino, E.F. Neurobiology of Phencyclidine. In: Pfeiffer, C.C., and Smythies, J.R., eds. *INTERNATIONAL REVIEW OF NEUROBIOLOGY ACADEMIC PRESS*, 1964. pp. 79-95

Drake RE, Ehrlich J. Suicide attempts associated with akathisia. *AM J PSYCHIATRY* 1985;142:499-501.

Drieu, K., "Multiplicity of Effects of Ginkgo Giloba Extract: Current Status and New Trends". *EFFECTS OF GINKGO BILOBA EXTRACTS ON ORGANIC CEREBRAL IMPAIRMENT*. John Libbey Eurotext Ltd., 1985.

Eadie, Betty Jean, *EMBRACED BY THE LIGHT*, Gold Leaf Press, Placerville, California, 1992.

Eastman CI, Mistleberger RE, Rechtschaffen A. Suprachiasmatic nuclei lessions eliminate circadian temperature and sleep rhythms in the rat. *PHSYIOL BEHAV* 1984;32:357-368.

Edman, G., Asberg, M., Levander, Sl, & Schalling, D. (1986). Skin conductance habituation and cerebrospinal fluid 5-hydroxyindoleaceticacid in suicidal patients. *ARCHIVES OF GENERAL PSYCHIATRY, 43,* 586-592.

Edmonds LC, Vance ML, Hughes JM. Morbidity form paraspinal dep corticosteroid injections for analgesia: Cushing's syndrome and adrenal suppression. *ANESTH ANALG* June 1991; 72(6):820-822.

Ehret, Arnold. *RATIONAL FASTING,* 1953.

Ehret, Arnold. *THE MUCUSLESS DIET HEALING SYSTEM.*

Emsley, John, "An Unexpectedly Strong Hydrogen Bond: AbInitio Calculations and Spectroscopic Studies of Amide-Fluoride Systems," *JOURNAL OF THE AMERICAN CHEMICAL SOCIETY,* Volume 103, pp. 24-28 (1981).

Epstein AW, Hill W. Ictal phenomena during REM sleep of a temporal lobe epileptic. *ARCH NEUROL* 1966;15:367-375.

Etons, Ursula, *ANGEL DUSTED, A Family's Nightmare,* 1979, MacMillan Publishing.

Ex-player's odd behavior due to steroid use, doctor says. (1988, February 14). *INDIANAPOLIS STAR*, p. B4.

Farnsworth, Dana L. *MENTAL ILLNESS*, In: *THE NEW BOOK OF KNOWLEDGE*, Grolier Inc., Danbury, Connecticut, 1987.

Fauman, M.A., and Fauman, B.J. Violence associated with phencyclidine abuse. *AM J PSYCHIATRY* 136:1584-1586, 1979.

Fava, M & Rosenbaum JF. Suicidality and fluoxetine: Is there a relationship?, *J CLIN PSYCH*, 1991;52;108-111.

Fava, M. & Rosenbaum, J.F. (1990, May) Suicidality and fluoxetine: Is there a relationship? (New Research Abstract #475). Presented at the Annual Meeting of the American Psychiatric Association, New York.

Feighner JP, Boyer WF, Tyler DL, et al: Adverse consequences of fluoxetine-MAOI combination therapy. *J CLIN PSYCHIATRY* 1990; 51:222-225.

Finnegan, John, *ADDICTIONS, A NUTRITIONAL APPROACH TO RECOVERY,*

1989, Elysian Arts, Mill Valley, California.

Fischer-Rizzi, Susanne. *COMPLETE AROMATHERAPY HANDBOOK,* Sterling Publishing, New York, 1990.

Fisher C, Kahn E, Edwards A et al. A psycho-physiological study of nightmares and night terrors. I Physiological aspects of the stage 4 terror. *J NERV MENT DIS* 1973; 157:75-98.

Fisher C, Byrne J, Edwards A et al. A psychophysiological study of nightmares. *J AM PSYCHOANAL ASSOC* 1970;1847-1882.

Forman, Jonathon, "What Looks Like a Neurosis May be a Fluorosis," *CLINICAL PHYSIOLOGY,* pp. 245-251 (Winter 1963)

Foss, G.L. (1937). Effect of testosterone propionate on a post-pubertal eunuch. *LANCET,* 2, 1301-1309.

Foster, S., "Ginkgo", Austin, Texas; American Botanical Council, 1990.

Frances H, Raisonan R, Simon P, et al: Lesions of the serotonergic system impair the facilitation of but not the tolerance to the effects of chronic clenbuterol administration. *PSYCHOPHARMACOLOGY* (Berlin) 91:496-499, 1987.

Franchi, F., Luisi, M., & Kicovic, P.M. (1978). Long-term study of oral testosterone undecanoate in hypogonadal males. *INTERNATIONAL JOURNAL OF ANDROLOGY,* 1, 270-278.

Franchimont, P., Kicovic, P.M., Mattei, A., & Roulier, R. (1978). Effects of oral testosterone in hypogonadal male patients. *CLINICAL ENDOCRINOLOGY,* 9, 313-320.

Freedman DX, Giarman NJ. LSD-25 and the status and level of brain serotonin. *ANN NY ACAD SCI* 90:98-107, 1962

Freedman DX. Hallucinogenic drug research - is so, so what? symposium summary and commentary. *PHARMACOL BIOCHEM BEHAV* 24:407-415, 1986.

Freedman DX. Effects of LSD-25 on brain serotonin. *J PHARMACOL EXP THER* 134:160-166, 1961.

Freinhar, J.P., & Alvarez, W. (1985). Androgen-induced hypomania. *JOURNAL OF CLINICAL PSYCHIATRY,* 46(8), 354-355.

Fricchione, G., Ayyala, M., & Holmes, V.F. (1989). Steroid withdrawal psychiatric syndromes. *ANNALS OF CLINICAL PSYCHIATRY,* 1(2), 99-108.

Fuller RW: Serotonergic stimulation of pituitary-adrenocortical function in rats. *NEUROENDOCRINOLOGY* 32:118-127, 1981.

Gaillard J-M. Biochemical pharmacology of paradoxical sleep. *BR J CLIN PHARM* 1983;16:205s-230s.

Garattinis K, Caccia S, Mennini T, et al: The mechanism of action of fenfluramine. *POSTGRAD MED* 1975; 5:27-34.

Gardner D, Cowdry R. Alprazolam-induced dyscontrol in borderline personality disorder. *AM J PSYCHIATRY,* 1985;142:98-100.

Gardner, Richard. *SEX ABUSE HYSTERIA, Salem Witch Trials Revisited,* 1991, Creative Therapeutics.

Gastaut H, Broughton RJ. A clinical and polygraphic study of episodic phenomena during sleep. *BIOL PSYCHIATRY* 1965;7:197-221.

Geller MR, Gourdji N, Christoff N, Fox E. The effects of sleep deprivation of the EEGs of epileptic children. *DEV MED CHILD NEUROL* 1969;11:771-776.

Gillin, JC. The sleep therapies of depression. *PROGRESS IN NEURO-PSYCHOPHARMACOLOGY & BIOLOGICAL PSYCHIATRY,* 7, 351-364, 1983.

Gillin JC, Kaplan J, Stillman R, et al. The psychedelic model of schizophrenia: the case of N,N-dimethyltryptamine. *AM J PSYCHIATRY* 133:203-208, 1976a.

Giroud M, d'Athis P, Guard O, Dumas R. Migraine and somnambulism: A survey of 122 migraine patients. *REV NEUROL* (Paris) 1986;142:42-46.

Glaser, G.H. (1953). Psychotic reactions induced by corticotropin(ACTH) and cortisone. *PSYCHOSOMATIC MEDICINE*, 15(4),289-291.

Glassman JN, Darko D, Gillin JC. Medication-induced somnambulism in a patient with schizoaffective dosorder. *J CLIN PSYCHIATRY* 1986;47(10):523-524.

Goldman, B., Bush, P., & Klatz, R. (1984). *DEATH IN THE LOCKER ROOM: STEROIDS AND SPORTS*. South Bend, IN: Icarus Press.

Goodwin GM, De Souza RJ, Wood AJ, et al: The enhancement by lithium of the 5HT1A mediated serotonin syndrome produced by 8-OH-DPAT in the rat: evidence for a post-synaptic mechanism. *PSYCHOPHARMACOLOGY* (Berlin) 1986; 90:488-493.

Gooren, L.J.F. (1987). Androgen level and sex functions in testosterone treated hypogonadal men. *ARCHIVES OF SEXUAL BEHAVIOR*, 16(6), 463-473.

Gorman, J.M., Liebowitz, M.R., Fyer, A.J. et al. (1087), An open trial of fluoxetine in the treatment of panic attacks. *J. CLIN. PSYCHOPHARMACOL.* 5:329-332.

Gottlieb P, Christensen O, Kramp P. On serious violence during sleepwalking. *BR J PSYCHIATRY* 1986;149:120-121.

Gottschalk L, *RESEARCH COMMUNICATIONS IN PSYCHOLOGY, PSYCHIATRY AND BEHAVIOR*, 1976.

Graedon, Joe, *THE NEW PEOPLE'S PHARMACY #3*, 1985, Bantam Books.

Greenberg R, Pearlman C. Delirium tremens and dreaming. *AM J PSYCHIATRY* 1967;124:37-46.

Greenblatt DJ, Preskorn S, Cotreau M: Fluoxetine impairs clearance of alprazolam but not of clonazepam. *CLIN PHARMACOL*, 1992.

Griffin, LaDean. *PLEASE DOCTOR I'D RATHER DO IT MYSELF... WITH VITAMINS AND MINERALS*, Hawkes Publishing, Salt Lake City, 1979.

Griffin, LaDean. *PLEASE DOCTOR I'D RATHER DO IT MYSELF... WITH HERBS*, Hawkes Publishing, Salt Lake City, 1979.

Griffin, LaDean. *IS ANY SICK AMONG YOU?*, Nature's Sunshine Publications, Springville, Utah, 1973.

Grimsley SR, Jann MW, Carter JG, et al: Increased carbamazepine plasma concentrations after fluoxetine coadministration. *CLIN PHARMACOL THER* 50:10-15, 1991.

Gross MM, Goodenough D, Tobin M et al. Sleep disturbances and halluninations in the acute alcoholic psychosis. *J NERV MENT DIS* 1966;142:493-514.

Grove, V.E. Painless self-injury after ingestion of "angel dust." *JAMA* 242:655, 1979.

Guidham, A. (1940). Treatment of mental disorders with male sex hormone. *BRITISH MEDICAL JOURNAL*, 1, 10-12.

Guilleminault C, Silvestri R. Disorders of arousal and epilepsy during sleep. In: Sterman MB, Shouse MN. Passouant P (eds.) *SLEEP AND EPILEPSY*. New York: Academic Press, 1982:513-531.

Guilleminault C, Raynal D, Takahashi S, Carskadon M, Dement W. Evaluation of short-term and long-term treatment of the narcolepsy syndrome with clomipramine hydrochloride. *ACTA NEUROL SCAND* 1976; 54:71-87.

Haas, H., "Brain Disorders and Vasoactive Substances of Plant Origin", *PLANTA MEDICA SUPPL*. 257-65.

Hall, R.C.W. (1980). *PSYCHIATRIC PRESENTATIONS OF MEDICAL ILLNESS*. New York: Medical and Scientific Books.

Hamaker, John D., *THE SURVIVAL OF CIVILIZATION,* California; Hamaker-Weaver, 1982.

Hamilton MS, Opler LA. Akathisia, Suicidality, and Fluoxetine, *J CLIN PSYCHIATRY.* 53:11, November 1992.

Hamilton, J.B. (1938). Precocious masculine behavior following administration of synthetic male hormone substance. *ENDOCRINOLOGY,* 21, 649-654.

Hanley HG, Stahl SM, Freedman DX: Hyperserotonemia and amine metabolism in autistic and retarded children. *ARCH GEN PSYCHIATRY* 34:521-531, 1977.

Hartman E. Two case reports: Night terrors with sleep-walking a potentially lethal disorder. *J NERV MENT DIS* 1983;171:503-550.

Hays, L.R., Littleton, S., & Stillner, V. (1990). Anabolic steroid dependence. *AMERICAN JOURNAL OF PSYCHIATRY,* 147(1), 122.

Hefez A, Metz L, Lavie P. Long-term effects of extreme situational stress on sleep and dreaming. *AM J PSYCHIATRY* 1987;144:344-347.

Hendricks JC, Lager A, O'Brien D, Morrison AR. Movement disorders during sleep in dogs and cats. *J AM VET MED ASSOC* 1989;194:686-689.

Hendricks JC, Morrison AR, Farnbach GL, Steinberg SA, Mann G. A disorder of rapid eye movement sleep in a cat. *J AM VET MED ASSOC* 1980;178:53-57.

Hendricks JC, Morrison AR, Mann GL. Different behaviors during paradoxical sleep without atonia depend on pontine lesion site. *BRAIN RES* 1982;239:81-105.

Hendricks JC, Bowker RM, Morrison AR. Functional characteristics of cats with pontine lesions during sleep and wakefulness and their usefulness for sleep research. In: *SLEEP* 1976. 3rd European Congress on Sleep Research, Montpellier, Basel:Karger, 1977:207-210.

Henley K, Morrison AR. A re-evaluation of the effects of lesions of the pontine tegmentum and locus coeruleus on phenomena of paradoxical sleep in the cat. *ACTA NEUROBIOL EXP* 1974;34:215-232.

Hermesh H, Molcho A, Munitz H. Successful propranolol therapy for neuroleptic-induced akathisia resistant to anticholinergic and benzodiazepine drugs. *CLIN NEUROPHARMACOL* 1988;11:369-372.

Herrmann, WM,& Beach,RC. (1976). Psychotropic effects of androgens: A review of clinical observations and new human experimental findings. *PHARMAKOPSYCHOLOGIE,* 9, 205-219.

Hickson, RC, Ball, KL, & Falduto, MT. (1989). Adverse effects of anabolic steroids. *MEDICAL TOXICOLOGY AND ADVERSE DRUG EXPERIENCE,* 4(4), 254-271.

Hishikawa Y, Sugita Y, Teshima Y et al. Sleep disorders in alcoholic patients with delirium tremens and transient withdrawal hallucinations - Reevaluation of the REM rebound and intrusion theory. In: Karacan I (ed). *PSYCHOLPHYSIOLOGICAL ASPECTS OF SLEEP.* Park ridge, New Jersey: Noyes Medical Publishers, 1981:109-122.

Hishikawa Y, Sugita Y, Iijima S, Teshima Y, Shimizu T. Mechanisms producint "stage 1-REM and similar dissociations of REM sleep and their relation to delirium. *ADV NEUROL SCI* (Tokyo) 1981;25:1129-1147.

Hobson JA, McCarley RW. The brain as a sleep state generator: an activation synthesis hypothesis of the dream process. *AM J PSYCHIATRY* 1977;134:1335-1348.

Hodge JV, Oates JA, Sjoerdsma A: Reduction of the central effects of tryptophan by a decarboxylase inhibitor. *CLIN PHARMACOL THER* 1964; 5:149-155.

Hoover DE. Additional cases of suicidal ideation associated with fluoxetine [letter]. *AM J PSYCHIATRY,* 1990;147:1570-1571

Houser, BB. (1979). An investigation of the

correlation between hormonal levels in males and mood, behavior and physical discomfort. *HORMONES AND BEHAVIOR*, 12, 185-197.

Hudson JI, Lipinski JF, Frankenburg FR, Grochocinski VJ, Kupfer DJ. Electroencephalographic sleep in mania. *ARCHIVES OF GENERAL PSYCHIATRY,* 45, 267-273, 1988.

Hunsinger RN, Wilson MC: A comparison of the fenfluramine-inducedserotonergicsyndrome in rats subacutely treated with either saline of d-amphetamine.*PHARMACOL RES COMMUN* 1984; 16:579-588.

Hunt, Douglas. *NO MORE CRAVINGS,* 1987, Warner Books, New York.

Hupapya LVM. Seven cases of sleepwalking induced by drugs. *AM J PSYCHIATRY* 1979; 136:985-986.

Huxley, Aldous. *THE DOORS OF PERCEPTION*, New York: Harper & Row, 1954.

Itil, TM, (1976). The neurophysiological models in the development of psychotropic hormones. In T.M. Itil, G. Laudahn, & W. Hermann (Eds.), *PSYCHOTROPIC ACTION OF HORMONES* (PP.53-77). New York: Spectrum.

Itil, TM, Cora, R, Akpinar, S, Herrmann, WM, & Patterson, CJ. (1974). "Psychotropic" action of sex hormones: Computerized EEF in establishing the immediate CNS effects of steroid hormones. *CURRENT THERAPEUTIC RESEARCH*, 16(11), 1147-1170.

Jacobovits, T. (1970). The treatment of impotence with methyltestosteronethyroid (100 patients-double blind study). *FERTILITY AND STERILITY,* 21(1), 32-35.

Jacobs, B. L., Henriksen, S.J., & Dement, W.C. (1972). Neurochemical bases of the PGO wave. *BRAIN RESEARCH,* 48, 406-411.

Jacobs, B.L. (1987). How hallucinogenicdrugs work. *AM. SCIENTIST,* 75, 386-392.

Johnson, Kenneth M. Neurochemical Pharmalcology of Phencyclidine in: Petersen, Robert C., Stillman, Richard C., eds. *PCP PHENCYCLIDINE ABUSE: AN APPRAISAL,* National Institute of Drug Abuse Monograph Series, Research 21, August, 1978.

Jones MT, Hillhouse E, Burden J. (1976): In: *FRONTIERS IN NEUROENDOCRINOLOGY,* Vol. 4, edited by Martini and WF Ganong, pp. 195-226. Raven Press, New York.

Jouven M, Delorme JF. Locus coeruleus et sommeil paradoxal. *CR SOC BIOL* 1965;159:895-899.

Joyce, C.R.B. and Welldon, R.M.C., "The Objective Efficacy of Prayer". *JOURNAL OF CHRONIC DISEASE,* Vol. 18, pp. 367-77, 1965.

Judd, FK, Burrows, GD, & Norman, TR. (1983). Psychosis after withdrawal of steroid therapy.*MEDICAL JOURNAL OF AUSTRALIA*, 2, 350-351.

Kahn A, Mozin MJ, Casmir F, Montauk L, Blum D. Insomnia and cow's milk allergy in infants. *PEDIATRICS* 1985;76:880-884.

Kales A, Constantin R, Soldatos R, Kales JD. Sleep disorders: Insomnia, sleepwalking, night terrors, nightmares, and enuresis.*ANN INTERN MED* 1987:106:582-592.

Kales A, Jacobson A, Paulson MJ et al. Somnambulism:Psychophysiologicalcorrelates. I. All-night EEG studies. *ARCH GEN PSYCHIATRY*1966;14:586-594.

Kales A, Soldatos CR, Caldwell AB et al. Sleepwalking. *ARCH GEN PSYCHIATRY* 1980;37:1406-1410.

Kales JD, Kales A, Soldatos CR, Chamberlin K, Martin ED, Sleepwalking and night terrors related to febrile illness. *AM J PSYCHIATRY* 1979;136:1214-1215.

Karson CN, Newton JE, Livingston R, Jolly JB, Cooper TB, Sprigg J, Komoroski RA. Human brain fluoxetine concentrations, *JOURNAL OF NEUROPSYCHIATRY AND*

CLINICAL NEUROSCIENCES, 5:322-329, 1993.

Kashkin, KB, & Kleber, HD. (1989). Hooked on hormones? An anabolic steroid addiction hypothesis. JOURNAL OF THE AMERICAN MEDICAL ASSOCIATION, 262(22), 3166-3170.

Katz, DL, & Pope, HG. (1990). Anabolic-androgenic steroid-induced mental status changes. In G.C. Lin & L. Erinoff (Eds.), ANABOLIC STEROID ABUSE (NIDA Research Monograph) (pp. 215-223). Rockville, MD: National Institute on Drug Abuse.

Kaufman, S. Hepatic phenylalanine hydroxylase and PKU. In: BRAIN MECHANISMS IN MENTAL RETARDATION, .A. Buchwald & M.A.B. Brazier (eds.), (1975), pp. 445-458, New York: Academic Press.

Kaufmann, M., Kahaner, K., Peslow, ED, Y Gershon, S (1982). Steroid Psychoses: Case report and brief overview. JOURNAL OF CLINICAL PSYCHIATRY, 43(2), 75-76.

Keckich WA. Violence as a manifestation of akathisia. JAMA 1978;240:2185

Kerman, EF. (1943). Testosterone therapy of involutional psychosis. ARCHIVES OF NEUROLOGY AND PSYCHIATRY, 49, 306-307.

Ketcham, Katherine; Mueller, M.D., Ann L. EATING RIGHT TO LIVE SOBER, New York, Writers House, 1983.

Kikuchi S. An electroencephalographic study of nocturnal sleep in temporal lobe epilepsy. FOLIA PSYCHIATR NEUROL JPN 1969;23:59-81.

Kilburn KH, Seidman BC, Warshaw R. Neurobehavioral and respiratory symptoms of formaldehyde and xylene exposure in histology technicians. ARCH ENVIRON HEALTH 1985;40:229-233.

Killing try is blamed on drugs. (1988, June 25). ROANOKE (VA) TIMES, pp. 3-5.

King RA, Riddle MA, Chappell PB, Hardin MT, Anderson GM, Lombroso P, Scahill L. Emergence of Self-Destructive Phenomena in Children and Adolescents during Fluoxetine Treatment, JOURNAL OF THE AMERICAN ACADEMY OF CHILD AND ADOLESCENT PSYCHIATRY, Vol. 30:2, pp. 179-186, 1991.

King RA & Noshpitz JD (1991), PATHWAYS OF GROWTH: ESSENTIALS OF CHILD PSYCHIATRY, Volume 2: Psychopathology. New York: Wiley.

Kline SS, Mauro LS, Scala-Barnett DM, et al: Serotonin syndrome versus neuroleptic malignant syndrome as a cause of death. CLIN PHARM 1989; 8:510-514.

Knowles J, Laverty S, Kuechler H. The effects of alcohol of REM sleep. J STUD ALCOHOL 1968;29:342-349.

Kochakian, CD. (1990). History of anabolic-androgenic steroids. In GC. Lin & L. Erinoff (Eds.), ANABOLIC STEROID ABUSE (NIDA Research Monograph) (pp. 25-29). Rockville, MD: National Institute on Drug Abuse.

Kopera, H. (1985). The history of anabolic steroids and a review of clinical experience with anabolic steroids. ACTA ENDOCRINOLOGICA, 110(Suppl.271), 11-18.

Kramer, Peter. Listening to Prozac, Viking, 1993.

Kreuz LE & Rose RM Assessment of aggressive behavior and plasma testosterone in a young criminal population. PSYCHOSOMATIC MEDICINE, 34, 321-332, 1972.

Lacomblez, L., "Comparative Effects of Ginkgo Biloba Extracts on Psychomotor Performances and Memory in Healthy Subjects", Department de Pharmacologie, Groupe Hospitalier, Pitie-Salpetriere, Division Ambroise Pare, Paris, THERAPIE, 46(1):33-36, Jan.-Feb., 1991.

Laguzzi, R.F., & Adrien, J. (1980). Inversion de l'insomnie produite par la parachlorophenylalanine chez le rat [Relief from insomnia produced by parachlorophenylalanine in the rat]. *ARCHIVES ITALIENNES DE BIOLOGIE,* 118, 109-123.

Landon J, Wynn V, Cooke JN, Kennedy A (1962) Effects of anabolic steroid methandienone, on carbohydrate metabolism in man. *METABOLISM,* 11, 501-512.

Lasher TA, Fleishaker JC, Steenwyk RC, Antal EJ. Pharmacokinetic pharmacodynamic evaluation of the combined administration of alprazolam and fluoxetine. *PSYCHOPHARMACOLOGY* (1991) 104:323-327.

Lasegue C. Le delire alcoolique n'est pas un delire, mais un reve. *ARCH GEN MED* 1881;88:513-536.

Leckman, J.F., Goodman, S.K., Riddle, M.A., Hardin, M.T. & Anderson, G.A., Letter to the Editor: low CSF 5HIAA and obsessions of violence: report of two cases. *PSYCHIATRY RES,* 1990.

Leckman JF & Scahill L. (1990). Possible exacerbation of tics by androgenic steroids. *NEW ENGLAND JOURNAL OF MEDICINE,* 322(23), 1674.

Lee AJ, Fernando JCR, Curzon F. Serotonergic involvement in behavioral responses to amphetamine at high dosage. *NEUROPHARMACOLOGY* 18:153-158, 1978.

Lee, Martin; Shlain, Bruce. *ACID DREAMS,* Grove Press Inc., New York, 1985.

Lemberger L, Bergstrom RF, Wolen RL, dt al: Fluoxetine: Clinical pharmalcology and physiologic disposition. *J CLIN PSYCHIATRY* 46:14-19, 1985.

Lemberger L, Rowe H, Bosomworth JC, et al: The effect of fluoxetine on the pharmacokinetics and psychomotor responses of diazepam. *CLIN PHARMACOL THER* 43:412-419, 1988.

Lemere F. The danger of amphetamine dependence. *AM J PSYCHIATRY* 1966;123:569-572.

Lerma J, Garcia-Austt E. Hippocampal theta rhythm during paradoxical sleep. Effects of afferent stimuli and phase relationships with phasic events. *EEG CLIN NEUROPHYSIOL* 1985;60:46-54.

Lerner, Steven E. & Burns, R. Stanley. Phencyclidine Use Among Youth: History, Epidemiology, and Acute and Chronic Intoxication, in: Petersen, Robert C., Stillman, Richard C., eds. *PCP PHENCYCLIDINE ABUSE: AN APPRAISAL,* National Institute of Drug Abuse Monograph Series, Research 21, August, 1978.

Lesieur P, Saavedra JM, Chiueh CC, et al: Serotonin versus dopamine in prolactin release. Paper presented at the annual meeting of the Society of Biological Psychiatry, Dallas, TX, May 15-19, 1985.

Lewis DA & Smith RE. (1983). Steroid-induced psychiatric syndromes. *JOURNAL OF AFFECTIVE DISORDERS,* 5, 319-322.

Lichtenstein MJ, Yarnell JW, Elwood PC, Beswick AD, Sweetnam PM, Marks V, Teale D, Riad-Fahmy D (1987) Sex hormones, insulin, lipids, and prevalent ischemic heart disease. *AMERICAN JOURNAL OF EPIDEMIOLOGY,* 126, 647-657.

Lieb J, Joseph JP, Engel J, Walker J, Crandall PH. Sleep state and seizure foci related to depth spike activity in patients with temporal lobe epilepsy. *ELECTROENCEPHALOGR CLIN NEUROPHYSIOL* 1980; 49:538-557.

Liebowitz, M.R., Hollander, E., Schneier, F. et al. (1989), Fluoxetine treatment of obsessive-compulsive disorder: an open clinical trial. *J. CLIN. PSYCHOPHARMACOL.* 9:423-427.

Ling MHM, Perry PJ & Tsuang MT. (1981). Side effects of corticosteroid therapy: Psychiatric aspects. *ARCHIVES OF GENERAL PSYCHIATRY,* 38, 471-477.

Linnoila M, Simpson D, Skinner T. Characteristics of therapeutic response to imipramine in cataplectic men. *AM J PSYCHIATRY* 1980;137:237-238.

393

Linnoila M, Virkkunen M, Scheinin M, Nuutila A, Rimon N, Goodwin FK. Low cerbrospinal fluid 5-hydroxyindoleacetic acid concentration differentiates impulsive from non-impulsive violent behavior. LIFE SCI 1983; 33: 2609-14.

Lipinski JF Jr, Mallya G, Zimmerman P, et al. Fluoxetine-induced akathesia: clinical and theoretical implications. J CLIN PSYCHIATRY, 1989:50:339-342

Lipinski, Mallya, Zimmerman, Pope, Journal of Clinical Psychiatry, September 1989

Lock JD, Gwirtsman HE, Targ EF. Possible adverse drug interactions between fluoxetine and other psychotropics. J CLIN PSYCHOPHARMACOL 10:383-384, 1990,

Long, James W., M.D., THE ESSENTIAL GUIDE TO PRESCRIPTION DRUGS 1992.

Lopez-Ibor Jr JJ, Saiz J, Perez de los Cobos JC. Biological correlations of suicide and aggressivity in major depressions (with melancholia): 5-HIAA and cortisol in cerebral spinal fluid, DST and therapeutic response to 5-hydrothrptophan. NEUROPSYCHOBIOLOGY 1985; 154 (suppl): 26-39.

Lopez-Ibor Jr JJ. The involvement of serotonin in psychiatric disorders and behaviour. BR J PSYCHIATRY 1988; 153 (suppl): 26-39.

Lubell A. (1989). Does steroid abuse cause or excuse violence? THE PHYSICIAN AND SPORTSMEDICINE, 17(2), 176-185.

Luisada, Paul V. The Phencyclidine Psychosis: Phenomenology and Treatment in: Petersen, Robert C., Stillman, Richard C., eds. PCP PHENCYCLIDINE ABUSE: AN APPRAISAL, National Institute of Drug Abuse Monograph Series, Research 21, August, 1978.

Luisada, Paul and Brown, Bernard. Clinical Management of Phencyclidine Psychosis. CLINICAL TOXICOLOGY, 9(4): 539-545, 1976)

Lytle, L.D., Messing, R.B., Fisher, L., & Phebus, L. (1975). Effects of long-term corn consumption on brain serotonin and the response to electric shock. SCIENCE, 190, 692-694.

Maccoby EE & Jacklin CN. THE PSYCHOLOGY OF SEX DIFFERENCES. Stanford, CA: Stanford University Press, 1974.

Mahowald MW, Schenck CH. REM sleep behavior disorder. In: Kryger M, Dement W, Roth T (eds). THE PRINCIPLES AND PRACTICE OF SLEEP MEDICINE. Philadelphia: Saunders, 1989:389-401.

Manier DH, Gillespie DD, Sanders-Bush E, et al: The serotonin/-noradrenaline link in brain. I. The role of noradrenaline and serotonin in the regulation of density and function of beta adrenoceptors and its alteration by desipramine. NAUNYN SCHMIEDEBERGS ARCH PHARMACOL 335:109-114, 1987.

Mann, J.J., Arango, V., & Underwood, M.D. (1990). Serotonin and suicidal behavior. ANNALS OF THE NEW YORK ACADEMY OF SCIENCES, 600, 476-485.

Mann, J.J., Stanley, M., McBride, A., & McEwen, B.S. (1986). Increased serotonin and adrenergic receptor binding in the frontal cortices of suicide victims. ARCHIVES OF GENERAL PSYCHIATRY, 43, 954-959.

Marshall KA; Chaplan SR. Adrenal suppression and paraspinal corticosteroids [letter; comment]. ANESTH ANALG Jun 1991;820-822.

Martin, J.R.; Berman, M.H.; Krewsum, I; and Small, S.F. Phencyclidine-induced stereotyped behavior and serotonergic syndrome in rat. LIFE DCI 24:1699-1704, 1979.

Martin PR, Adinoff B, Bone GAH, et al. Fluvoxamine treatment of alcoholic chronic organic brain syndromes. CLIN PHARMACOL THER 41:211, 1987.

Marwah, Joe & Pitts, David K. Psychopharmacology of Phencyclidine in: Clouet, Doris H., Ph.D. ed. PHENCYCLIDINE: AN UPDATE, National Institute of Drug Abuse Research Monograph Series 64, 1986.

Maryland v. Michael David Williams. (1986, April). Circuit Court record for St. Mary's County, pp. 5630-5635.

Masand P, Gupta S, Dewan M. Suicidal ideation related to fluoxetine treatment [letter]. *N ENGL J MED* 1991:324:420

Masson, Jeffrey Moussaieff. *AGAINST THERAPY, Emotional Tyranny and the Myth of Psychological Healing*, 1988, Macmillan Publishing Company.

Matossian MK. Ergot and the Salem witchcraft affair, (1982), *AMERICAN SCIENTIST*, 70, 355-357.

Matsumoto AM. (1988). Is high dosage testosterone an effective male contraceptive agent? *FERTILITY AND STERILITY*, 50, 324-328.

Mawson, A.R., & Jacobs, K.W. (1978). Corn, tryptophan, and homocide. *JOURNAL OF ORTHOMOLECULAR PSYCHIATRY*, 7, 227-230.

Mayanagi Y. The influence of natural sleep on focal spiking in experimental temporal lobe epilepsy in the monkey. *ELECTROENCEPHALOGR CLIN NEUROPHYSIOL* 1977;43:813-824.

Mazur A & Lamb TA. (1980). Testosterone, status, and mood in human males. *HORMONES AND BEHAVIOR*, 14, 236-246.

McCall RB. Neurophysiological effects of hallucinogens on serotonergic neuronal systems. *NEUROSCI BIOBEHAV REV* 6:509-514, 1982.

McCarron, Margaret M. Phencyclidine Intoxication, in: Clouet, Doris H., Ph.D. ed. *PHENCYCLIDINE: AN UPDATE*, National Institute of Drug Abuse Research Monograph Series 64, 1986.

McCarron, M.M.; Schulze, B.W.; Thompson, G.A.; Conder, M.C.; and Goetz, W.A. Acute phencyclidine intoxication: Incidence of clinical findings in 1,000 cases. *ANN EMERG MED* 10:237-242, 1981a.

McCarron, M.M.; Schulze, B.W.; Thompson, G.A.; Conder, M.C.; and Goetz, W.A. Acute phencyclidine intoxication: Clinical patterns, complications, and treatment. *ANN EMERG MED* 10:290-297, 1981b.

McGraw JM (1990). The psychology of anabolic steroid use. *JOURNAL OF CLINICAL PSYCHIATRY*, 51(6), 260.

Meltzer HY: Neuroendocrine abnormalities in schizophrenia: prolactin, growth hormone, and gonadotropins, in *NEUROENDOCRINOLOGY AND PSYCHIATRIC DISORDER*. Edited by Brown GM. New York, Raven Press, 1984, pp 1-28.

Meltzer HY: Biological studies in schizophrenia. *SCHIZOPHRENIA BULLETIN* 13:77-111. 1987.

Meltzer HY, Flemming R, Robertson A: The effect of buspirone on prolactin and growth hormone secretion in man. *ARCH GEN PSYCHIATRY* 40:1099-1102, 1983.

Meltzer HY, Lowery M, Robertson A et al: Effect of 5-hydroxytryptophan serum cortisol levels in major affective disorders. III. Effect of antidepressants and lithium carbonate. *ARCH GEN PSYCHIATRY* 41:391-397, 1984a.

Meltzer HY, Lowy MT: The serotonin hypothesis of depression, in *PSYCHOPHARMACOLOGY: THE THIRD GENERATION OF PROGRESS*. Edited by Meltzer HY. New York, Raven Press, 1987, pp 513-526.

Meltzer HY, Perline R, Tricou BJ, et al: Effect of 5-hydroxytryptophan serum cortisol levels in major affective disorders. II. Relation to suicide, psychosis, and depressive symptoms. *ARCH GEN PSYCHIATRY* 41:379-387, 1984b.

Meltzer HY, Simonovic M, Ravitz AJ: Effect of psychotomimetic drugs on rat and human prolactin and growth hormone levels, in *HANDBOOK OF PSYCHIATRY AND ENDOCRINOLOGY*, Edited by Beumont PJV, Burrows GD. New York, Elsevier Biomedical, 1982a, pp 215-238.

Meltzer HY, Umberkoman-Wiita B, Robertson A, et al: Effect of 5-hydrotryptophanon serum cortisol levels in major affective disorders. I. Enhanced responce in depression and mania. *ARCH GEN PSYCHIATRY* 41:366-374, 1984c.

Meltzer HY, Witta B, Tricou BJ, et al: Effect of serotonin precursors and serotonin agonists on plasma hormone levels, in *SEROTOIN IN BIOLOGICAL PSYCHIATRY.* Edited by Ho BT, Schooler JC, Usdin E. New York, Raven Press, 1982b, pp 117-136.

Mendelsohn, Robert S., Editor, *THE PEOPLE'S DOCTOR NEWSLETTER,* Vol. 12, No. 3 (undated, circa. April, 1988), p. 6-7.)

Mendelson, Jack, M.D., & Mello, Nancy Ph.D. *THE ENCYCLOPEDIA OF PSYCHOACTIVE DRUGS - THE DANGEROUS ANGEL,* 1985, Chelsa House Publishers, New York.

Miller RA. Discussion of fluoxetine and suicidal tendencies. *AMER J PSYCHIATRY.* 147; 1571, 1990.

Mintz, Morton, Cohen, Jerry S. *AMERICA, INC., Who Owns And Operates The United States,* 1971, The Dial Press, New York.

Mintz, Morton, *BY PRESCRIPTION ONLY, A report on the roles of the united States Food and Drug Administration, the American Medical Association, pharmaceutical manufacturers, and others in connection with the irrational and massive use of prescription drugs that may be worthless, injurious, or even lethal.* - revised edition, originally published as *THE THERAPEUTIC NIGHTMARE,* 1967, Beacon Press, Boston.

Mohun, Janet, *Understanding Drugs - DRUGS, STEROIDS AND SPORTS,* Franklin Watts, New York/London/Toronto/Sydney, 1988.

Montgomery, S.A. & Fineberg, N. (1989), Is there a relationship between serotonin receptor subtypes and selectivity of response in specific psychiatric illnesses? *BR J PSYCHIATRY* 155:(Suppl. 8)63-70.

Montgomery SA, Pinder RM. Do some antidepressants promote suicide? *PSYCHOPHARMACOLOGY,* 1987;92:265-266.

Montplaisir J, Laverdiere M, Saint-Hilaire JM, Walsh J, Bouvier G. SLeep and temporal lobe epilepsy: a case study with depth electrodes. *NEUROLOGY* (Minneap.), 1981;31:1352-1356.

Montplasisir J, Laverdiere M, Saint-Hilaire JM. Sleep and focal epilepsy: Contribution of depth recording. In: Sterman MB, Shouse MN, Passouant P (eds). *SLEEP AND EPILEPSY.* New York: Academic Press, 1982:301-314.

Montplasisir J, Laverdiere M, Saint-Hilaire JM. Nocturnal sleep recording in partial epilepsy: a study with depth electrodes. *J CLIN NEUROPHYSIOL* 1987;4(4):383-388.

Morgane, P.J., & Stern, W.C. (1974). Chemical anatomy of brain circuits in relation to sleep and wakefulness. In E.D. Weitzman (Ed.), *ADVANCES IN SLEEP RESEARCH* (Vol. 1, pp. 1-131). Flushing, NY: Spectrum.

Morgane, P.J. (1981). Serotonin: Twenty-five years later. *PSYCHOPHARMACOLOGY BULLETIN,* 17, 13-17.

Morrison A. Paradoxical sleep and alert wakefulness: Variations on a theme. In: Chase MH, Weitzman ED (eds). *SLEEP DISORDERS: BASIC AND CLINICAL RESEARCH.* New York: S.P. Medical and Scientific Books, 1983:95-122.

Morrison AR, Reiner PB. A dissection of paradoxical sleep. In: McGinty DJ, Drucker-Colin R, Morrison A, Parmeggiani PL (eds). *BRAIN MECHANISMS OF SLEEP.* New York: Raven Press, 1985:97-110.

Moss DC (1988, October 1). And now the steroid defense? *AMERICAN BAR ASSOCIATION JOURNAL,* pp. 22-24.

Moyer KE. Sex differences in aggression. In RC Friedman, RM Richart & RL VandWiele (eds.), *SEX DIFFERENCES IN BEHAVIOR* (pp.335-372). New York: Wiley, 1974.

Muijen, M., Roy, D., Silverstone, T.,

Mehmet, A. & Christie, M.(1988), A comparative clinical trial of fluoxetine, manserin and placebo in depressed outpatients. *ACTA PSYCHIATR SCAND,* 78:384-390.

Munch, J.C. Phencyclidine: pharmacology and toxicology. *BULLETIN ON NARCOTICS,* 26(4):131-133, October-December, 1974.

Nabeshima, T.; Yamaguchi, K.; Hiramatsu, M.; Amano, M.; Furukawa, H.; and Kameyama, T. Serotonergic involvement in phencyclidine-induced behaviors. *PHARMACOL BIOCHEM BEHAV* 21:401-408, 1984.

Nardo, Don. *DRUGS AND SPORTS,* 1990, Lucent Books, San Diego, California.

Nelson, J. C., Bowers, M.B. & Sweeney, D.R. (1979), Exacerbation of psychosis by tricyclic antidepressants in delusional depression. *AM J PSYCHIATRY,* 136:574-576.

NEWSWEEK, Halcion, February 17, 1992, p. 58

NEWSWEEK, The insanity of steroid abuse. (1988, May 23). p. 75.

Niedermeyer E. Sleep electroencephalograms in petit mal. *ARCH NEUROL* 1965;12:625-630.

Nuwer, Hank, *STEROIDS,* An Impact Book, New York/London/Toronto/Sydney,1990.

O'Carroll R & Bancroft J. (1985). Androgens and aggression in man: A controlled case study. *AGGRESSIVE BEHAVIOR,* 2, 1-7.

Oates JA, Sjoerdsma A: Neurologic effects of tryptophan in patients receiving a monoamine oxidase inhibitor. *NEUROLOGY* 1960; 10:1076-1078.

Oliver, B., Mos, J., Tulp, M., Schipper, J., den Daas, S. & van Oortmerssen, G. (1990), Serotonergic involvement in aggressive behavior in animals. In: *VIOLENCE AND SUICIDALITY: PERSPECTIVES IN CLINICAL AND PSYCHOBIOLOGICAL RESEARCH,* eds. H.M. van Praag, R. Plutchik & A. Apter. New York: Brunner/Mazel, pp. 79-137.

Olweus DO, Mattsson A, Schalling D, & Low H. (1988). Circulating testosterone levels and aggression in adolescent males: A causal analysis. *PSYCHOSOMATIC MEDICINE,* 50, 261-272.

Omura T, Ishimura Y, Fujii-Kuriyama Y. *CYTOCHROME P-450, Second Edition,* VCH Publishers, Weinheim, New York, Basel, Cambridge, 1993.

Opler LA. Fluoxetine and preoccupation with suicide [letter]. *AM J PSYCHIATRY* 1991;148:1259.

Oswald I. Sleep and dependence on amphetamine and other drugs. In: Kales A, ed. *SLEEP: PHYSIOLOGY AND PATHOLOGY.* Philadelphia; Lippincott, 1969; pp. 317-330.

Oswald I. Effects on sleep of amphetamine and its derivatives. In: Costa E, Garattini S (eds). *AMPHETAMINES AND RELATED COMPOUNDS.* New York: Raven Press, 1970:865-871.

Oswald I, Evans J; *BR J PSYCHIATRY,* 1985; 27:62-67.

Oswald I, Evans J. On serious violence during sleep-walking. *BR J PSYCHIATRY,* 1985;147:688-691.

Oswald I, Lewis SA, Dunleavy DLF, Brezinova V, Briggs M. Drugs of dependence but not of abuse: fenfluramine and imipramine. *BR MED J* 1971;3:70-73.

Oswald I, Thacore WR. Amphetamine and phenmetrazine addiction. Physiological abnormalities in the abstinence syndrome. *BR MED J* 1983;2:427-431.

Owens, S. Michael & Mayersohn, Michael. Modulation of Phencyclidine (PCP) Pharmacokinetics With PCP-Specific Fab Fragments in: Clouet, Doris H., Ph.D. ed. *PHENCYCLIDINE: AN UPDATE,* National Institute of Drug Abuse Research Monograph Series 64, 1986.

Papp LA, Gorman JM. Suicidal preoccupation during fluoxetine treatment. *AMER J*

PSYCHIATRY 147;1380(1990).

Pardoll, D.J., & Belinson, L. (1941). Androgen therapy in psychosis: Effect of testosterone propionate in male involutional psychotics. *JOURNAL OF CLINICAL ENDOCRINOLOGY*, 1, 138-141.

Partington MW, Tu JB, Wong Cy: Blood serotonin levels in severe mental retardation. *DEV MED CHILD NEUROL* 15:616-627, 1973.

Passouant P, Cadihac J, Ribstein M. Les privations de sommeil avec mouvements oculaires par les anti-depresseurs. *REV NEUROL* 1972;127:173-192.

Patry G, Lyagoubi S, Tassinari CA. Subclinical electrical statue epilepticus induced by sleep in children. *ARCH NEUROL* 1971;24:242-252.

Pearson HJ. Interaction of fluoxetine with carbamazepine. *J CLIN PSYCHIATRY* 51:126, 1990.

Peck, Rodney G. *DRUGS AND SPORTS*, The Drug Abuse Prevention Library, The Rosen Publishing Group, Inc., New York, 1992.

Pessah MA, Roffwarg HP. Spontaneous middle ear muscle activity in man: A rapid eye movement sleep phenomenon. *SCIENCE* 1972;178:773-776.

Petersen, Robert C., Stillman, Richard C., eds. *PCP PHENCYCLIDINE ABUSE: AN APPRAISAL*, National Institute of Drug Abuse Monograph Series, Research 21, August, 1978.

Petraglia F, Facchinetti F, Martignoni E, et al: Serotoninergic agonists increase plasma levels of B-endorphin and B-lipotropin in humans. *J CLIN ENDOCRINAL METAB* 59:1138-1142, 1984.

Petus M, Netter JC, Rance F, Chateauneuf R, Bildstein G, Cabalet C, Sermet J, Delprat A. Iatrogenic Cushing syndrome in infants. Report of a case with dwarfism. *ANN PEDIATR PARIS*. Jan 1990; 48-50.

Phelps, M.D., Janice Keller; Nourse, M.D.,

Alan E. *HIDDEN ADDICTION AND HOW TO GET FREE*, Massachusetts, Little, Brown & Co., 1986.

Phoenix CJ, Goy RW, Gerall AA, Young WC (1959). Organizing action of prenatally administered testosterone propionate on the tissues mediating mating behavior in the female guinea pig. *ENDOCRINOLOGY*, 65, 369-382.

PHYSICIAN'S DESK REFERENCE (PDR), 1990, p.906.

Pickard GE, Turek FW. The suprachiasmatic nuclei. Two circadian clocks? *BRAIN RES* 1983;268:201-210.

Poitras R. A propos d'episodes d'amnesies anterogrades associes a l'utilisation du triazolam. *UNION MED CAN* 1980;109:427-429.

Pollack, S. *FORENSIC PSYCHIATRY IN THE DEFENSE OF DIMINISHED CAPACITY*. Los Angeles: University of Southern California, 1976.

Pope HG, Katz DL (1990). Homicide and near-homicide by anabolic steroid users. *JOURNAL OF CLINICAL PSYCHIATRY, 51, 28-31.*

Pope HG, Katz DL (1987). Bodybuilder's psychosis. *LANCET*, 1, 863.
Pope HG, Katz DL (1988). Affective and psychotic symptoms associated with anabolic steroid use. *AMERICAN JOURNAL OF PSYCHIATRY,* 145(4), 487-490.

Potter WZ, Scheinin M, Golden RN, et al. Selective antidepressants lack specificity on norepinephrine and serotonin metabolites in cerebrospinal fluid. *ARCH GEN PSYCHIATRY* 42:1171-1177, 1985.

Pratt KL, Mattson RH, Weikers NJ, Williams R. EEG activation of epileptics following sleep deprivation: A prospective study of 114 cases. *E L E C T R O E N C E P H A L O G R C L I N NEUROPHYSIOL* 1968;24:11-15.

Pujol, J.F., Buguet, A., Froment, J.L., Jones, B., & Jouvet, M. (1971). The central metabolism of serotonin in the cat during insomnia: A neurophysiological and biochemical study after administration of p-chlorophenylalanineor desruction of the raphe system. BRAIN RESEARCH, 29, 195-212.

Rada RT, Laws DR, Kellner R (1976). Plasma testosterone and aggressive behavior. PSYCHOSOMATIC MEDICINE, 38(4), 257-268.

Rada RT, Kellner R, Winslow WW (1976). Plasma testosterone and aggressive behavior. PSYCHOSOMATICS, 17, 138-141.

Rai, G.S., "A Double-blind, Placebo Controlled Study of Ginkgo Biloba Extract in Elderly Outpatients with Mild to Moderate Memory Impairment", CURR MED RES OPIN 12(6):350-355, 1991.

Rampling, D. (1978), Aggression; a paradoxical response to tricyclic antidepressants.AM J PSYCHIATRY, 135:359-386.

Rauch PH, Stern TA. Life-threatening injuries resulting from sleepwalking and night terrors. PSYCHOSOMATICS 1986;27:62-64.

Restak, Richard M. THE BRAIN: THE LAST FRONTIER, New York: Doubleday, 1979.

Riddle, M.A., Brown, N., Dzubinski, D., Jetmalani, A.N., Law, Y. & Woolston, J.L. (1989), Case Study: Fluoxetine overdose in an adolescent. J AM ACAD CHILD ADOLESC PSYCHIATRY, 28:587-588.

Riddle, M.A., King, R.A., Hardin, M.T., Scahill, L., Ort, S.L. & Leckman, J.F. (1990b, October), BEHAVIORAL SIDE EFFECTS OF FLUOXETINE (New Research). Presented at the Annual Meeting of the American Acadamy of Child and Adolescent Psychiatry, Chicago.

Riddle, M.A., Hardin, M.T., King, R. A., Scahill, L. & Woolston, J.L. (1990a), Fluoxetine treatment of children and adolescents with Tourette's and obsessive-compulsive disorders: preliminary clinical experience.J AM ACAD CHILD ADOLESC PSYCHIATRY,29:45-48.

Ritvo ER, Yuwiler A, Geller E, et al: Increased blood serotonin and platelets in early infantile autism. ARCH GEN PSYCHIATRY 23:566-572, 1970.

Robbins, John. DIET FOR A NEW AMERICA, Stillpoint Publishing, Wallpole, NH, 1987.

Robbins, John. MAY WE ALL BE FED - DIET FOR A NEW WORLD, Wm Morrow & Co., New York, 1992.

Roby DS, Greenberg JO. Sleep deprivation and electroencephalographicabnormalities. J CLIN PSYCHIATRY 1978;39:542-543.

Rodgers, Joann Ellison, THE ENCYCLOPEDIA OF PSYCHOACTIVE DRUGS, DRUGS AND SEXUAL BEHAVIOR, Snyder, Solmon, ed., 1988, Chelsa House Publishers.

Rome HP, Braceland FJ (1952). Psychological response to corticotropin, cortisone, and related steroid substances.JOURNAL OF THE AMERICANMEDICALASSOCIATION,148(1), 27-30

Rosenblatt JE, Rosenblatt NC. More about spontaneous postmarketing reports of bupropion-related seizures. CURRENTS IN AFFECTIVE ILLNESS 11:18-20, 1992.

Rossi GF, Colicchio G, Pola P. Interictal epileptic activity during sleep: A stereo-EEG study in patients with partial epilepsy. EEG CLIN NEUROPHYSIOL 1984;58:97-106.

Rothschild, Anthony J., Locke, Carol A., "Reexposure to Fluoxetine After Serious Suicide Attempts by Three Patients: The Role of Akathisia", JOURNAL OF CLINICAL PSYCHIATRY, 52:12, December 1991.

Rothman, David. Shiny Happy People, The problem with "cosmetic psychopharmacology." THE NEW REPUBLIC February 14, 1994, p. 34.

Rowan AJ. Veldhuisen RJ, Nagelkerke NJD. Comparative evaluation of sleep deprivation and sedated sleep EEG's as diagnostic aids in epilepsy. ELECTROENCEPHALOGR CLIN

NEUROPHYSIOL 1982;54:357-364.

Roy, A., DeJong, J., & Linnoila, M. (1989). Cerebrospinal fluid monoamine metabolites and suicidal behavior in depressed patients. ARCHIVES OF GENERAL PSYCHIATRY, 46, 609-612.

Roy A, Linnoila M: Suicidal behavior impulsiveness and serotonin. ACTA PSYCHIATR SCAND 78:529-535, 1988.

Roy A, Linnoila M: Suicide and alcoholism, in: BIOLOGY OF SUICIDE. Edited by Maris R. New York, 1986, p 244-273.

Roy A, Linnoila M: CSF studies on alcoholism and related behaviors. PROGR NEUROPSYCHOPHARMACOL BIOL PSYCHIATRY 113:505-511, 1989.

Roy, A. & Linnoila, M. (1990), Monoamines and suicidal behavior. In: VIOLENCE AND SUICIDALITY: PERSPECTIVES IN CLINICAL AND PSYCHOBIOLOGICAL RESEARCH, H.M. van Pragg, R. Plutchik & A. Apter. New York: Brunner/Mazel, pp. 141-183.

Ryan AJ (1981). Anabolic steroids are fool's gold. FEDERATION PROCEEDINGS, 40, 2682-2688.

Ryman, Daniele. AROMATHERAPY, The Complete Guide to Plant and Flower Essences for Health and Beauty, Bantam Books, New York, 1991.

Sack DA, Nurnberger J, Rosenthal NE, Ashburn E, Wehr TA. Potentiation of antidepressant medications by phase advance of the sleep-wake cycle. AMERICAN JOURNAL OF PSYCHIATRY, 142, 606-608, 1985.

Sakai K, Sastre J-P, Kanamori N, Jouvet M. State-specific neurons in the ponto-medullary reticular formation with special reference to the postural atonia during paradoxical sleep in the cat. In: Pomepiano O, Ajamone Marsan C (eds). BRAIN MECHANISMS AND PERCEPTUAL AWARENESS. New York: Raven Press, 1981:405-429.

Salmon UJ, Geist SH (1943). Effects of androgens upon libido in women. JOURNAL OF AMERICAN ENDOCRINOLOGY, 3, 235-238.

SALT LAKE TRIBUNE, "Study Says Prozac Doesn't Raise Risk of Birth Defects", May 5, 1993.

Sato S, Dreifus F, Penry JK. The effect of sleep on spike-wave discharges in absence seizures. NEUROLOGY (Minneap.), 1973;23:1335-1345.

Schaffler, K., and Reeh, P., "Long-Term Drug Administration Effects of Ginkgo Biloba on the Performance of Healthy Subjects Exposed to Hypoxia", EFFECTS OF GINKGO BILOBA EXTRACTS ON ORGANIC CEREBRAL IMPAIRMENT, John Libbey Eurotext Ltd., 1985.

Schain RJ, Freedman DX: Studies on 5-hydroxyindole metabolism in autistic and other mentally retarded children. J PEDIATR 58:315-320, 1961.

Scheflin, Alan W; Opton, Edward M Jr. THE MIND MANIPULATORS, Paddington Press Ltd., New York and London, 1978.

Schenck CH, Bundlie SR, Patterson AL, Mahowald MW. Rapid eye movement sleep behavior disorder: A treatable parasomnia affecting older adults. JAMA 1987;257:1786-1789.

Schenck CH, Bundlie SR, Ettinger MG, Mahowald MW. Chronic behavioral disorders of human REM sleep: A new category of parasomnia. SLEEP 1986;9:293-308.

Schmid, N.D., Ronald F. TRADITIONAL FOODS ARE YOUR BEST MEDICINE, New York; Ballentine, 1987.

Schmidt G. Eie verbrechenin schlaftrunkenkeit. Z NEUROL PSYCHIATRIE 1943;176:208-254.

Schulte, Jerome L. "Homicide and Suicide Associated With Akathisia and Haloperidol," AMERICAN JOURNAL OF FORENSIC PSYCHIATRY, Vol. 6, p. 3-7, 1985.

Schwab, H.J. A trial attorney's manual on diminished capacity. In: Pollack, S., ed. *FORENSIC PSYCHIATRY IN THE DEFENSE OF DIMINISHED CAPACITY.* Los Angeles: University of Southern California, 1976.

Schweizer E, Dever A, Clary C. Suicide upon recovery from depression: a clinical note. *J NERV MENT DIS,* 1988;176:633-636.

Scollo-Lavizzari G, Scollo-Lavizzari GR. Sleep, sleep deprivation, photosensitivity and epilepsy. *EUR NEUROL* 1974; 11:1-21

Scollo-Lavizzari G, Pralle W, De la Cruz N. Activation effects of sleep deprivation and sleep in seizure patients. *EUR NEUROL* 1975;13:1-5.

Selye, Hans, M.D., *THE STRESS OF LIFE,* McGraw Hill, 1976.

Shaw ED, Mann JJ, Weiden PJ, et al. A case of suicidal and homocidal ideation and akathisia in a double-blind neuroleptic crossover study [letter]. *J CLIN PSYCHOPHARMACOL* 1986;6:196-197.

Sheally, C. Norman. *90 DAYS TO SELF-HEALTH, Biogenics: How to Control All Types of Stress by Yoursef Through a Complete Health Program of Autogenics, Diet, Vitamins and Exercise,* Dial Press, New York, 1977.

Shear MK, Frances a Weiden P. Suicide associated with akathisia and depot fluphenazine treatment. *J CLIN PSYCHOPHARMACOL* 1983;3(4):235-236.

Shelton, Herbert M. *FASTING CAN SAVE YOUR LIFE,*

Shelton, Herbert M. *HEALTH FOR ALL,* Health Research Publications, Molkelumne Hill, California.

Shelton, Herbert M. *HYGENIC SYSTEM,* Health Research Publications, Molkelumne Hill, California, 1934.

Shimizu T, Inami Y, Sigita Y, Iijima S, Teshima Y, Matsuo R, Yashshima A, Okawa M, Hishikawa Y. REM without muscle atonia (stage 1-REM) and its relation to delirius

behavior during sleep. *SLEEP RES* 1987;16:503.

Shimizu T, Ookawa M, Ijuma S et al. Effect of clomipramine on nocturnal sleep of normal human subjects. *ANN REV PHARMACOPSYCHIATR RES FOUND* 1985;16:138.

Sholomskas AJ. Mania in a panic disorder patient treated with fluoxetine. *AMER J PSYCHIATRY* 147;1090-91(1990).

Shoulson I, Chase TN. Fenfluramine in man: hypophagia associated with diminished serotonin turnover. *CLIN PHARMACOL THER* 17:616-621, 1975.

Shouse MN, Sterman MB. (1981b) *EXP. NEURO.* 71:563.

Shouse MN, Sterman MB. "Kindling" a sleep disorder: Degree of sleep pathology predicts kindled seizure susceptibility in cats. *BRAIN RES* 1983;271(1):196-200.

Shukla D. Intracranial hemorrhage associated with amphetamine use. *NEUROLOGY* 1982;32:917-918.

Siegel, Bernie, M.D., *LOVE, MEDICINE & MIRACLES,* New York; Harper & Row, 1986.

Siegal, Ronald K. Phencyclidine and Ketamine Intoxication: A Study of Four Populations of Recreational Users in: Petersen, Robert C., Stillman, Richard C., eds. *PCP PHENCYCLIDINE ABUSE: AN APPRAISAL,* National Institute of Drug Abuse Monograph Series, Research 21, August, 1978.

Siegel, Ronald K. Phencyclidine, Criminal Behavior, and the Defense of Diminished Capacity, in: Petersen, Robert C., Stillman, Richard C., eds. *PCP PHENCYCLIDINE ABUSE: AN APPRAISAL,* National Institute of Drug Abuse Monograph Series, Research 21, August, 1978.

Siegel, R.K. PCP and violent crime: The people vs. peace. *J PSYCHEDELIC DRUGS* 12(3-4):317-330, 1980.

Silverman D. Sleep as a general activation procedure in electroencephalography. *ELECTROENCEPHALOGR CLIN NEUROPHYSIOL* 1956;8:317-324.

Silverstein, Alvin, Virginia & Robert. *STEROIDS...BIG MUSCLES, BIG PROBLEMS,* Enslow Publishers, Inc., New Jersey, 1992.

Siminoski K, Goss P, Drucker DJ. The Cushing syndrome induced by medroxyprogesterone acetate. *ANN INTERN MED.* Nov 1, 1989;111(9):758-760.

Simon NG, Whalen RE, Tate MP (1985). Induction of male-typical aggression by androgens but not by estrogens in adult female mice. *HORMONES AND BEHAVIOR*, 19, 204-212.

Simonds, J.F., and Kashani, J. Specific drug use and violence in delinquent boys. *AM J DRUG ALCOHOL ABUSE* 7(3&4):305-322, 1980.

Slothower, Jodie. "Mean Mental Muscles: The Psychological Price of Steroids.," *HEALTH,* January 1988, p. 20.

Smith, R.C.; Meltzer, J.Y.; Arora, R.C.; and Davis, J.M. Effects of phencyclidine on 3H-catecholamine and 3H-serotonin uptake in synaptosomal preparations from rat brain. *BIOCHEM PHARMACOL* 26:1435-1439, 1977.

Snyder, Solomon H. *DRUGS AND THE BRAIN,* New York, Freeman & Company, 1986.

Soloff PH, George A, Nathan RS, et al. Paradoxical effects of amitriptyline of borderline patients. *AM J PSYCHIATRY,* 1986;142:98-100.

Sourial N, Fenton F (1988). Testosterone treatment of an XXYY male presenting with aggression: A case report. *CANADIAN JOURNAL OF PSYCHIATRY,* 33, 846-850.

Solviter, R.S., E. G. Drust and J. E. Connor. Evidence that serotonin mediates some behavioral effects of amphetamine. *J PHARMACOL EXP THER* 206:348-352, 1978.

Spiller HA, Morse S, Muir C. Fluoxtine ingestion: A one year retrospective study. *VET HUM TOXICOL.* 32;153-55, 1990.

Spring GK. Neurotoxicity with combined use of lithium and thioridazine. *J CLIN PSYCHIATRY* 40:135, 1979,

Stahl SM, Ciaranello RD, Berger PA. Platelet serotonin in schizophrenia and depression, in *SEROTONIN IN BIOLOGICAL PSYCHIATRY.* Edited by Ho BT, Schoolar JC, Usdin E. New York, Raven Press, 1982, pp 183-198.

Stahl SM, Woo DJ, Mefford IN, et al. Hyperserotonemia and platelet serotonin uptake and release in schizophrenia and affective disorders. *AM J PSYCHIATRY* 140:26-30, 1983.

Stalder M, Pometta D, Suenram A (1981) Relationship between plasma insulin levels and high density lipoprotein cholesterol levels in healthy men. *DIABETOLOGIA,* 21, 544-548.

Stark P, Fuller RW, Wong DT: The pharmacologic profile of fluoxetine. *J CLIN PSYCHIATRY* 46 (No 3, suppl 2):7-13, 1985.

Stein MH. Tardive dyskiinesia in a patient taking halperidol and fluoxetine [letter]. *AM J PSYCHIATRY* 1991;148:683.

Steiner W, Fontaine R: Toxic reaction following the combined administration of fluoxetine and L-tryptophan: five case reports. *BIOL PSYCHIATRY* 1986; 21:1067-1071.

Stenn PG, Klaiber EL, Vogel W, Broverman DM. (1972) Testosterone effects upon photic stimulation of the electrocephalogram (EEG) and mental performance of humans. *PERCEPTUAL AND MOTOR SKILLS,* 34, 371-378.

Stephen E. Langer, *SOLVED: THE RIDDLE OF ILLNESS,* Connecticut, Keats, 1984.

Steriade M, Hobson JA. Neuronal activity during the sleep-wake cycle. *PROG NEUROBIOL* 1976;6:155-376.

Sternbach, Harvey, M.D. *"THE SEROTONIN SYNDROME,"* AM J PSYCHIATRY, 148:6, June 1991.

Sternbach H: Danger of MAOI therapy after fluoxetine withdrawal (letter). *LANCET* 1988; 2:850.

Sternbach H. Fluoxetine-associated potentiation of clacuim-channel blockers. *J CLIN PSYCHOPHARMACOL* 11:390, 1991.

Sterman MB, Shouse M, Passouant P. (eds.) *SLEEP AND EPILEPSY*, Academic Press, 1982.

Steur, Ernst N H Jansen. Increase of Parkinson Disability After Fluoxetine Medication, *NEUROLOGY,* 1993;43:211-213.

Stevens, Jay, *STORMING HEAVEN, LSD and The American Dream*, 1987, Harper and Row , p. 73-84.

Strom-Paikin, Joyce E., *MEDICAL TREASON, Nurses on Drugs,* 1988, New Horizon Press.

Strupp, BJ, Himmelstein, S, Bunsey, M, Levitsky, DA, Kesler, M. Cognitive profile of rats exposed to lactational hyperphenylalaninemia: Correspondence with human mental retardation. *DEVELOPMENTAL PSYCHOBIOLOGY*, (1990), 23, 195-214.

Stumpf WE, Sar M. (1976) Steroid hormone target sites in the brain: The differential distribution of estrogen, progestin, androgen and glucocorticosteroid. *JOURNAL OF STEROID BIOCHEMISTRY*, 7, 1163-1170.

Stunkard AJ, Grace WJ, Wolfe HG. The night-eating syndrome. *AM J MED* 1955;7:76-78.

Susman EJ, Inoff-Germain G, Nottelmann ED, Loriaux DL, Cutler GB, Chrousos GP. (1987) Hormones, emotional dispositions, and aggressive attributes in young adolescents. *CHILD DEVELOPMENT*, 58, 1114-1134.

Susman EJ, Nottelmann ED, Inoff-Germain G, Dorn LD, Chrousos GP. (1987) Hormonal influences on aspects of psychological development during adolescence *JOURNAL OF YOUTH AND ADOLESCENCE*, 14(3), 245-264.

Svare BB. (1983) *HORMONES AND AGGRESSIVE BEHAVIOR*. New York: Plenum Press.

Svare BB. (1990) Anabolic steroids and behavior: A preclinical research prospectus. In GC Lin & L Erinoff (Eds.), *ANABOLIC STEROID ABUSE (NIDA RESEARCH MONOGRAPH)*, pp 224-241. Rockville, MD: National Institute on Drug Abuse.

Tachibana M, Tanaka K, Hishikawa Y, Kaneko Z. A sleep study of acute psychotic states due to alcohol and meprobamate addiction. *ADV SLEEP RES* 1975;2:177-205.

Taillandier, J., "Ginkgo Biloba Extract in the Treatment of Cerebral Disorders Due to Againg", *ROKAN (GINKGO BILOBA), RECENT RESULTS IN PHARMACOLOGY AND CLINIC*, E.W. Funfgeld, Ed. Berlin, Germany: Springer-Verlag, 1988.

Takahashi S, Kanai H, Miyamoto Y: Reassessment of elevated serotonin levels in blood platelets in early infantile autism. *J AUTISM CHILD SCHIZOPHR* 6:317-326, 1976.

Talmadge, Katherine S. *A DRUG ALERT BOOK - FOCUS ON STEROIDS*, 1991, Twenty-First Century Books, Frederick, Maryland.

Tate JL. Extrapyramidal symptoms in a patient taking haloperidol and fluoxetine. *AM J PSYCHIATRY* 1989;146:399-400.

Tate JL. Extrapyramidal symptoms in a patient taking haloperidol and fluoxetine [letter]. *AM J PSYCHIATRY* 1989;146:1352-1353.

Taylor WN (1987a) Anabolic steroids: A plea for control. *CHIROPRACTIC SPORTS MEDICINE*, 1(2), 47-52.

Taylor, J.E., "The Effects of Chronic, Oral Ginkgo Biloba Extract Administration on Neurotransmitter Receptor Binding in Young and Aged Fisher 344 Rats", *EFFECTS OF FINKGO BILOBA EXTRACT ON ORGANIC CEREBRAL IMPAIRMENT*, John Libbey Eurotext Ltd., 1985.

Taylor WN (1987b) Commentary: Synthetic anabolic-androgenic steroids: A plea for controlled substance status. *THE PHYSICIAN AND SPORTS MEDICINE*, 15(5), 140-150.

Taylor, Gordon Rattray. *THE BIOLOGICAL TIME BOMB*, New York & Cleveland; The World Publishing Co., 1968.

Tec L (19740 Nandrolone in anorexia nervosa. *JOURNAL OF THE AMERICAN MEDICAL ASSOCIATION*, 229(11), 1423.

Teicher MH et al. (1990b), Suicidal preoccupation during fluoxetine treatment (letter), *AM. J. PSYCHIATRY,* 147:207-210.

Teicher, M.H., Glod, C. & Cole, J.O. (1990a), Emergence of intense suicidal preoccupationduring fluoxetine treatment. *AM. J. PSYCHIATRY,* 147:207-210.

Tennant F, Black DL, Voy RO (1988) Anabolic steroid dependence with opioid-type features. *NEW ENGLAND JOURNAL OF MEDICINE*, 319(9), 578-c.

Thomas, Clayton. *TABER'S CYCLOPEDIC MEDICAL DICTIONARY*, F.A. Davis Company, Philadelphia, 1985.

Thomas DR, Nelson DR, Johnson AM. Biochemical effects of the antidepressant paroxetine, a specific 5-hydroxytryptamine uptake inhibitor. *PSYCHOPHARMACOLOGY* (Berlin) 93:193-200, 1987.

Thomas, Gordon. *JOURNEY INTO MADNESS, The True Story of CIA Mind Control and Medical Abuse,* 1989, Bantam Books, New York, Toronto, London, Sidney, Auckland.

Thorpy, Michael J. *HANDBOOK OF SLEEP DISORDERS,* 1992.

Tilzey A, Heptonstall J, Hamblin T (1981) Toxic confusional state and choreiform movements after treatment with anabolic steroids. *BRITISH MEDICAL JOURNAL,* 283, 349-350.

Tinklenberg, J. Drugs and crime. In: *DRUG USE IN AMERICA: PROBLEM IN PERSPECTIVE.* The technical papers of the Second Report of the National Commission on Marihuana and Drug Abuse. March 1973. Vol. 1, pp. 242-299.

Tollelson GD. Fluoxetine and suicidal ideation. *AMER J PSYCHIATRY* 147; 1691-92, 1990.

Tongue, S.R. and Leonard, B.E. The effects of some hallucinogenicdrugs upon the metabolism of 5-hydroxytryptaminein the brain. *LIFE SCI*, 8:805-814, 1969.

Touchon J. Effect of awakening on epileptic activity in primary generalized myoclonic epilepsy. In: Sterman MB, Shouse MN, Passouant P (eds.). *SLEEP AND EPILEPSY.* New York: Academic Press, 1982:269-286.

Train GJ, Winkler EG (1962) Homicidal psychosis while under ACTH. *PSYCHOSOMATICS,* 3, 317-322.

Traskman L, Asberg M, Bertilsson L, et al. Plasma levels of chlorimipramine and its desmethylmetabolite during treatment of depression. *CLIN PHARMACOL THER* 26:600-610, 1079.

Traskman, L., Asberg, M., Bertilsson, L., & Sjostrand, L. (1981). Monoaminemetabolitesin CSF and suicidal behavior. *ARCHIVES OF GENERAL PSYCHIATRY,* 38, 631-636.

Treben Maria, *HEALTH THROUGH GOD'S PHARMACY,* Austria; Wilhelm Ennsthaler, Steyr, 1987.

Treben, Maria, *HEALTH FROM GOD'S GARDEN,* Vermont; Healing Arts, 1988.

Trulson, Michael E., *THE ENCYCLOPEDIA OF PSYCHOACTIVEDRUGS, LSD, Visions or Nightmares,* Snyder, Solomon, ed., 1985, New York, Chelsa House Publishers.

Trulson ME, Jacobs BL, Morrison AR. Raphe unit activity during REM sleep in normal cats and in pontine lesioned cats displaying REM sleep without atonia. *BRAIN RES* 1981;226:75-91.

Trulson ME, Jacobs BL: Behavioral evidence for rapid release of CNS serotonin by PCA and fenfluramine. *EUR J PHARMACOL* 1976; 36:149-154.

Tu J, Partington MW: 5-hydroxyindole levels in the blood and CSF in Down's syndrome, phenylketonuria and severe mental retardation. *DEV MED CHILD NEUROL* 14:457-466, 1972.

U.S. NEWS AND WORLD REPORT, November 8, 1993, p. 76-79.

Udry JR, Billy JOG, Morris NM, Groff TR, Raj MH (1985) Serum androgenic hormones motivate sexual behavior in adolescent boys. *FERTILITY AND STERILITY,* 43 (1), 90-94.

Valzelli, L., & Bernasconi, S. (1979). Aggressiveness by isolation and brain serotonin turnover changes in different strains of mice. *NEUROPSYCHOBIOLOGY,* 5, 129-135.

Valzelli, L., Bernasconi, S., & Garattini, S. (1981). p-Chlorophenylalanine-induced muricidal aggression in male and female laboratory rats. *NEUROPSYCHOBIOLOGY,* 7, 315-320.

Valzelli, L., Bernasconi, S., & Dalessandro, M. (1983). Time-courses of P-CPA-induced depletion of brain serotonin and muricidal aggression in the rat. *PHARMACOLOGICAL RESEARCH COMMUNICATIONS,* 15, 387-395.

Valzelli L & Garattini S. (1972). Biochemical and behavioural changes induced by isolation in rats. *NEUROPHARMACOLOGY,* 11, 17-22.

Valzelli, L., & Garattini, S. (1982). Biochemical and behavioural changes induced by isolation in rats. *NEUROPHARMACOLOGY,* 11, 17-22.

van de Poll NE, van Zanten S, de Jonge FH (1986) Effects of testosterone, estrogen, and dihydrotestosterone upon aggressive and sexual behavior of female rats. *HORMONES AND BEHAVIOR,* 20, 418-431.

van Praag HM. Neurotransmitters and CNS Disease. *J AFFECT DIS* 1982; 4: 275-90.

van Praag HM. (Auto) aggression and CSF 5-HIAA indepression and schizophrenia. *PSYCHOPHARMACOLOGICAL BULL* 1982; 22: 669-673.

Van Putten, Theodore, "The Many Faces of Akathisia," *COMPREHENSIVE PSYCHIATRY,* Vol. 16, No. 1 (January/February 1975), pgs. 43-47.

Van Putten T, Marder SR. Behavioral toxicity of antipsychotic drugs. *J CLIN PSYCHIATRY* 1987;48(9, suppl):13-19.

Van Putten T, Mutalipassi LR, Malkin MD. Phenothiazine-induced decompensation. *ARCH GEN PSYCHIATRY* 1974;30:102-105.

VEGETARIAN TIMES, Vegetarians Live Longer, 190:14, June 1993.

Venkataraman S, Naylor MW, King CA. Mania Associated with Fluoxetine Treatment in Adolescents, *J AM ACAD CHILD ADOLESC PSYCHIATRY.* 31:2, March 1992.

Vertes RP. Brainstem control of the events of REM sleep. *PROG NEUROBIOL* 1984;22:241-288.

Virkkunen, M., DeJong, J., Bartko, J., Goodwin, F.K., & Linnoila, M. (1989). Relationship of psycholbiological variables to recidivism in violent offenders and impulsive fire setters. *ARCHIVES OF GENERAL PSYCHIATRY,* 46, 600-603.

Virkkunen, M., Nuutila, A., Goodwin, F.K., & Linnoila, M. (1987). Cerebrospinal fluid monoamine metabolite levels in male arsonists. *ARCHIVES OF GENERAL PSYCHIATRY,* 44, 241-247.

Vogel HCA. *THE NATURE DOCTOR,* translated from the original German version of *DER KLEINE DOKTOR,* 1991, Keats

Publishing, New Canaan, Connecticut.

Vogel W, Klaiber EL, Broverman DM (1985) A comparison of the antidepressant effects of a synthetic androgen (mesterolone) and amitriptyline in depressed men. *JOURNAL OF CLINICAL PSYCHIATRY*, 46(1), 6-8.

von Ammon Cavanaugh S. Drug-drug interactions of fluoxetine with tricyclics. *PSYCHOSOMATICS* 31:273-276, 1990.

Walker JM, Berger RJ. Sleep as an adaptation for energy conservation functionally related to hibernation and shallow torpor. *PROGR BRAIN RES* 1980;53:255-278.

Wang T, Okano, Y, Eisensmith, R, Huang, SZ, Zeng, YT, Wilson, HYL, Woo, SL Molecular genetics of phenylketonuria in Orientals: linkage disequilibrium between a termination mutation and haplotype 4 of the phenylalanine hydroxylase gene. *AMERICAN JOURNAL OF HUMAN GENETICS*, (1989), 45, 675-680.

Weber JJ, Seizure Activity Associated With Fluoxetine Therapy, *CLINICAL PHARMACY*. April, 1989.

Weddington WW, Banner A. Organic affective syndrome associated with metoclopramide: case report. *J CLIN PSYCHOPHARMACOL* 1986;47:208-209.

Weiden P. Akathisia from prochlorperazine [letter]. *JAMA* 1985:253:635

Weissman, M.M., Klerman, G.L., Markowitz, J.S. & Ouellette, R. (1989), Suicidal ideation and suicide attempts in panic disorder and attacks. *N. ENG. J. MED.* 321:1209-1214.

Weitbrecht, W.V., and Jansen, W., "Double-blind and Comparative (Ginkgo Biloba vs Placebo) Theraputic Study in Geriatric Patients with Primary Degenerative Dementia - A Preliminary Evaluation", *EFFECTS OF GINKGO BILOBA EXTRACT ON ORGANIC CEREBRAL IMPAIRMENT*, John Libbey Eurotext Ltd., 1985.

Werner AA, Johns GA, Hoctor EF, Ault CC,

Kohler LH, Weis MW (1934) Involutional melancholia: A probable etiology and treatment. *JOURNAL OF THE AMERICAN MEDICAL ASSOCIATION*, 103, 13-16.

Wilson IC, Prange AJ, Lara PP (1974) Methyltestosterone with imipramine in men: Conversion of depression to paranoid reaction. *AMERICAN JOURNAL OF PSYCHIATRY*, 131(1), 21-24.

Winters, W.D., and Ferrar-Allado, T. The cataleptic state induced by ketamine: A review of the neuropharmacology of anesthesia. *NEUROPHARMACOLOGY*, 11:303-315, 1972.

Wirshing WC, Rosenberg J, Van Putten T, et al. Fluoxetine and suicidality: a consequence of akathisia. In: *NEW RESEARCH PROGRAM AND ABSTRACTS OF THE 144TH ANNUAL MEETING OF THE AMERICAN PSYCHIATRIC ASSOCIATION;* May 11-16, 1991; New Orleans, La. Abstract NR 13:52.

Wish, Eric D. PCP and Crime: Just Another Illicit Drug? in: Clouet, Doris H., Ph.D. ed. *PHENCYCLIDINE: AN UPDATE,* National Institute of Drug Abuse Research Monograph Series 64, 1986.

Woodard TL, Burghen GA, Kitabehi AE, Wilimas JA (1981) Glucose intolerance and insulin resistance in splastic anemia treated with oxymetholone. *JOURNAL OF CLINICAL ENDOCRINOLOGY AND METABOLISM*, 53, 905-908.

Wooley DW, Campbell NK. Exploration of the central nervous system serotonin in humans. *ANN NY ACAD SCI* 90:108-117, 1962.

Wooley DW, Shaw E. A biochemical and pharmacological suggestion about certain mental disorders. *PROC NATL ACAD SCI USA* 40:228-231, 1954.

Worwood, Valerie, *THE COMPLETE BOOK OF ESSENTIAL OILS AND AROMATHERAPY,* 1992.

Wu FCW, Bancroft J, Davidson DW, Nichol K (1982) The behavioral effects of testosterone undecanoate in adult men with Klinefelter's

Syndrome: A controlled study. *CLINICAL ENDOCRINOLOGY*, 16, 489-497.

Yamawaki S, Yanagawak K, Hotta I, et al: Effect of long-term lithium treatment on serotonin syndrome in rats. *YAKUBUTSU SEISHIN KODO* 1986; 6:247-252.

Yaryura-Tobias, J.A. (1977). Obsessive-compulsive disorders: A serotonergic hypothesis. *JOURNAL OF ORTHOMOLECULAR PSYCHIATRY*, 6, 317-326.

Yaryura-Tobias, J.A., & Neziroglu, F.A. (1981). Aggressive behavior, clinical interfaces. In L. Valzelli & L. Morgese (Eds.), *Aggression and violence: A psycho/biological approach* (pp. 195-210). Milan, Italy: Edizioni Saint Vincent.

Yellowlees D. Homicide by a somnambulist. *J MENT SCI* 1878;24:451-458.

Yesalis CE, Vicary J, Buckley W, Streit A, Katz D, Wright J (1990) Indications of psychological dependence among anabolic-androgenic steroid abusers. In G. C. Lin & L. Erinoff (eds.), *ANABOLIC STEROID ABUSE (NIDA RESEARCH MONOGRAPH)*, pp 196-214, Rockville MD: National Institute on Drug Abuse.

Yesalis CE, Wright JE, Bahrke MS (1989) Epidemiological and policy issues in the measurement of the long term health effects of anabolic-androgenic steroids. *SPORTS MEDICINE*, 8(3), 129-138.

Yesalis, Charles E., ed., *ANABOLIC STEROIDS IN SPORT AND EXERCISE*, 1993, Human Kinetics Publishers, Inc., Champaign, Illinois.

Yi SJ, Gifford AN, Johnson KM. Effect of cocaine and 5HT receptor antagonists on 5HT-induced dopamine release from rat striatal synaptosomes. *EUR J PHARMACOL* 1991;199:185-189.

Yiamouyiannis, John, *FLORIDE THE AGING FACTOR*, 1986.

Young GB, Blume WT, Wells GA, Mertens WC, Eder S. Differential aspects of sleep epilepsy. *CAN J NEUROL SCI* 1985;12:317-320.

Zohar, J., Insel, T.R., Zohar-Kadouch, R.C., Hill, J.L., & Murphy, D. L. (1988). Serotonergic responsivity in obsessive-compulsive disorder. *ARCHIVES OF GENERAL PSYCHIATRY*, 45, 167-172.

407

INDEX

410

411

412

414

417

418

423

424